Lifestyle and Epidemiology - The Double Burden of Poverty and Cardiovascular Diseases in African Populations

Edited by Kotsedi Daniel Monyeki and Han C.G. Kemper

Published in London, United Kingdom

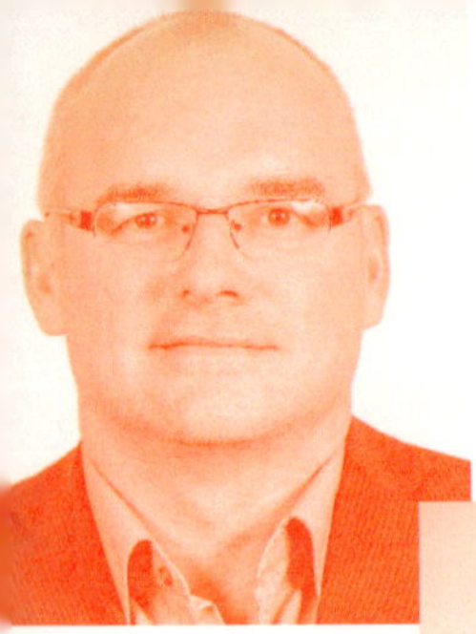
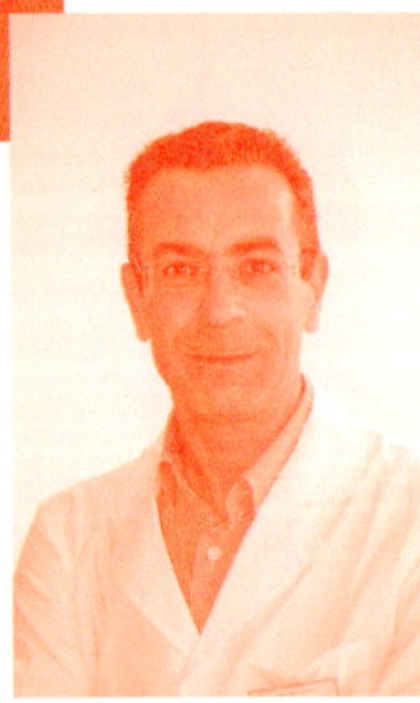
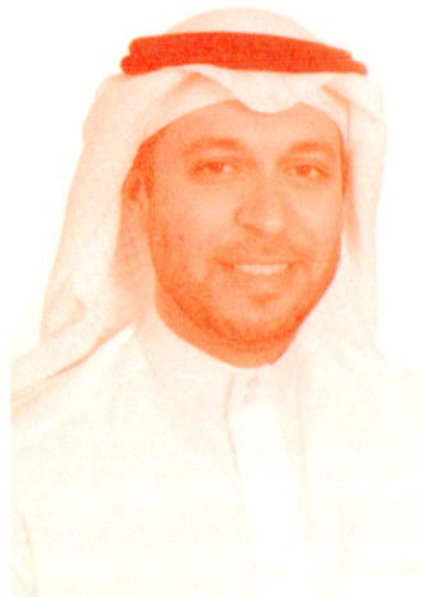
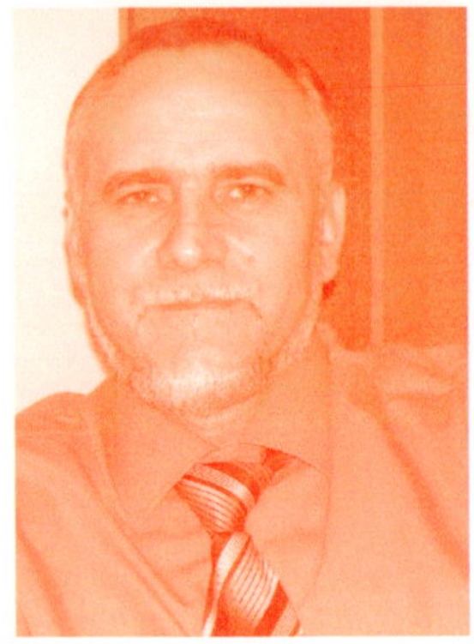
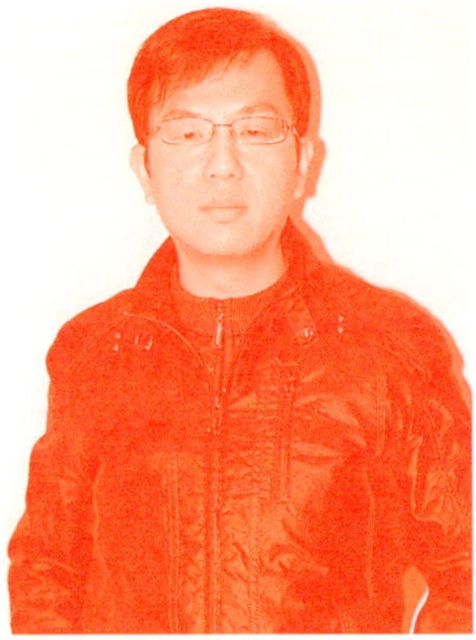
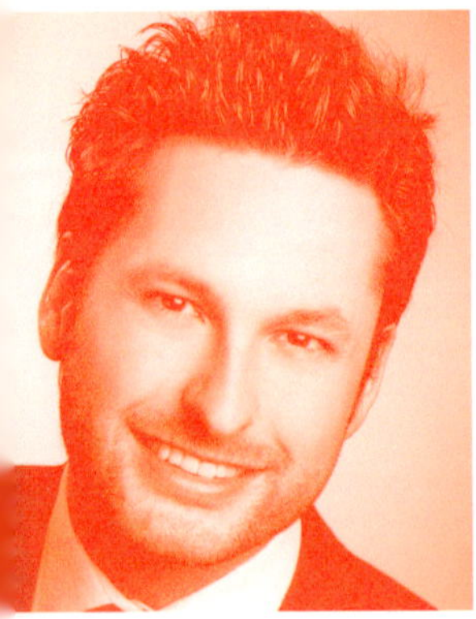
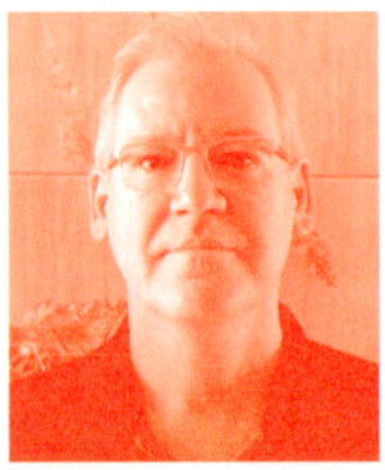

IntechOpen

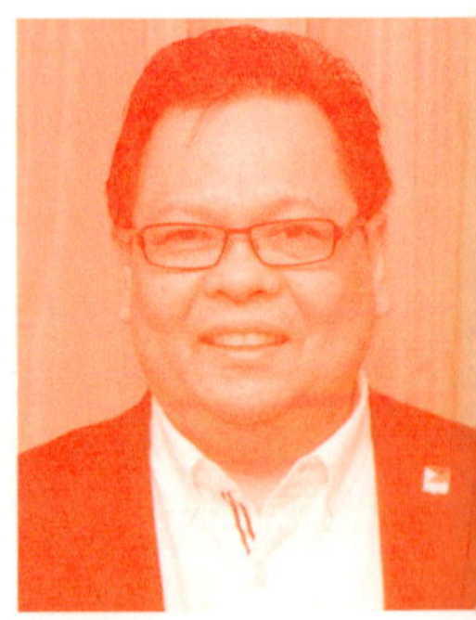
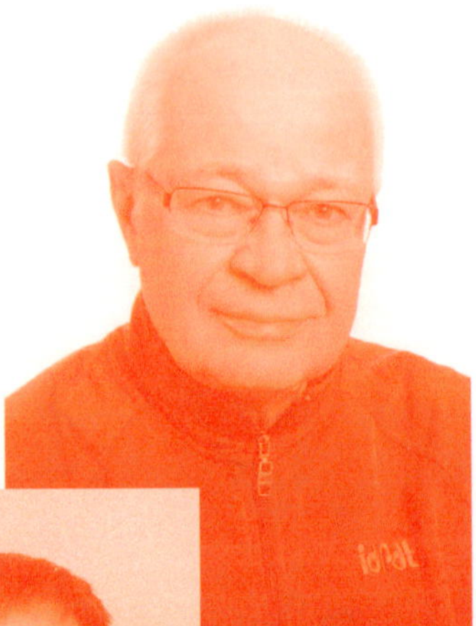
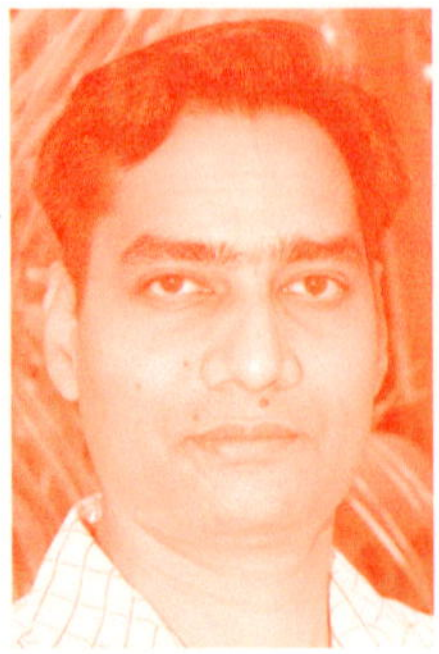
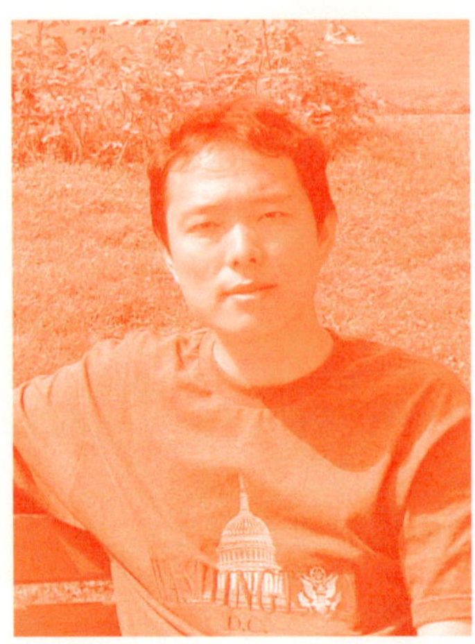
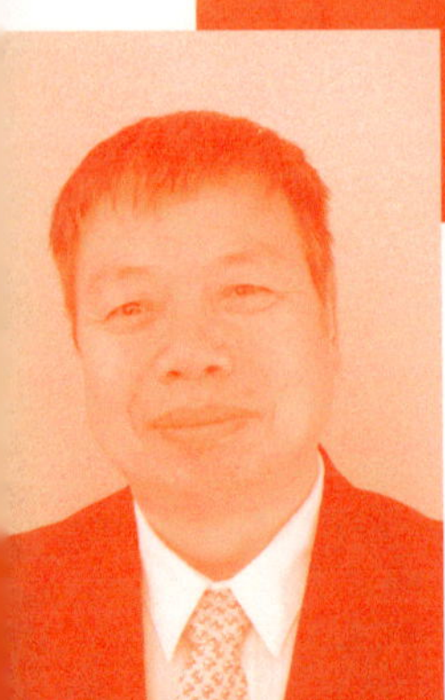
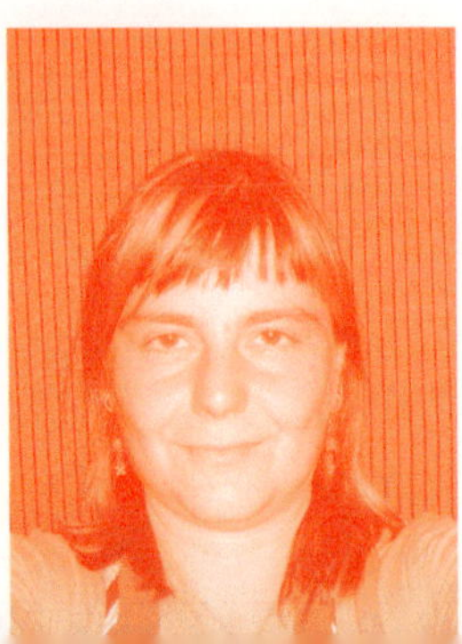

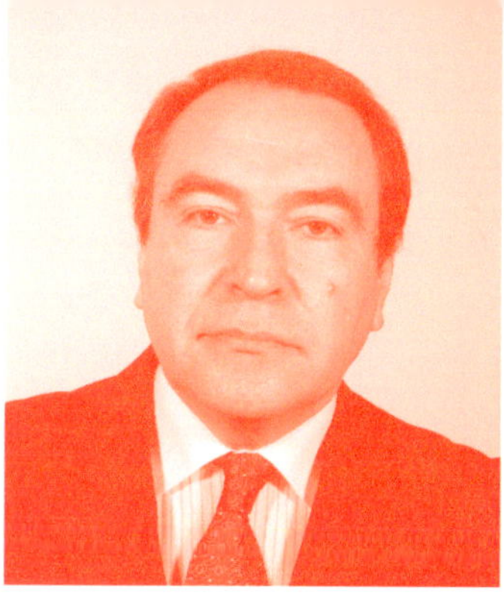
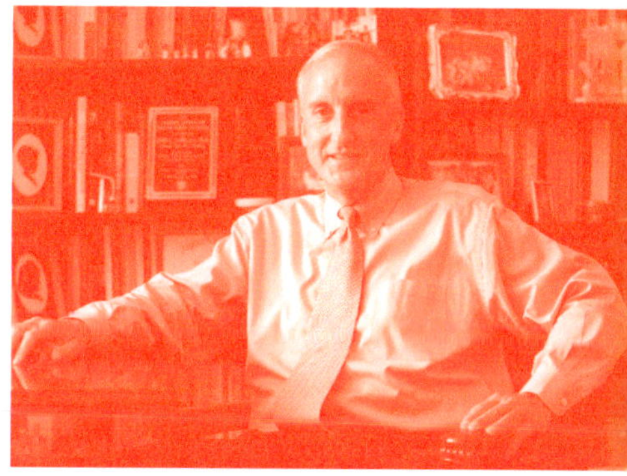
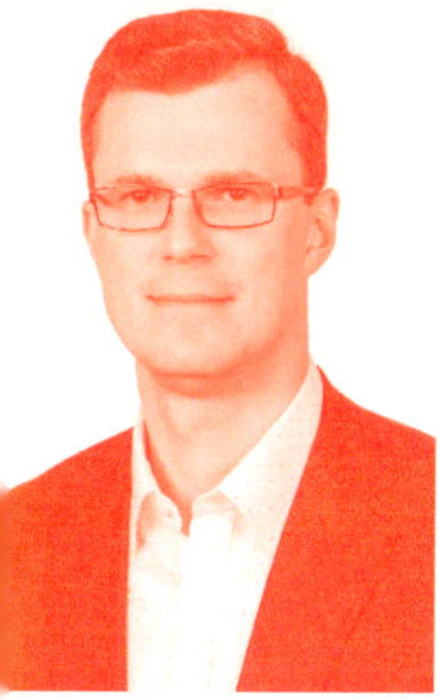
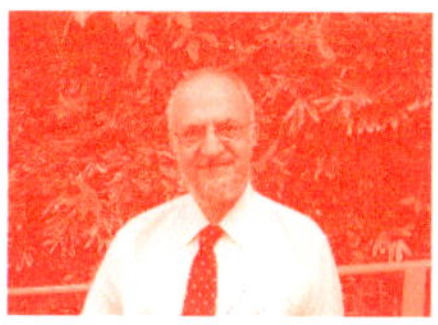
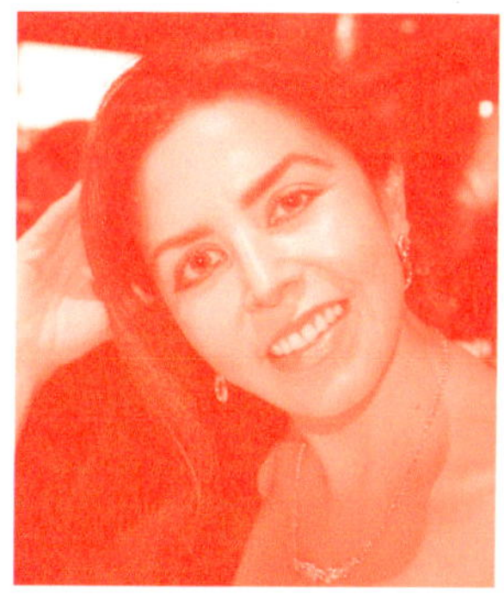

Supporting open minds since 2005

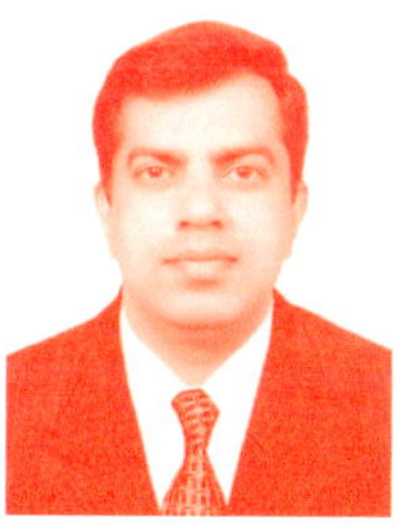
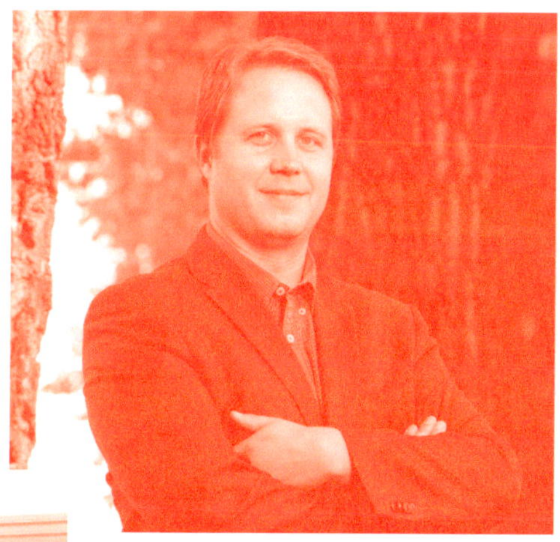
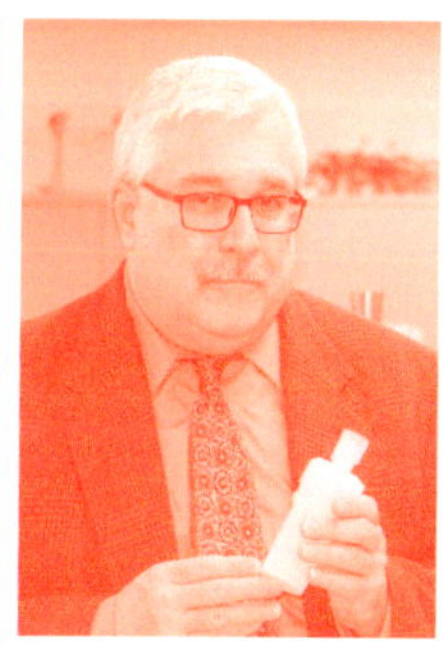
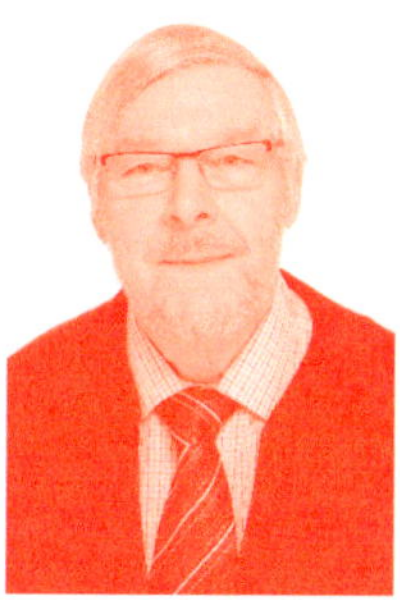
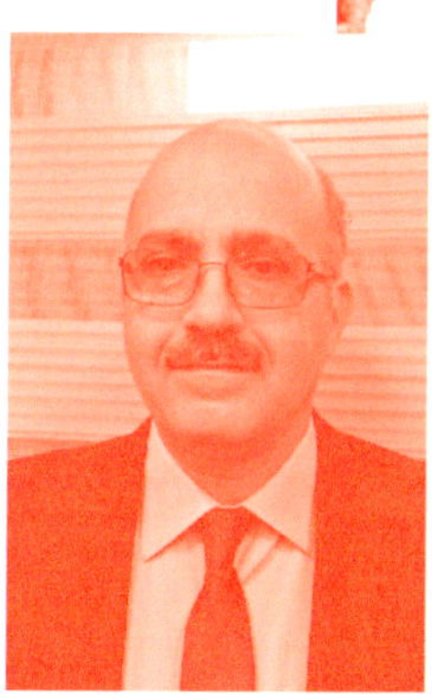
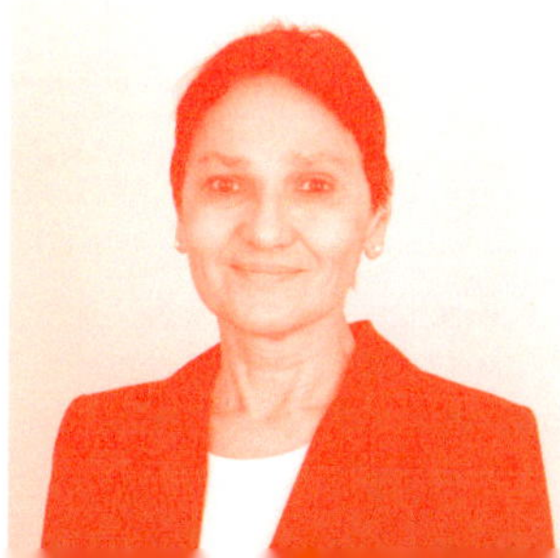
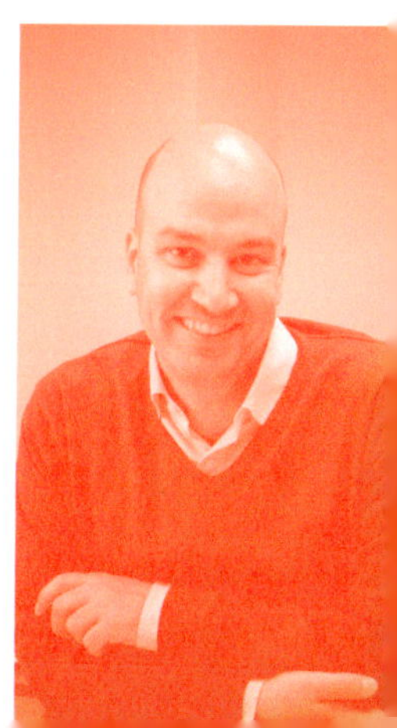

Lifestyle and Epidemiology - The Double Burden of Poverty and Cardiovascular Diseases in African Populations
http://dx.doi.org/10.5772/intechopen.92932
Edited by Kotsedi Daniel Monyeki and Han C.G. Kemper

Contributors
Muzi Maseko, Bongubuhle Mlambo, Edgar Phukubje, Thamsanqa Nyundu, Joel Noutakdie Tochie, Frank Nzali, Mazou Ngou Temgoua, Simeon Pierre Choukem, Maseabata Ramathebane, Lineo Maja, Molungoa Sello, Emmanuel Limbole Bakilo, Dadi Serge Nkarnkwin Kasanza, Lucette Womba Tshomba, Gilot Ngoma, Venance Atheno Simele, Mireille Kika, Jean Booto, Reagan Wiyaka, Martine Ekeba, Janet Michel Michel, Marcel Tanner, Ahmed Anas Guerboub, Ghizlaine Belmejdoub, Tebogo Maria Maria Mothiba, Kudzaishe Mangombe, Ronald Musizvingoza, Naomi Wekwete, Amos Milanzi, Charles Lwanga, Shisana M. Baloyi, Kebogile Mokwena, Stella Chewe Sabi, Wilna Oldewage-Theron, Christa Grobler, Mamare Adelaide Bopape, Betty Sebati, Kotsedi Daniel Monyeki, James Hlengani Siweya, Mafoloa Suzan Monyeki, Julius Chacha Mwita, Brian Godman, Charity Ngoatle, Moloko Matshipi, Phuti Makgae, Abayomi Olusola Ayodapo, Ibisola Babalola, Rosina Nkwana, Gift Makaleng, Mabitsela Mphasha, Debbie Habedi, Julia Manyelo

First published in London, United Kingdom, 2021 by IntechOpen
IntechOpen is the global imprint of INTECHOPEN LIMITED, registered in England and Wales, registration number: 11086078, 5 Princes Gate Court, London, SW7 2QJ, United Kingdom
Printed in Croatia

British Library Cataloguing-in-Publication Data
A catalogue record for this book is available from the British Library

Additional hard and PDF copies can be obtained from orders@intechopen.com

Lifestyle and Epidemiology - The Double Burden of Poverty and Cardiovascular Diseases in African Populations
Edited by Kotsedi Daniel Monyeki and Han C.G. Kemper
p. cm.
Print ISBN 978-1-83962-736-1
Online ISBN 978-1-83962-737-8
eBook (PDF) ISBN 978-1-83962-745-3

For EU product safety concerns:
IN TECH d.o.o. Prolaz Marije Krucifikse Kozulić 3, 51000 Rijeka, Croatia, info@intechopen.com or visit our website at intechopen.com.

Meet the editors

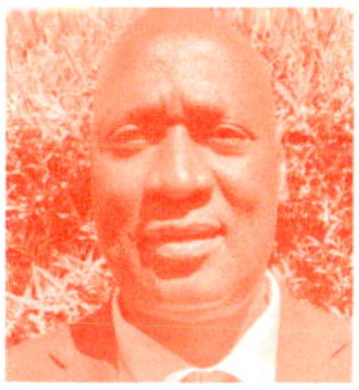

Kotsedi Daniel Monyeki, MA, MPH, Ph.D., is a full professor in the Department of Physiology and Environmental Health, University of Limpopo, South Africa. In 2020, he was rated as a South African National Research Foundation C2 researcher. He has a background in kinesiology and physical education (human movement science). He received an MPH from the University of Cape Town, South Africa. His research interests are in non-communicable diseases, physical activity, and epidemiology. He has been the principal investigator of the Ellisras Longitudinal Study (ELS) since 1996, which inaugurated a biannual international conference in 2017. The ELS project plays a pivotal role in creating awareness of chronic diseases and prevention among members of local communities. Dr. Monyeki is an editorial board member for the *Journal of Human Hypertension*. He has authored and published eight book chapters, three technical reports, and 135 peer-reviewed journal articles. He has presented 131 research papers at national and international conferences. He has supervised and co-supervised graduates and postgraduates at the University of Limpopo and Amsterdam Medical University Center, Amsterdam, the Netherlands.

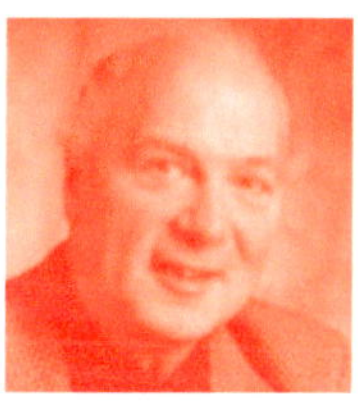

Prof Emeritus Han C.G. Kemper, Ph.D., Hon D, obtained a Ph.D. from the Free University of Brussels, Belgium, in 1968. He also has three honorary degrees from universities in London (University of Surrey), Budapest (Semmelweiss University), and Riga (Radins University). In 1985 he was appointed a full professor at the Faculty of Human Movement Sciences, University of Amsterdam and Vrije University, Amsterdam. Dr. Kemper has supervised twenty-five Ph.D. students over the course of his career. In 1996 he joined the VU University Medical Center in the EMGO+ Institute for Care and Health Research (Amsterdam Public Health Research Institute at Amsterdam UMC). He was the principal investigator of the Amsterdam Growth and Health Longitudinal Study (AGAHLS) from 1974 until 2004. With his research group he has published more than 350 articles in both national and international journals and ten books (or chapters in books) about AGAHLS. From 1996 until 1998 he gave intensive courses for scientific staff members at the University of Limpopo, Polokwane, SA. Since then, he has worked closely with Dr. Monyeki in his Ellisras Longitudinal Study. Dr. Kemper was associate editor of the international journal *Pediatric Exercise Science* from 1988 until 2018. In 2002 he received a citation award from the prestigious American College of Sports Medicine, St. Louis, MO, USA, based upon his publication records in the field of sports and exercise sciences.

Contents

Preface

The profile of non-communicable diseases (NCDs) is changing rapidly in the rural South African population due to COVID-19, poverty, and other social factors. The South African National Development Plan vision for 2030 highlights key recommendations to reduce the prevalence of NCDs by 28% by the year 2030. Similarly, the World Heart Federation set the year 2025 to reduce the prevalence of NCDs by 25%. However, the onset of the COVID-19 pandemic in early 2020 has already significantly impacted efforts towards attaining these national and global targets. Some individuals and families have been pushed into extreme poverty in low social-economic contexts. Therefore, there is an urgent need to tackle the triple burden of NCDs, poverty, and COVID-19. Unfortunately, literacy levels on the triple burden of disease and recommended lifestyle changes remain extremely low among individuals, families, and communities. Communities must seek new innovative ways of addressing issues facing the population with regard to obesity, overweight, hypertension, general health, smoking, alcohol abuse and low physical activity in line with a healthy living lifestyle. To succeed in changing the lifestyle of an individual first requires eradication of illiteracy by health professionals, academics, and scholars in terms of providing primary health information to these sectors of the community through personal interaction.

To that effect, the first and second Ellisras Longitudinal Study and Other Non-communicable Diseases Studies International Conferences (ELSONCDICs) were organized during the period 28–29 November 2017 and 3–5 December 2019, respectively, at the University of Limpopo and Ellisras/Lephalale. The purpose of these ELSONCDICs was (1) to provide a unique inclusive platform for discussion by ordinary members of the Ellisras community, expert scholars, students, and experienced professionals from places all over the world offering a truly special international networking experience; and (2) to provide a comprehensive and interactive programme in which participants can cultivate their cross-cultural and communication skills while shining a light on different topics related to poverty, COVID-19, and NCDs. 3) to let the programme have a long lasting effect on the conference participants as well as the Ellisras/Lephalale communities as the knowledge gained will be taken back to our respective communities and families. An adjunct to the ELSONCDICs is the Phashasha newsletter, which is based on major NCD findings of other studies including the ELS. The language used in the Phashasha newsletter can be understood by ordinary people in the community, ensuring that the correct choice of lifestyle is an achievable goal. Preparations for the third ELSONCDIC scheduled for 22–24 November 2022 at the University of Limpopo and Ellisras/Lephalale are well underway.

Lifestyle and Epidemiology - The Double Burden of Poverty and Cardiovascular Diseases in African Populations is a product of these initiatives. The book is divided into six sections: Section 1, ”Poverty and Cardiovascular Diseases”; Section 2, “Risk Factors for Cardiovascular Diseases”; Section 3, “Lifestyle and Cardiovascular Diseases”; Section 4, “Metabolic Syndrome and Reproductive Health”; Section 5, “Type 2 Diabetes”; Section 6, “Care and Treatment of Cardiovascular Diseases and Diabetes”

Although the book is a group effort, there are two persons who are the driving force behind its success: Han CG Kemper, Emeritus Professor at the Amsterdam Medical University Centre, Amsterdam, the Netherlands, and Hlengani J Siweya, Professor and Executive Dean of the Faculty of Science and Agriculture, University of Limpopo, South Africa. They provided support and sound leadership to the ELSONCDICs, which culminated in this book. They had a vision and the stamina essential in longitudinal research and community empowerment. Both scientists have substantial international exposure; they are also champions of motivation, inspiration, and fundraising. Through them we have learned that "success is not a position but a direction."

Kotsedi Daniel Monyeki
Physiology and Environmental Health Department,
University of Limpopo,
South Africa

Han C.G. Kemper
Amsterdam Medical University Centre,
Amsterdam, The Netherlands

Section 1

Poverty and Cardiovascular Diseases

Chapter 1

Poverty Is Not Poverty: The Reality on the Ground Including the Rural-Urban Divide and How We Can Turn the Tide on NCDs

Janet Michel and Marcel Tanner

Abstract

Cardiovascular diseases (CVDs) tend to occur in younger sub-Saharan African (SSA) populations, about 20 years earlier as compared to high income countries (HIC). Weak health systems and infrastructure, scarce cardiac professionals, skewed budget away from non-communicable diseases (NCD), high treatment costs and reduced access to health care. On top of that, hypertension diagnosis, treatment and control are low, less than 40%, less than 35% and 10-20% respectively. SSA has 23% of the worlds rheumatic disease, while 80% of CVD deaths occur in low to middle income countries. Poverty is not poverty. The rural–urban divide is one reality that has to be acknowledged among others, particularly in Africa. Being poor, while owning land and having the possibility to grow crops and rear livestock, goats and chickens, is different from being an unemployed young man or young woman, renting one room, in a crowded township with dilapidated infrastructure, intermittent or untreated water and surrounded by leaking sewers. Understanding the dynamics in different contexts is important for us to identify and address the different challenges affecting health in general, and heart health of people in these contexts in particular. For example, the detection, treatment and control rates of hypertension are higher in semi-urban as compared to rural areas. Detection rates for both men and women are suboptimal particularly in rural areas. Diet, sedentary life, loneliness and stress, insecure environments rather and unsafe places to walk are issues more common in urban settings. The conditions in which people are born, live, grow and work affect their health. The rural conditions are very different from the urban ones. The quality of air, access and types of food, stress levels, isolation, loneliness and fear not to mention violence, vary. All these factors affect heart health in one way or the other. Addressing heart health issues therefore ought to be context specific. The burdens might be treble or more for some -economically, environmentally (climate change, political instability), socially and historically-apartheid and colonialism.

Keywords: land ownership, traditional foods, environment, spirituality, social or relationship poverty, time poverty, economic poverty, insects, wild vegetables, forms of poverty, health as an asset

1. Introduction

1.1 Defining poverty

Poverty is defined as a state of being inferior in quality or insufficient in amount [1]. Poverty is also defined as not having socially acceptable material possessions or money [2]. The second definition raises the question of who defines what is socially acceptable. Absolute poverty on the other hand is defined as a complete lack of means to meet basic needs like food, clothing and shelter [2]. Relative poverty is defined as an inability of a person to meet a minimum level of living standards compared to others in the same time and place, taking into account context (society or country) [3]. Context matters and it matters a lot [3]. It is imperative to note that none of the above definitions explicitly mentions that a lack of access to education or health care services is poverty. The very means that take a person out of poverty are not mentioned when defining poverty. In most African contexts, one has to be healthy first and foremost, before gaining access to education, and access or entitlement to land.

2. Universal health coverage (UHC)

Billions world-wide live in squalid conditions of disease, hunger and desperation-a state of pandemic poverty [4]. Poverty eradication has become a buzz word but commitment to addressing systemic causes of poverty is lacking [4]. The inextricable link between poor health, poverty and development is well documented [5]. Hunger can lead to poor health, social unrest, conflict and displacement [5]. The decision to migrate itself is not easy and many illegal migrants face challenges to access health care in transit and even years after settling [6].

UHC is defined as ensuring that everyone has access to health care services of high quality without suffering financial impoverishment. The services range from health promotion, prevention, treatment, rehabilitative and palliative care [7–9]. Good health allows children to access school and learn and adults to be productive and earn. UHC, good health therefore is a determinant for people to escape poverty.

2.1 Health the foundation block in eradicating poverty

We reckon, it is imperative for societies and governments to identify health as a tool and resource against poverty that needs to be protected and guarded. Poverty is defined by the United Nations as a violation of human dignity through not having choices and opportunities. It includes not having basic capacity to participate effectively in a society, not having enough food, clothing, not having access to education or health care, not having land, a job or access to credit facilities [10]. Health, the very condition that defines whether we can attend school or till the

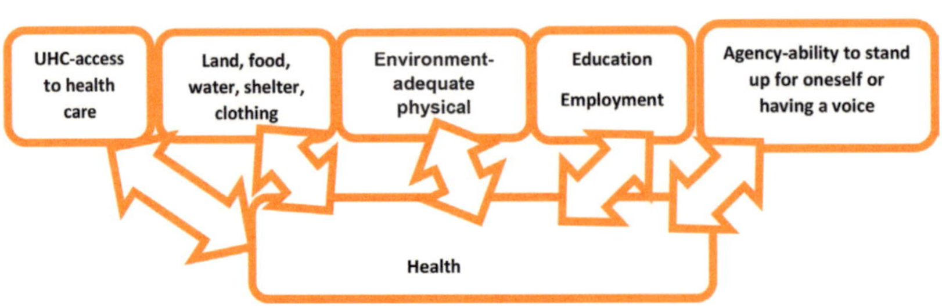

Figure 1.
What health unlocks.

land, is not emphasised enough in the definitions of poverty. Having land but being in poor health or having access to education but being in poor health is a form of poverty. Health, is therefore the basic block in life which gives one access to education, work, food, clothes and shelter. From a public health perspective, health ought to be identified as a basic block that is essential for the eradication of poverty. One prerequisite to accessing everything else in life though seems to be health. Health poverty affects all the other domains. See **Figure 1** above.

3. Forms of poverty

Poverty may include social, economic and political elements as seen above [11]. An unemployed young person, who has migrated to a foreign land, leaving behind friends and family, and now illegally living in a crowded township room, might be socially, economically and health poor all at once.

4. Strategies used to address poverty

How best to help the poor is a longstanding debate [12–17]. Governments and other organisations try to reduce economic poverty by a) providing basic needs to people who are unable to earn a sufficient income like the child grant in South Africa. Barriers are corruption, a dwindling tax base in a society that is driven by the informal sector and ultimately sustainability. Less than half of South Africas' rather population eligible for work is formally employed [18].

4.1 Start by protecting the physically healthy and making them aware of their wealth-health

The physically healthy, the very assets of our economies, are currently not sufficiently being made aware of their wealth-health, and neither are they supported sufficiently to value their own health nor are they protected from environmental pollution, water pollution, unsanitary conditions, and the lack of access to health care services. Many black South Africans live in crowded squalor illegally and with no or limited access to land.

5. Time poverty

Many public health facilities are overcrowded. Someone who needs to be seen by a doctor has to calculate many hours of waiting. Many people are forced to take a day or two from work making them time impoverished. Additional hours are also lost daily during the commute to and fro the work, leaving them both time and economically poor [18].

5.1 Sickness strips one of agency making one unable to stand up for oneself or have a voice

Poverty exposes one to violence, since it renders one powerless and excluded from society, living in marginal or fragile environments, with limited access to clean water or sanitation [10]. One can have access to education but being hungry will affect outcomes [12]. Children can be sent to school in poor health, suffering from e.g. anaemia, bilharzia or worms and this will affect outcomes [12]. So, health is a fundamental building block.

6. Conditions in which we are conceived, born, grow, live and work affect our health

24 years since independence apartheid in South Africa has persisted in an economic form [18]. Many families live in airless hovels constructed using splintered boards and metal sheets [18]. Post-apartheid, land is still largely in the hands of the white elites with most black South Africans still living in the townships [18] and one needs political ties to survive and thrive in business [18], closing this door to many.

Health is determined by the conditions in which we are born, grow, live and work [19]. We take this a step further and say health is determined by the conditions in which we are **conceived**, born, grow, live, work etc. One South African domestic worker said;

> *"Our children are being born in the same situation I was born" [18] - Credit Jao Silvia, New York Times.*

In rural settings, people often have land, are surrounded with friends and neighbours, have time, have spiritual groups usually and the environment is less crowded and less filthy. Many have access to seasonally available fruit and vegetables. In the urban setting, many blacks have no access to land, live in crowded unsanitary, unsafe environments and neighbourhoods, isolated and often cannot practice spirituality, and many live from hand to mouth-informal sector. The usual diets are high in carbohydrates and saturated fats.

7. Conditions in which most south Africans live

The impact of former apartheid policies on the health system have been documented and these inequalities have grown along class rather than racial lines recently [20] and these issues still have effects on children being conceived under these conditions to date. The well to do have access to quality health care services from the private health sector, while 80 percent access health care from the overburdened public health sector [21]. Rapid urbanisation is also partly to blame for the increase in coronary heart and artery disease and metabolic disorders [22]. Some people moved from a shack during apartheid to another shack [18] post-apartheid. The living conditions have not changed much. Several hours a day are spent commuting [18] to places of work making them time poor. A foetus conceived while mum is in poor health, malnourished etc., will be affected by these conditions even later on in life -health consequences. The health of the mother affects the heath of the baby. A healthy mum is predictive of a healthy infant. This might sound like chicken egg debate, which was first-and health is the chicken.

8. Access to land

No land no collateral [18], is another glaring issue in South Africa. Many South Africans have no access to land. Investment in ensuring that people have access to land, ensuring safe water supplies through digging more wells, boreholes and improving sanitation- the very conditions that promote people to be and stay healthy is fundamental. Land ownership is one instrument that is pivotal in addressing both rural and urban poverty [16]. In good health people can then access education, employment etc.

> *"We never dismantled apartheid. The patterns of enrichment and impoverishment are still the same." Ayabonga Cawe, former economist Oxfam [18].*

9. Fossil fuel, sedentary life unsafe places

Causes of cardio vascular diseases (CVDs) in SA are high BP, smoking, drinking, poor eating habits, obesity and lack of physical activity [22, 23] and psychosocial stress (depression, anxiety, hostility) [24]. Cardiovascular risk factors disproportionately affect the socio-economically disadvantaged [25] and we can speculate how this comes about.

People use fire for cooking, breathing in fumes, barefoot they walk on ground littered with broken glass, needles, tins and daily they exchange armed robbery updates [18]. Is this conducive for health? Police frequently descend on these informal settlements tearing down these shacks without warning [18]. In some settlements human waste forms puddles [18]. While in some predominantly white areas toilets are stocked with soap, toilt paper, staffed with janitors and security guards [18], many townships are ghettos of isolation [18]. Diet, sedentary life, loneliness and stress and how people deal with it e.g., drinking and smoking are prevalent issues in townships. People often do not know where to get the next meal and the insecure environments prevents physical activities like walking forcing people to take taxis home or to school (no safe places to walk). Attending worship is also affected by these unsafe places. Some services are in the evening. Spirituality has been proven to give meaning and purpose to stressful life events leading to more positive emotions like well-being, happiness, optimism and fewer negative emotions. The psychological benefits of spirituality affect immune, inflammatory, endocrine and even autonomic functions. These unsafe contexts further deprive people of these benefits further affecting heart health [24].

9.1 How do people get diseases in theses contexts?

- Living in filthy overcrowded and unsanitary conditions
- Lack of food
- Lack of knowledge- leading to exposures
- Having knowledge but no options e.g., forced to scavenge from dump sites

9.2 How are the sick further affected in these contexts?

- Lack of financial means to buy drugs, pay for transport, lack of knowledge to eat healthy (ongoing care and regular checks) and the condition gets worse.
- Living conditions, not safe to exercise, or walk, limited access to clean water and sanitation
- No means to follow recommendations made by medical staff (medical education to change) e.g., Eat broccoli when you cannot afford this or live-in rural areas where such foods do not exist-unrealistic recommendations by medical personnel that do not take context into account
- People get medicine and are sent back to the very environment that caused the disease, leaving the stressors unaddressed e.g. the crime ridden township that caused disease.

How to destress, a different approach that includes preventive and promotive health is needed. There is a direct link between stress and heart health. High emotional stress, isolation and loneliness have been linked to atrial and ventricular arrhythmias [24].

10. Causes of heart diseases in SA

Causes of CVD in SSA are hypertension, cardiomyopathy, rheumatic heart disease and congenital heart disease [26]. One multicentre study on PHC in SA revealed that primary care is dominated by NCDs and the most common diagnosis and reason to attend PHC being hypertension and HIV ranking third [25]. Death rates from non-communicable diseases in SA now exceed those of TB and HIV combined [25] and cardiovascular diseases are leading the NCDs. Obesity (68% of women and 31% of men) is another culprit [25]. The high burden of HIV directs most health care spending towards antiretroviral treatment, limiting funds for NCDs particularly in primary health care setting.

10.1 Neglected causes of cardiovascular diseases and their causes

Neglected CVDs in SSA are endomyocardial fibrosis, congenital heart diseases, and rheumatic heart disease [26]. Rheumatic fever affects children in low resource settings where poverty is rife, overcrowding and poor sanitary conditions and limited access to health care services. Rhematic heart disease can be prevented by preventing streptococcal infections or treating them early when they occur [27].

Congenital heart disease: Genes and environmental factors are associated with congenital heart diseases. Maternal health is critical particularly during the first trimester [28]. New-born heart health is affected by maternal health during pregnancy and the environmental conditions in which the mother lives. Causes of endomyocardial fibrosis are virus infections and toxic insults among others [29, 30]. See **Table 1** below.

It is important to point out that social determinants of health are alluded to in the national development plan 2030 [31]. The realisation and implementation of these policies however, remain a challenge.

Condition	Cause	Available interventions
Congenital heart disease	Genes and environmental factors	Preventive Promotive Curative-medical and surgical treatment Rehabilitative
Endomyocardial fibrosis	Virus infections and toxic insults	Preventive Promotive Curative-treatment Rehabilitative
Rheumatic heart disease	Poverty, overcrowding, poor sanitary conditions and limited access to health care services	Preventive Promotive Curative-treatment with antibiotics Rehabilitative

Table 1.
Neglected causes of cardiovascular diseases and their causes.

11. South African plans to decrease NCD related premature mortality

SA has plans to decrease NCD related premature mortality by 25% by end of 2020. This includes population and individual based strategies.

11.1 Population based strategies to prevent NCDs

- Legislation for reduction of sodium in processed foods [32]
- Taxation of sugar sweetened beverages [32] and alcohol
- Tightening of anti-tobacco regulations [25]

11.2. Individual level strategies (crucial)

- Detection, treatment and control of cardiovascular disease risk [25]
- Emphasis -assertive treatment, targeting antihypertensive and statin treatment guidelines [25]
- Training of nurses (lest we forget) on correct measurement and aggressive management of NCDs, active detection, prevention, control of cardio-vascular diseases to avert expenses on hospitalizations [25].

12. Public health lip service?

Both the population based and individual based strategies above, are focussing mainly on treatment rather than prevention. Why wait for the population to fall sick? Simple, cost effective and culturally adapted behaviour and educational interventions rather needed (**Figure 2**) [23].

Health of the population should be protected- a central tenet of public health. The health care in SA is hospicentric rather than preventive and promotive. Only 10% of health expenditure is spent on promotive health? The system seems to foster the idea that people should get ill first before being assisted.

Step 1: Health is an asset -acknowledgement and identification of that).

Step 2: Health needs to be preserved.

Step 3: Health gives us access to everything else in the society, education, jobs, security etc.

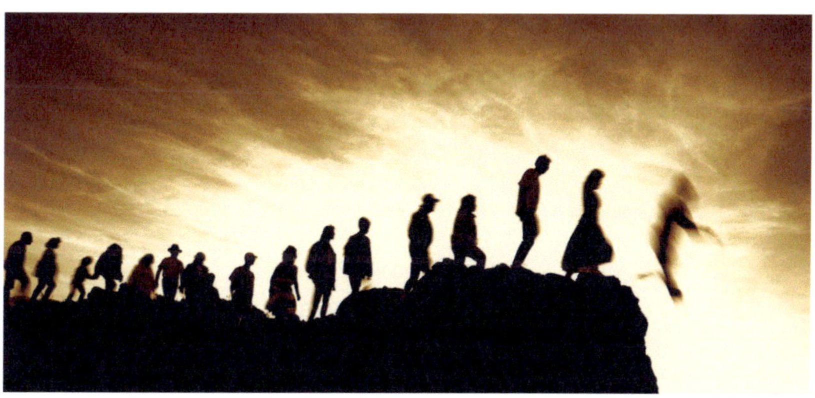

Figure 2.
We are waiting for people to fall sick as depicted below.

13. If I am healthy, I am rich (health rich)

Making people aware that being healthy is an asset can go a long way. In the HIV context too, little money is spent on preventive strategies. Some young people are not aware that being healthy, HIV negative is an asset worthy to be protected. Some seem not afraid of HIV saying if they get it, they will get onto treatment. The value of health as an asset seems not widely and explicitly valued?

The environments in which many South Africans live are characterised by land poverty, environmental poverty, social or relational poverty, economic poverty, political poverty (lack of voice for some) and spiritual poverty, all of which lead to health poverty including cardiovascular health issues. See **Table 2** below.

Forms of poverty	Effects
Environmental poverty	Causes stress, toxic exposures, violence
Time poverty	Causes stress, loss of income
Spiritual poverty	Causes stress and hopelessness
Land poverty	Limits access to loans, one cannot grow own food
Social or relational poverty	Causes loneliness
Economic poverty	Reduces access to food and basics including health care
Political poverty	Lack of voice, stress
Health poverty	Decreases access to land, education, jobs, relationships, spirituality and increases health complications

Table 2.
How do these factors affect heart health?

14. Interconnectedness of the different forms of poverty

The interconnectedness of the different forms of poverty and their effect on health ought to be mentioned [33]. Systems thinking is therefore called for if health issues are to be addressed effectively. See **Figure 3** below.

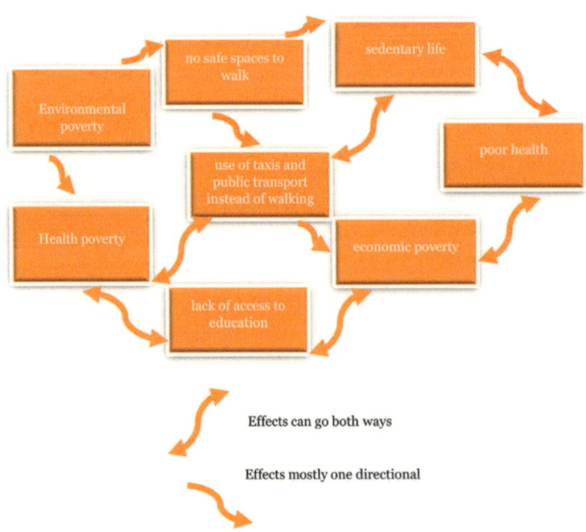

Figure 3.
Interconnectedness and the need for systems thinking.

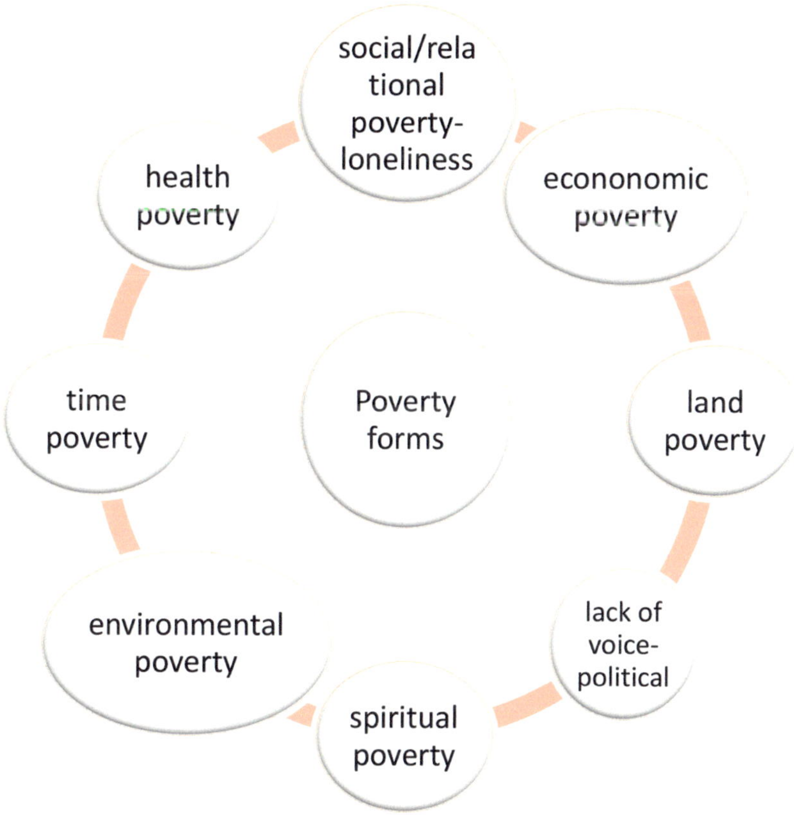

Figure 4.
Forms of poverty.

Figure 4 shows how connected the different forms of poverty are and how they affect health.

15. Adapting current medical interventions and training to reflect context

As depicted above, **Figure 5**, the current interventions work differently for the poor and the rich. The poor often have no choice to change their environment, be it living or working environment, they live in unsafe neighbourhoods where it is unsafe to walk let alone access to a gym. Many church services are held at night. The poor are not safe to attend these spiritual opportunities depriving them of a freely available healing tool-spirituality. They eat what is cheap and this is often high in unsaturated fats, and they often miss check-ups due to transport costs etc.

It is therefore easier for the well to do who get diagnosed with cardiovascular diseases to get back to the optimal health line. The current CVD interventions are pro rich. How can we make them pro poor? Doing so would mean addressing environmental and psychosocial factors and economic and health system factors. Context matters. The training of medical personnel should incorporate locally available nutrition that promotes health without making the poor sink into deeper poverty if they want to stay healthy. The currently recommended healthy diet should be high in fibre, green vegetables, fruit the year round, fish and low

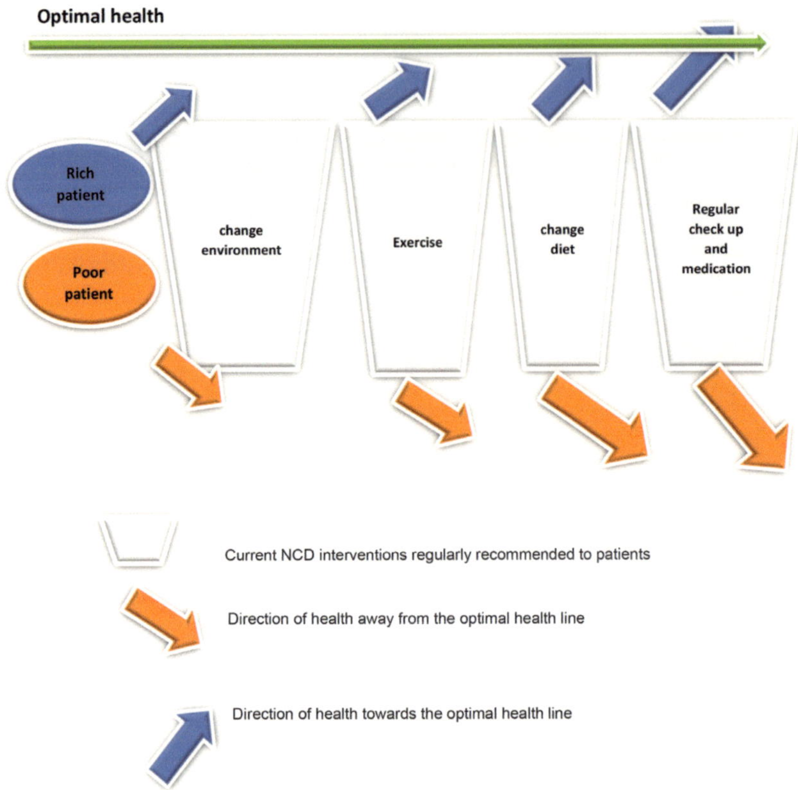

Figure 5.
The current interventions and their effect on health including heart health depending on whether one is rich or poor.

processed foods and fat [24]. Can the average township person afford this? Locally available foods e.g., seasonal fruits, wild vegetables, peanut butter and insects are all good for heart health and should be widely promoted and made easily available.

16. Conclusion

Health is an asset. The conditions in which we are born, grow, live and work affect our health. Countries do not necessarily need wealth to gain health e.g. Sri Lanka had a maternal mortality rate of 2% in the 1930s not comparable to any country today [34]. Sri Lanka reduced maternal mortality to 0.6% today, spending less each year as they learnt what worked and did not work [34]. Similarly, countries in SSA could adapt their approach through first identification of health as asset and then investing in preventive and promotive health while still ensuring efficacy and efficiency of curative services. Addressing the different forms of poverty, utilising a systems thinking lens, could contribute to healthier societies.

Author details

Janet Michel[1,2]* and Marcel Tanner[2,3]

1 Insel University Hospital, University of Bern, Switzerland

2 Department of Epidemiology and Public Health, Swiss Tropical and Public Health Institute (Swiss TPH), Basel, Switzerland

3 University of Basel, Basel, Switzerland

*Address all correspondence to: janetmichel71@gmail.com

References

[1] Poverty definition. From: https: //www.google.com/search?q=poverty+definition&oq =poverty+definition&aqs=chrome.69i57.6680j0j15&sourceid=chrome&ie=UTF-8. Accessed October 9, 2020.

[2] Migration and inclusive societies. UNESCO 2019. From: https://en.unesco.org/themes/fostering-rights-inclusion/migration. Accessed October 9, 2020

[3] Bressers JTA. From public administration to policy networks: Contextual interaction analysis. Rediscovering Public Law Public Adm Comp Policy Anal Tribute Peter Knoepfel 2009:123-142.

[4] Poverty and Development. From: https://www.globalpolicy.org/social-and-economic-policy/poverty-and-development.html. Accessed January 5, 2021

[5] Health, Poverty and Development. From: https://www.globalpolicy.org/social-and-economic-policy/poverty-and-development/health-poverty-and-development Accessed January 5, 2021

[6] Legido-Quigley H, Pocock N, Tan ST, Pajin L, Suphanchaimat R, Wickramage K, et al. Healthcare is not universal if undocumented migrants are excluded. BMJ 2019;366:l4160.

[7] Carrin G, James C, Evans DB. WHO | Achieving universal health coverage: developing the health financing system. WHO 2005. From: http://www.who.int/health_financing/documents/cov-pb_e_05_1-universal_cov/en/. Accessed October 23, 2019.

[8] Universal health coverage (UHC) implementation | Global Health 2035 2018. From: http://globalhealth2035.org/our-work/domestic-health-investments/universal-health-coverage-uhc-implementation. Accessed December 29, 2018.

[9] Kruk ME. Universal health coverage: a policy whose time has come. BMJ 2013;347:f6360.

[10] Gordon D. Indicators of Poverty & Hunger 2005. From: https://www.un.org/esa/socdev/unyin/documents/ydiDavidGordon_poverty.pdf. Accessed 6 January 2020

[11] Ending Poverty 2018. From: https://www.un.org/en/sections/issues-depth/poverty/. Accessed October 9, 2020.

[12] Kristof N. How Can We Help the World's Poor? N Y Times 2009.

[13] Postrel V. The Poverty Puzzle (Published 2006). N Y Times 2006.

[14] Drezner DW. "The End of Poverty": Brother, Can You Spare $195 Billion? N Y Times 2005.

[15] Moyo D, Ferguson N. Dead Aid: Why Aid Is Not Working and How There Is a Better Way for Africa. Reprint Edition. Farrar, Straus and Giroux; 2009.

[16] Is Aid Killing Africa? Dambisa Moyo talks about Dead Aid on ABC. From: https://www.abc.net.au/foreign/uk---is-aid-killing-africa/1624286. Accessed 6 January 2021

[17] Collier P. The Bottom Billion: Why the Poorest Countries are Failing and What Can Be Done About It: From: https://www.amazon.com/Bottom-Billion-Poorest-Countries-Failing/dp/0195373383. Accessed October 10, 2020.

[18] Goodman PS. End of Apartheid in South Africa? Not in Economic Terms. N Y Times 2017.

[19] Bloomsbury.com. The Health Gap. Bloomsbury Publ n.d. https://www.bloomsbury.com/uk/

the-health-gap-9781408857991/. Accessed June 2, 2019.

[20] Mcintyre D, Mcleod H. The challenges of pursuing private health insurance in low- and middle-income countries: lessons from South Africa. In: Sagan A, Mossialos E, Thomson S, editors. Priv. Health Insur. Hist. Polit. Perform., Cambridge: Cambridge University Press; 2020, p. 377-413.

[21] Socio-economic inequalities in the multiple dimensions of access to healthcare: the case of South Africa. From: https://bmcpublichealth.biomedcentral.com/articles/10.1186/s12889-020-8368-7. Accessed January 5, 2021.

[22] Zuhlke L. Why heart disease is on the rise in South Africa. The Conversation. From: http://theconversation.com/why-heart-disease-is-on-the-rise-in-south-africa-66167. Accessed December 2, 2020.

[23] Cappuccio FP, Miller MA. Cardiovascular disease and hypertension in sub-Saharan Africa: burden, risk and interventions. Intern Emerg Med 2016; 11:299-305.

[24] Lucchese FA, Koenig HG. Religion, spirituality and cardiovascular disease: research, clinical implications, and opportunities in Brazil. Braz J Cardiovasc Surg 2013; 28:103-128.

[25] Schutte AE. Urgency for South Africa to prioritise cardiovascular disease management. Lancet Glob Health 2019;7: e177–e178.

[26] Yuyun MF, Sliwa K, Kengne AP, Mocumbi AO, Bukhman G. Cardiovascular Diseases in Sub-Saharan Africa Compared to High-Income Countries: An Epidemiological Perspective. Glob Heart 2020; 15:15.

[27] Rheumatic Heart Disease. From: https://www.who.int/news-room/fact-sheets/detail/rheumatic-heart-disease. Accessed December 2, 2020.

[28] Stanford Children's Health From: https://www.stanfordchildrens.org/en/topic/default?id=factors-contributing-to-congenital-heart-disease-90-P01788. Accessed December 2, 2020

[29] Liu T, Song D, Dong J, Zhu P, Liu J, Liu W, et al. Current Understanding of the Pathophysiology of Myocardial Fibrosis and Its Quantitative Assessment in Heart Failure. Front Physiol 2017;8.

[30] Tartaglione AM, Venerosi A, Calamandrei G. Early-Life Toxic Insults and Onset of Sporadic Neurodegenerative Diseases—an Overview of Experimental Studies. In: Kostrzewa RM, Archer T, editors. Neurotoxin Model. Brain Disord.-Long Outcomes Behav. Teratol., Cham: Springer International Publishing; 2016, p. 231-264.

[31] National development plan 2030. National Development Plan 2030 Our Future-make it work. 2020. From: https://www.gov.za/documents/national-development-plan-2030-our-future-make-it-work. Accessed 6 January 2021.

[32] World Heart Federation. World Heart Federation 2020. From: https://www.world-heart-federation.org/. Accessed 6 January 2021

[33] Senge PM. The fifth discipline: the art and practice of the learning organization. London: Random House Business Books; 1999.

[34] Saving millions for just a few dollars: cost-effective health measures for poor nations. World Hunger News 2006. From: https://www.worldhunger.org/saving-millions-for-just-a-few-dollars-cost-effective-health-measures-for-poor-nations/. Accessed October 10, 2020.

Chapter 2

Poverty and Cardiovascular Diseases in Sub-Saharan Africa

Julius Chacha Mwita and Brian Godman

Abstract

There is a rise in cardiovascular diseases (CVDs) in sub-Saharan Africa (SSA). Even though SSA is home to 14% world's inhabitants, it is home to more than half of the global poor. The objective of this chapter is to evaluate the interconnection between CVD and poverty in SSA. We found that the relationship between poverty and CVD is bidirectional. The intersection between poverty and CVD cuts through primordial, primary prevention and secondary prevention interventions. In the context of poverty in SSA, CVD prevention is a challenge due to competing demands to address the never conquered infectious diseases exacerbated by the current COVID-19 pandemic. With a weak healthcare system and out of pocket payment for the costs of CVD care, a significant proportion of individuals with CVD and their households are consequently impoverished. Besides, CVD affects a younger and productive population in SSA than in the rest of the world. Thus, CVD-related loss of productivity progressively pushes an additional number of individuals into poverty, requiring urgent attention.

Keywords: cardiovascular diseases, medicines, poverty, sub-Saharan Africa

1. Introduction

Cardiovascular diseases (CVDs) include coronary heart disease, cerebrovascular diseases, peripheral arterial disease, rheumatic and congenital heart disease, and deep vein thrombosis [1]. Except for coronary heart disease on the rise in urban areas, hypertension, stroke, cardiomyopathies, and rheumatic heart disease are the most common CVDs across sub-Saharan Africa (SSA) [2, 3]. CVDs account for 30% of global deaths, and about 80% of them occurring in low- and middle-income countries (LMICs), including SSA [2, 4]. By 2030, projections show that CVD alone will cause more SSA deaths than infectious diseases, maternal and perinatal conditions, and nutritional disorders combined [5]. Consequently, an increasing priority area for future activities. The rising burden of CVD in SSA is due to increasing population exposure to various modifiable risk factors that account for at least three-quarters of all the CVDs [3]. The risk factors include unhealthy diets, physical inactivity, hypertension, obesity, diabetes, dyslipidaemia, and tobacco use [4]. Given the poverty and multiple competing health priorities across SSA, similar to several other LMICs, both prevention and treatment of CVDs get less attention [3]. With the high patient co-payments in many SSA countries, CVDs impose a significant health and economic burden on individuals and families in the region than in higher-income countries [6]. Above and beyond, poverty may contribute to an increased burden of CVD by its effect on several social and cultural factors responsible for the increasing burden of CVD [7]. Consequently, this report looked at CVD and poverty interconnection in SSA and the implications for the future.

2. Poverty in sub-Saharan Africa

SSA is home to 14% of the 7.8 billion world's inhabitants but contributes to more than half of the global poor [8, 9]. Using the 1-dimensional measurement of poverty that focuses on income or wealth, over 40% of SSA residents live below the poverty line of $1.90 per person per day [9]. This poverty level is far above the average poverty rate of 13% in other regions of the world [10]. While the rest of the world has observed a significant decline in extreme poverty, SSA observed a rise in the number of people living in extreme poverty from 278 million in 1990 to 413 million in 2015 [9, 11]. Even those who live above the $1.90 poverty, a significant proportion of them are still very poor due to deprivations in various aspects of well-being [9, 11]. Using deprivation from education, health, and assets as multi-dimensional measures of poverty, about half (51%) of the poor population in the world lives in SSA [12]. Therefore, most sub-Saharan inhabitants lack sufficient income and basic needs, including quality health and education [12]. Most of the causes of poverty in SSA are not different from the rest of the world. They include colonialism, war and political instability, national debts, discrimination and social inequality, and vulnerability to natural disasters [13]. The impact of colonialism, the slave trade and resource extraction from SSA likely contributed in some ways to the persistent poverty in the region [14]. The existence of a significant inequality in income distribution and access to productive resources, essential social services, opportunities, markets exacerbate the already existing poverty despite the autonomy of African countries following their independence [15]. Women and children are the most affected groups with inequalities and natural catastrophic events such as drought, flooding, and frequent disease epidemics in the region [14, 15]. In these events, the already impoverished people are often displaced, lose their belongings, and remain in the vicious cycle of poverty [15].

Similarly, violent regional conflicts, forced displacement and political instability in a significant number of SSA countries interfere with safety, stability and security needed for investment and economic growth [13]. The situation is made worse by weak national institutions permissive to corruption and resource misallocation in many SSA countries [9]. As a result, these countries carry significant debts that have high-interest rates and are linked to conditions that may be unfavourable to the development of local economies [13]. The impact of HIV and AIDS is also significant as the disease affected the working-age population leading to a reduction in economic productivity [16]. In the context of all these factors, it remains unclear if the region will end poverty in all its forms by 2030 as per the Sustainable Development Goal 1 (SDG 1) [17].

3. The effect of poverty of CVD in Africa

With poverty, SSA has the lowest healthcare expenditure, the lowest life expectancy, and inadequate access to health care services, safe water, education, and sanitation facilities [18, 19]. Although poverty is among the reasons behind the region's high burden of infectious diseases such as malaria, tuberculosis and human immunodeficiency virus (HIV), it is also a reason behind the rising burden of CVDs [4]. Economic development in SSA leads to urbanisation and increased tobacco consumption, harmful alcohol use, unhealthy diets, and physical inactivity [2]. While the wealthy population can revise their lifestyle, lack of access to both preventative and remedial health care among the poor partly explains the high burden of CVD risk factors [20, 21]. Besides poor access to healthcare services for CVD prevention and control, low education significantly affects a good understanding of the disease process and promoting a healthy lifestyle among the poor [22]. With poverty encompassing low income and consumption, poor education, health, nutrition, and other human development parameters, its effect on CVD is complex [23]. It affects different stages, ranging from primordial prevention that targets the emergence of CVD risk factors, primary prevention in the presence of CVD risk factors, and educational programmes on modifiable CVD risk factors.

Unfortunately, data on the overall burden of CVD and its association with poverty are scarce in SSA [24]. With the weak state of the health systems in many SSA countries, typical patient record systems are not sufficiently functional to support accurate morbidity and mortality data documentation [25]. Given the high burden of environmentally induced risk behaviours and limited access to good-quality and affordable health care, the CVD burden, morbidity, and mortality are disproportionately higher among the poor than the affluent population in the region [20–22, 26–28]. Only a few countries (e.g., Botswana) have a universal healthcare system that extends coverage to poor communities [28]. Besides, CVD modifiable risk factors such as hypertension, diabetes, and cholesterol disorders remain undiagnosed or untreated in a significant proportion of the poor communities in SSA [28–33]. The situation is concerning because early detection and effective management of risk factors can substantially reduce most CVD [34]. Over and above the behavioural and physiological risk factors, anger, anxiety and depression are important risk factors for CVD [35]. Poor housing, sanitation and limited access to healthcare are psychosocial stressors that may lead to anger, anxiety and depression in the poor urban sub-Saharan populations [35]. Psychosocial stressors lead to an increased behavioural risk factors for CVD such as tobacco consumption, harmful alcohol use, unhealthy diets, and physical inactivity [2]. Also, most of these populations live in overpopulated unplanned urban settlements, which are often not conducive for establishing healthy behaviours [2, 18, 19]. These communities can hardly afford healthy food and have high illiteracy levels [20, 21].

Hence, poverty leads to CVD through multiple ways that lie within and outside the health sector. Consequently, broad partnerships across various sectors are needed to achieve the 25% reduction in premature NCD mortality by 2025 (the 25 by 25 goal) in SSA [36].

Although not related to the epidemiological transition, rheumatic heart disease (RHD) is another poverty-related CVD that has remained unconquered in SSA [30, 37]. The disease is responsible for over 95% of the 492 042 global deaths per year among the young population in SSA and other impoverished communities in Oceania, South Asia, Central Asia, and the Middle East [38]. SSA (5·7 cases per 1000), the Pacific and indigenous Australia and New Zealand (3·5 cases per 1000), and south-central Asia (2·2 cases per 1000) are the regions with the highest prevalence of RHD [38]. The disease results from acute rheumatic fever (ARF) - an abnormal immunological response to Group A Streptococcal (GAS) infection of the throat [39]. Risk factors of ARF include poverty, overcrowding and reduced access to medical care, all prevalent in SSA [38, 40]. Primary prevention of ARF involves early detection and antibiotic treatment of streptococcal pharyngitis [38, 41]. Early detection and treatment of streptococcal pharyngitis require functional health care services and a community with enough health literacy and appropriate health-seeking behaviour. With rampant poverty and the absence of universal healthcare, the treatment of streptococcus pharyngitis is poorly practised in many SSA countries [42]. Consequently, RHD remains prevalent in SSA versus other countries and an appreciable cause of premature mortality with a mean age of death as low as 25 years [43]. While medical and surgical management can reduce morbidity and mortality, poverty reduction and improvement of overall living standards are crucial in reducing the overall burden and complications of RHD [44].

4. The effect of CVD on poverty in Africa

CVDs occur approximately two decades earlier in SSA than in the rest of the world [5]. In the context of poverty and weak healthcare systems, patients with CVD in SSA have higher all-cause mortality and shorter lifespans than in the other parts of the world due to often limited access to healthcare. Over 50% of these patients die between 30 and 69 years of age, approximately ten years or more below the equivalent group in higher-income countries [45]. Consequently, death and disability attributable to CVD occur in the middle and economically productive age, affecting young families and the much-needed workforce in the region [45, 46]. Available evidence implicates stroke as the cause of the majority of CVD-related mortality in SSA [46]. With the absence of universal health coverage and robust health insurance systems among most SSA countries, patients and their families bear the costs of CVD care costs [47]. In some instances, patients forego treatment due to costs [47]. The impoverishing effect of out-of-pocket payments is increasingly pushing many individuals and families into poverty with family members affected by CVD [6].

5. Poverty, illiteracy, and indigenous knowledge system effect on CVD

Given the high cost and inaccessibility of biomedical care and medications for CVD, traditional healers are central to CVD treatment among patients in SSA [48, 49]. The spiritual underpinning of chronic diseases such as CVD, cultural beliefs, and taboos are reasons behind the preference of traditional healers over biomedicine as the first choice in some parts of SSA [50]. Consequently, it is not uncommon for individuals in the region to seek help from traditional healers to treat diabetes, hypertension, and stroke [51–53]. The belief that traditional healers are experts in treating and curing CVDs and their risk factors delays the transfer to biomedical care despite the clinical deterioration in some patients [50]. Those who transfer to biomedical care are less likely to maintain treatment compliance equivalent to traditional medicines. These culturally driven practices present the greatest threat to the treatment and control of CVDs and their risk factors [50]. Some cultural ideas partly explain the persistently low knowledge of CVDs, risk factors, and clinical symptoms in the SSA population [54]. Therefore, governments and other key stakeholder groups understanding these cultural-driven beliefs and practices are essential in devising strategies to improve health literacy in managing and controlling CVDs [55].

6. Effect of poverty on diagnosis treatment and control/eradication of CVD

With the growing burden of NCDs worldwide, the 2011 United Nation (UN) high-level meeting adopted a political declaration on NCDs that aimed at a 25% reduction in premature mortality from the four main NCDs (cardiovascular diseases, chronic respiratory diseases, cancers, and diabetes) by 25% relative to their 2010 levels by 2025 (the 25 × 25 target) [36]. In 2015, the UN SGD-3 was adopted to reduce by one-third premature mortality from NCDs by 2030 [17]. To realise the SGD-3 target on health, a reduction in tobacco use, harmful alcohol use, salt intake, obesity, raised blood pressure, increased blood glucose and diabetes, and physical inactivity is essential [56]. Besides, treating people at high risk of CVD and ensuring a sustainable availability of medicines to treat NCDs and avoid potential complications is also critical [56]. The above measures are challenging to implement because of the regional poverty, underfunded healthcare systems and the absence of clear policies and strategies [57]. To overcome these challenges, governments and other key stakeholder groups need to instigate several measures that may reduce CVD morbidity and mortality, especially among the poor. These include researching to assess the optimal way to help diagnose CVD early and educate patients of the benefits of biomedical versus traditional medical approaches alongside lifestyle changes. In cognisance of the high levels of illiteracy among many of these patients, approaches such as pictograms are helpful in enhancing understanding [36, 58]. In addition, for governments to produce up-to-date guidelines that are robust and easy to use in electronic formats, with regular monitoring of prescribing patterns to improve the future quality of prescribing [59, 60]. This recognises that adherence to prescribing guidelines is seen as a better marker of the quality of prescribing than current WHO/INRUD criteria [61]. Alongside this, seek to instigate policies to enhance access to low-cost medicines, thereby reducing costly co-payments. This can potentially be achieved with the help of donors and pharmaceutical companies and exploring the potential for local manufacturing of multiple sourced medicines building on concerns during the COVID-19 pandemic [61]. In the meantime, exploration of the potential for aggressive procurement programmes since we have seen in Europe that such programmes have resulted in the prices of generic medicines used to manage CVD as low as 2% of pre-patent prices [62]. Issues of transport costs to clinics to effectively treat patients with CVD also needs to be researched further as lack of contact can be a significant barrier to adherence to medicines for NCDs [63]. In addition, exploring different methods to improve the convenience of medicine dispensing that reduces time off work building on current initiatives in South Africa and wider [27].

7. Conclusions

There are concerns about the rising burden of CVD in SSA, adding to the prevalent infectious diseases in the region. The increase in CVD is due to behavioural and metabolic risk factors resulting from the epidemiologic transition in the region. The intersection between poverty and CVD cuts through primordial, primary prevention and secondary prevention interventions. In the context of poverty in SSA, CVD prevention is a challenge due to competing demands to address the never conquered infectious diseases. With a weak healthcare system and out of pocket payment for the costs of CVD care, a significant proportion of individuals with CVD and their households are pushed into poverty. Besides, CVD affects a younger and productive population in SSA than in the rest of the world.

Consequently, CVD-related loss of productivity will push an additional number of individuals into poverty. Because of this, appropriate strategies are needed to address the rising burden of CVD across SSA, and these should include activities to address poverty issues. Activities include providing available funding and resources for effective screening for NCDs, especially CVD and diabetes, given high rates of patients not being diagnosed. Alongside this, improving the access and availability of medicines, especially where co-payments are an appreciable issue among patients. Multiple channels exist, including activities of donors as well as increasing local production. Alongside this, enhance educational input, especially for patients with low educational levels, to improve adherence rates to suggested lifestyle changes and prescribed medicines, which can be appreciable concerns. This includes a more significant role for pharmacists and nurse practitioners in SSA ambulatory care clinics to help diagnose and manage CVDs. Access and other schemes can also help to enhance the affordability of chronic medications to prevent and manage CVDs, building on current schemes. Should there continue to be high poverty levels and lack of healthcare, including medicines, CVDs will continue to be a growing issue. This is not in the best interest of any key stakeholder group or higher income countries seeking to benefit from growing African populations. We will continue to monitor the situation.

Acknowledgements

There was no funding for this work.

Conflict of interest

The authors declare no conflict of interest.

Author details

Julius Chacha Mwita[1*] and Brian Godman[2,3]

1 University of Botswana, Gaborone, Botswana

2 Strathclyde Institute of Pharmacy and Biomedical Sciences, Glasgow, United Kingdom

3 School of Pharmacy, Sefako Makgatho Health Sciences University, Pretoria, South Africa

*Address all correspondence to: mwitajc@ub.ac.bw

References

[1] World Health Organization. April 2, 2021]; Available from: https://www.who.int/health-topics/cardiovascular-diseases/#tab=tab_1.

[2] World Health Organization regional committee for Africa. Noncommunicable Diseases. 2014 April 2, 2021]; Available from: https://www.afro.who.int/health-topics/noncommunicable-diseases.

[3] Regional Committee for Africa. Cardiovascular diseases in the African region: current situation and perspectives: Report of the Regional Director. 2011 April 2, 2021]; Available from: https://apps.who.int/iris/handle/10665/1871.

[4] Bigna, J.J. and J.J. Noubiap, The rising burden of non-communicable diseases in sub-Saharan Africa. The Lancet Global Health, 2019. 7(10): p. e1295-e1296. doi: 10.1016/S2214-109X(19)30370-5

[5] Yuyun, M.F., et al., Cardiovascular Diseases in Sub-Saharan Africa Compared to High-Income Countries: An Epidemiological Perspective. Glob Heart, 2020. 15(1): p. 15. doi: 10.5334/gh.403

[6] Salari, P., et al., The catastrophic and impoverishing effects of out-of-pocket healthcare payments in Kenya, 2018. BMJ Glob Health, 2019. 4(6): p. e001809. doi: 10.1136/bmjgh-2019-001809

[7] Beaglehole, R. and R. Bonita, Global public health: a scorecard. The Lancet, 2008. 372(9654): p. 1988-1996.

[8] United Nations - Department of Economic Social Affairs and Population Division. World population prospects 2019. 2019 [cited I: Comprehensive Tables ST/ESA/SER.A/426]; Available from: https://population.un.org/wpp/Publications/Files/WPP2019_Volume-I_Comprehensive-Tables.pdf.

[9] World Bank Poverty and shared prosperity 2018: piecing together the poverty puzzle. 2018. https://openknowledge.worldbank.org/bitstream/handle/10986/30418/9781464813306.pdf.

[10] World Bank. Year in Review: 2018 in 14 Charts. 2018 April 12, 2021]; Available from: https://www.worldbank.org/en/news/feature/2018/12/21/year-in-review-2018-in-14-charts.

[11] World Bank Poverty and Shared Prosperity 2020: Reversals of Fortune. 2020. https://openknowledge.worldbank.org/bitstream/handle/10986/34496/9781464816024.pdf.

[12] United Nations Development Programme and Oxford Poverty and Human Development Initiative. Global MPI 2020–Charting pathways out of multidimensional poverty: Achieving the SDGs. United Nations Development Programme (UNDP) and Oxford Poverty and Human Development Initiative (OPHI) 2020; Available from: http://hdr.undp.org/en/2020-MPI.

[13] Williams, D. What are the Causes of Poverty. 2016; Available from: https://borgenproject.org/what-causes-global-poverty/.

[14] Austin, G., African economic development and colonial legacies. 2010: Institut de hautes études internationales et du développement.

[15] Kabuya, F.I., Fundamental causes of poverty in Sub-Saharan Africa. IOSR Journal of Humanities and Social Science, 2015. 20(6): p. 78-81.

[16] Haacker, M., The economic consequences of HIV/AIDS in Southern Africa. 2002,

[17] United Nations. Transforming our world: the 2030 Agenda for Sustainable Development. 2015 March 5, 2021]; Available from: https://sustainable development.un.org/content/documents/21252030%20Agenda%20for%20Sustainable%20Development%20web.pdf.

[18] Chang, A.Y., et al., Past, present, and future of global health financing: a review of development assistance, government, out-of-pocket, and other private spending on health for 195 countries, 1995-2050. The Lancet, 2019. 393(10187): p. 2233-2260. doi: 10.1016/S0140-6736(19)30841-4

[19] Addae-Korankye, A., Causes of poverty in Africa: A review of literature. American International Journal of Social Science, 2014. 3(7): p. 147-153.

[20] Schultz, W.M., et al., Socioeconomic Status and Cardiovascular Outcomes: Challenges and Interventions. Circulation, 2018. 137(20): p. 2166-2178. doi: 10.1161/circulationaha.117.029652

[21] Jones, C.A., et al., Cardiovascular disease risk among the poor and homeless - what we know so far. Curr Cardiol Rev, 2009. 5(1): p. 69-77. doi: 10.2174/157340309787048086

[22] Mensah, G.A., et al., Mortality from cardiovascular diseases in sub-Saharan Africa, 1990-2013: a systematic analysis of data from the Global Burden of Disease Study 2013. Cardiovascular journal of Africa, 2015. 26(2 H3Africa Suppl): p. S6. doi: 10.5830/CVJA-2015-036

[23] World Bank World development report 2000/2001: Attacking poverty. 2000. http://documents1.worldbank.org/curated/en/230351468332946759/pdf/226840WDR00PUB0ng0poverty0200002001.pdf.

[24] Murray, C.J., et al., The global burden of disease: a comprehensive assessment of mortality and disability from diseases, injuries, and risk factors in 1990 and projected to 2020: summary/edited by Christopher J. L. Murray, Alan D. Lopez. World Health Organization. 1996: World Health Organization.

[25] Roth, G.A., et al., Global and regional patterns in cardiovascular mortality from 1990 to 2013. Circulation, 2015. 132(17): p. 1667-1678. doi: 10.1161/CIRCULATIONAHA.114.008720

[26] Rosengren, A., et al., Socioeconomic status and risk of cardiovascular disease in 20 low-income, middle-income, and high-income countries: the Prospective Urban Rural Epidemiologic (PURE) study. The Lancet Global Health, 2019. 7(6): p. e748-e760. doi: 10.1016/S2214-109X(19)30045-2

[27] Meyer, J.C., et al., Ongoing initiatives to improve the quality and efficiency of medicine use within the public healthcare system in South Africa; a preliminary study. Frontiers in pharmacology, 2017. 8: p. 751.

[28] Mwita, J.C., et al., Glycaemic, blood pressure and low-density lipoprotein-cholesterol control among patients with diabetes mellitus in a specialised clinic in Botswana: a cross-sectional study. BMJ open, 2019. 9(7): p. e026807.

[29] Asmelash, D. and Y. Asmelash, The Burden of Undiagnosed Diabetes Mellitus in Adult African Population: A Systematic Review and Meta-Analysis. J Diabetes Res, 2019. 2019: p. 4134937. doi: 10.1155/2019/4134937

[30] Keates, A.K., et al., Cardiovascular disease in Africa: epidemiological profile and challenges. Nature Reviews Cardiology, 2017. 14(5): p. 273-293. doi: 10.1038/nrcardio.2017.19

[31] Mwita, J.C., et al., Undiagnosed and diagnosed diabetes mellitus among

hospitalised acute heart failure patients in Botswana. SAGE open medicine, 2017. 5: p. 2050312117731473. doi: 10.1177/2050312117731473

[32] Godman, B., et al., Ongoing and planned activities to improve the management of patients with Type 1 diabetes across Africa; implications for the future. Hospital practice, 2020. 48(2): p. 51-67.

[33] Mwita, J.C., et al., Hypertension control and other cardiovascular risk factors among diabetic patients at Muhimbili National Hospital, Tanzania. East African journal of public health, 2013. 10(1): p. 337-342.

[34] Agyemang, C. and B.-J. van den Born, Limited access to CVD medicines in low-income and middle-income countries: poverty is at the heart of the matter. The Lancet Global Health, 2018. 6(3): p. e234-e235. doi: 10.1016/S2214-109X(18)30048-2

[35] Wekesah, F.M., et al., Understanding of and perceptions towards cardiovascular diseases and their risk factors: a qualitative study among residents of urban informal settings in Nairobi. BMJ Open, 2019. 9(6): p. e026852. doi: 10.1136/bmjopen-2018-026852

[36] Organization, W.H., Global NCD target: reduce premature deaths from NCDs. 2016, World Health Organization.

[37] Pazdernik, M., et al., Screening for RHD in Botswana: A young Czech team introduces echocardiography screening for rheumatic heart disease (RHD) in Botswana. 2019, Oxford University Press.

[38] Carapetis, J.R., et al., The global burden of group A streptococcal diseases. Lancet Infect Dis, 2005. 5(11): p. 685-694. doi: 10.1016/s1473-3099(05)70267-x

[39] Guilherme, L., J. Kalil, and M. Cunningham, Molecular mimicry in the autoimmune pathogenesis of rheumatic heart disease. Autoimmunity, 2006. 39(1): p. 31-39. doi: 10.1080/08916930500484674

[40] Mayosi, B.M., et al., Rheumatic heart disease in Africa: the Mosi-o-Tunya call to action. The Lancet Global Health, 2014. 2(8): p. e438-e439. doi: 10.1016/S2214-109X(14)70234-7

[41] Coffey, P.M., A.P. Ralph, and V.L. Krause, The role of social determinants of health in the risk and prevention of group A streptococcal infection, acute rheumatic fever and rheumatic heart disease: A systematic review. PLoS Negl Trop Dis, 2018. 12(6): p. e0006577. doi: 10.1371/journal.pntd.0006577

[42] Karthikeyan, G. and B.M. Mayosi, Is primary prevention of rheumatic fever the missing link in the control of rheumatic heart disease in Africa? Circulation, 2009. 120(8): p. 709-713. doi: 10.1161/circulationaha.108.836510

[43] Günther, G., J. Asmera, and E. Parry, Death from rheumatic heart disease in rural Ethiopia. Lancet, 2006. 367(9508): p. 391. doi: 10.1016/S0140-6736(06)68128-2

[44] Remenyi, B., et al., Position statement of the World Heart Federation on the prevention and control of rheumatic heart disease. Nature Reviews Cardiology, 2013. 10(5): p. 284-292. doi: 10.1038/nrcardio.2013.34

[45] in Disease and Mortality in Sub-Saharan Africa, D.T. Jamison, et al., Editors. 2006, The International Bank for Reconstruction and Development/The World Bank Copyright © 2006, The International Bank for Reconstruction and Development/The World Bank.: Washington (DC).

[46] Moran, A., et al., The Epidemiology of Cardiovascular Diseases in

Sub-Saharan Africa: The Global Burden of Diseases, Injuries and Risk Factors 2010 Study. Progress in Cardiovascular Diseases, 2013. 56(3): p. 234-239. doi: https://doi.org/10.1016/j.pcad.2013.09.019

[47] Murphy, A., et al., The household economic burden of non-communicable diseases in 18 countries. BMJ Glob Health, 2020. 5(2): p. e002040. doi: 10.1136/bmjgh-2019-002040

[48] Aikins, A.d.-G., Healer shopping in Africa: new evidence from rural-urban qualitative study of Ghanaian diabetes experiences. BMJ, 2005. 331(7519): p. 737. doi: 10.1136/bmj.331.7519.737

[49] Winston, C.M. and V. Patel, Use of traditional and orthodox health services in urban Zimbabwe. Int J Epidemiol, 1995. 24(5): p. 1006-1012. doi: 10.1093/ije/24.5.1006

[50] BeLue, R., et al., An overview of cardiovascular risk factor burden in sub-Saharan African countries: a socio-cultural perspective. Globalization and Health, 2009. 5(1): p. 10. doi: 10.1186/1744-8603-5-10

[51] Lunyera, J., et al., Traditional medicine practices among community members with diabetes mellitus in Northern Tanzania: an ethnomedical survey. BMC Complementary and Alternative Medicine, 2016. 16(1): p. 282. doi: 10.1186/s12906-016-1262-2

[52] Hughes, G.D., et al., The prevalence of traditional herbal medicine use among hypertensives living in South African communities. BMC Complementary and Alternative Medicine, 2013. 13(1): p. 38. doi: 10.1186/1472-6882-13-38

[53] Bham, Z. and E. Ross, Traditional and western medicine: cultural beliefs and practices of South African Indian Muslims with regard to stroke. Ethn Dis, 2005. 15(4): p. 548-554.

[54] Boateng, D., et al., Knowledge and awareness of and perception towards cardiovascular disease risk in sub-Saharan Africa: A systematic review. PLoS One, 2017. 12(12): p. e0189264. doi: 10.1371/journal.pone.0189264

[55] Magnani, J.W., et al., Health literacy and cardiovascular disease: fundamental relevance to primary and secondary prevention: a scientific statement from the American Heart Association. Circulation, 2018. 138(2): p. e48-e74.

[56] Kontis, V., et al., Contribution of six risk factors to achieving the 25× 25 non-communicable disease mortality reduction target: a modelling study. The Lancet, 2014. 384(9941): p. 427-437.

[57] Nyaaba, G.N., et al., Tracing Africa's progress towards implementing the Non-Communicable Diseases Global action plan 2013-2020: a synthesis of WHO country profile reports. BMC Public Health, 2017. 17(1): p. 297. doi: 10.1186/s12889-017-4199-6

[58] Sletvold, H., L.A.B. Sagmo, and E.A. Torheim, Impact of pictograms on medication adherence: A systematic literature review. Patient education and counseling, 2020. 103(6): p. 1095-1103.

[59] Mashozhera, S., et al., Compliance to hypertensive prescribing guidelines and blood pressure control in elderly patients in Namibia: findings and implications. Journal of Pharmaceutical Health Services Research, 2021. 12(1): p. 53-60.

[60] Niaz, Q., et al., Compliance to prescribing guidelines among public health care facilities in Namibia; findings and implications. International journal of clinical pharmacy, 2020. 42: p. 1227-1236.

[61] Niaz, Q., et al., Validity of World Health Organisation prescribing

DOI: http://dx.doi.org/10.5772/intechopen.98575

indicators in Namibia's primary healthcare: findings and implications. International journal for quality in health care, 2019. 31(5): p. 338-345.

[62] Woerkom, M.v., et al., Ongoing measures to enhance the efficiency of prescribing of proton pump inhibitors and statins in The Netherlands: influence and future implications. Journal of comparative effectiveness research, 2012. 1(6): p. 527-538.

[63] Nashilongo, M., et al., Assessing adherence to antihypertensive therapy in primary health care in Namibia: findings and implications. Cardiovascular drugs and therapy, 2017. 31(5): p. 565-578.

Chapter 3

Poverty, Compromised Dietary Intake and Health Implications among South Africa's Sub-Populations: A Conceptual Analysis

Stella Chewe Sabi

Abstract

Hunger and malnutrition-related problems have been identified as proxies for extreme poverty. Poverty and hunger currently affect >400 million people in Sub-Saharan Africa, the poorest region in the world. South Africa, being the most unequal society in Africa, is no exception to the crisis of food poverty and health implications among sub-population groups. Research shows that individuals or households that experience food insecurity have staple diets that are energy-dense, thereby compromising their health lifestyle. This qualitative study reviewed the evidence of the potential impact of poverty on compromised-dietary intake and healthy lifestyle using 53 publications among them scientific studies, policy documents, government documents and electronic sources. Contextual analysis was used to arrive at discussions, conclusions and recommendations. Major findings reveal that the historically disadvantaged including undocumented immigrants are highly vulnerable to compromised dietary intake and non-communicable diseases due to persistent inequality in the country. As the global extreme poverty is expected to rise in 2020/2021 due to COVID-19 pandemic which is negatively affecting the global health and economic system, vulnerable groups with little to no social protection such as financial social grants from the state in middle income countries like South Africa, will be more affected. The findings conclude by providing valuable information for state actors and non-state actors to protect the most vulnerable to acute food insecurity and chronic poverty.

Keywords: compromised dietary-intake, public health concern, non-communicable diseases, undernutrition, vulnerable groups

1. Introduction and background

Poverty and hunger related issues have been paramount concern of humanity. Poverty has been identified as a complex problem affecting nearly 700 million people across the globe, of whom 422 million or > 70% live in the world's poorest region—Sub-Saharan Africa [1]. Current estimates by the World Bank are that between 2020 and 2021, the pandemic nature of the severe acute respiratory syndrome coronavirus 2 (SARS-CoV-2), fondly known as COVID-19 disease which is ravaging the global health and economic system would result in increased extreme poverty by 100 million people with Sub-Saharan Africa accounting for 40 million individuals [1]. Extreme poverty refers to the socio-economic condition of people living below the international poverty line of $1.90 a day. This population will experience abject poverty in addition to being vulnerable to acute food insecurity, and compromised health lifestyle. It is worth noting that the global concern for food security as a necessity for quality health, dates back to early years of twentieth century post-World Wars (World War I and World War II in 1930s and 1940s, respectively) during which most societies afflicted with non-communicable diseases resulted from several factors including famine which led to their compromised health lifestyle. It was not until 1935, that the first survey report on global nutrition and public health by the League of Nation's Health Division, documented the extent of malnutrition and hunger in the world. The report revealed a critical food shortage in low and middle-income countries [2]. The League of Nations' survey report is fundamental to the present discourse on dietary intake and health implications because it resulted in the Organization's fundamental discussions on action-oriented developmental policies including the need for coordinated nutrition-related policies in several countries [2].

Contemporary episodes of famine and global food insecurity dates back to early 1970s during the world food crisis when food production and consumptions significantly dropped. This prompted the General Assembly of the United Nations to convene the member states to take specific actions to determine the global food challenge using the comprehensive approach of development agenda and international economic operation [3]. The conference, attended by 135 member states from developed and developing countries (including countries in Sub-Saharan Africa) was concluded through the adoption of the following declaration; "Universal Declaration on Eradication of Hunger and Malnutrition" [3]. The participating states were invited within the context of the United Nations Economic and Social Council Resolution [3]. Thenceforth, the issue of food and nutrition security has been prominent on the global development agenda. In other words, the process of eradicating chronic hunger and poverty and the implication on wellbeing has been a priority since the last quarter of the twentieth century.

However, contemporary research on the history of global food security revealed that for much of the twentieth century, food security was broadly viewed through the lenses of accelerating food production as remedy to famine and international food insecurity. Within this context, the equal relation between health and agriculture would enhance the international economies [2]. Such a perspective, also promoted the need for meeting human basic needs through fundamental policy objectives using commercial agriculture as means to economic development [2]. Consequently, between 1950s to 1970, the world recorded an increase in food production (particularly staple food and/or cereal); concurrently, production per capita improved by 50% and 20%, respectively [2]. Research on the history of food security [2] also reveals that, the period between late 1960s to early 197os saw an annual food aid distribution by high income countries such as the United States to middle income and low-income countries, dropping from an estimated 17 million tons to only 7 million tons. By 1972, several regions of the world among them Sub-Sahara Africa witnessed bad climate conditions such as drought that resulted in famine or general food insecurity. As a consequence, the global food production in staple food such as cereal, sharply fell by 30 million tons [2].

While such substantial measures in post-World Wars were undertaken by the international communities, and three decades after the 1970s' Universal Declaration on Eradication of Hunger and Malnutrition, the chronic poverty and undernutrition continued to engulf developing regions such as Sub-Sahara Africa, the Middle East and South Asia. Accordingly, the World Development Report [4] revealed that while Sub-Sahara Africa constituted only 11.1% of the global population, the region had 16.1% of the worlds' chronically impoverished. By 1992, more than 780 million people in developing countries were undernourished [5].

Reassuringly, at the dawn of the new millennium (21 century), the past decades of the aforementioned poverty related conditions prompted the United Nations General Assembly to devise eight fundamental goals, of which— eradicating extreme poverty and hunger was set as a priority goal. The Millennium Development Goals (MDGs) were international development goals that resulted from the UN Millennium Summit in 2000 after the adoption of the United Nations Millennium Declaration. These ambitious goals would be achieved by 2015 [6]. However, in 2015, the global report on the state of food insecurity in the world revealed that some 795 million people were undernourished and/or food insecure largely due to poverty [7] of which, >400 million were from Sub-Sahara Africa. This is despite the region's significant progress in reducing extreme poverty from >50% in 1990 to about 41% in 2013 [8]. Thus, the MDGs were preceded by the 17 Sustainable Development Goals that would be implemented from 2016 to 2030 [6]. The Sustainable Development Goals were devised by the United Nations' General Assembly. Expectantly, the process of eradicating extreme poverty and hunger have been reprioritized on the SDGs agenda.

The aim of this study is to determine the nexus between poverty and compromised dietary intake, and the implication on health in selected sub-population groups in a developing country, within the socio-economic context of South Africa. The choice of South Africa as a focal point is suitable because of the nation's complex history that traverse 150 years of colonialism and about 50 years (1948–1994) of the oppressive apartheid regime whose white minority rule and its radical racialized policies significantly disadvantaged the country's majority (>90%) mostly people of black ancestry who were left in abject poverty [9]. The scars of the historically unjust policies remain visible as evidenced by the black majority or the historically disadvantaged population [10] being the most vulnerable to socio-economic issues such as poverty, food insecurity and poor health— making the country one of the most unequal societies in the world. Historically disadvantaged simply means South African citizens that live in poverty due to the unjust systematic racism of the apartheid policy or Act 110 of 1983 Constitution of the Republic of South Africa that disenfranchised them.

2. Clarification of concepts

2.1 Food security and insecurity

As a concept, food security was coined in 1970s following the global economic crisis and the subsequent United Nations Conference that aimed to combat the global food insecurity. Although there is no universally accepted definition of food security, one internationally recognized definition is authored by the World Food Programme of the United Nations which posits that "food security exists when all people, at all times, have physical, social and economic access to sufficient, safe and nutritious food to meet their dietary needs and food preferences for an active and healthy life" [11]. Within this context, a household or, an individual's ability to obtain sufficient and nutritious food to stay healthy is crucial. The definition of food security was also documented as the principle achievement of the 1996 World Food Summit [2] because it operationalized food security as a condition that exists at different levels of society including international, national, community, and household or individual level.

Therefore, food security includes factors such as availability, accessibility, utilization and stability. Within the context, availability refers to the quantity of food commodities that result from mass food production that is sufficient enough to feed the entire human population; food accessibility happens when all people have access to sufficient food or an individual's economic power to access or acquire sufficient food for consumption. This implies that high food prices can negatively affect food access. Furthermore, food, utilization refers to an individual's means to acquire safe-nutritious food that meets their basic nutritional needs. Under this notion, nutritious food and food safety includes one's food preference, its conservation and preparations, and "nutrient absorptions in the human body" [2]. Food utilization also refers to the process by which a human body detects the nutrients or calories stemming from macronutrients and micronutrients, feeding practices, and food preparations. This concept is critical to the current discourse as it unveils the importance of dietary intake as one of the key factors to a healthy lifestyle. It could be reasoned that, individuals with compromised-dietary intake are likely to meet the challenge of being unhealthy.

Among conditions that are associated with compromised-dietary intake are cardiovascular diseases such as heart failure, stroke, heart attack, cardiac arrest, obesity, and other non-communicable diseases such as malnutrition and iron deficiency anemia. An individual's nutritional status is determined by biological absorption of the food consumed [12, 13]. In this regard, the basic nutritional knowledge and good dietary habits, clean and safe water, sanitation, and health care should be considered when ensuring food security. Likewise, the food utilization aspect authenticates that nutrition is directly associated with food security and as such, there is food insecurity when the human population is not adequately nourished.

Food stability is another fundamental element when analyzing the notion of food security [12, 14]. From this perspective, an individual is food secure provided that there is stability in the other three elements of food security (availability, accessibility and utilization of the food) over time. Within this context, food security can neither be limited to a particular moment such as, a month or a year but that it should be sustainable. In other words, where there is lack of food stability, transitory or chronic food insecurity occurs. Thenceforth, if a household has adequate and nutritious food intake today, they are regarded food insecure whenever they lack a sustainable food supply because, their health or nutritional status risk being compromised by inadequate food consumption. In cases where there is credit crisis that influence food prices, food security at all levels (international, national community or household) may be difficult to achieve. For instance, the sharp rise in global food crisis in post 2000, resulted in accelerating food prices, anxiety and food riots in some parts of the world [15]. Furthermore, unfavorable weather conditions such as floods and famine, economic factors, or political instability may impact negatively on household or individual food security status.

3. Contextualizing poverty as a proxy for food insecurity and compromised health

Poverty is a multifaceted phenomenon that derives from the word poor— or the inability to meet basic human necessities [16]. Being a such phenomenon, poverty has various dimensions of human deprivation in terms of food consumption, health, education, dignity, security, decent employment, and voice [17].

As a concept, poverty includes the state of being vulnerable to adverse shocks. This implies that people who are poor, are burdened with having little to lack of resources such as goods, finances or means for their livelihood. In economic terms, poverty means that the income level from employment is so low that one's basic needs such as food security is highly compromised. Literature shows that poverty is increasingly recognized as a prime determinant of food insecurity. From this perspective, food poverty is the extent to which individuals live without basic resources such as money to acquire a stable supply of adequate food, and the ability to make appropriate decisions to live and maintain a lifestyle [18, 19]. Research on association between poverty related conditions such as food insecurity and mental health revealed that, individuals who are food secure are less likely to experience anxiety disorder than their food insecure counterparts [20]. Anxiety about the availability of food can affect one's social and/or mental well-being, by creating feelings of depression and irritability [21].

As a concept, food insecurity is the state of being without reliable access to sufficient safe and nutritious food for consumption to enhance normal growth and to live an active and healthy life [22]. The phenomenon is one of the leading cause of chronic hunger in Sub-Saharan Africa. As highlighted in the foregoing, food insecurity may be caused an absence of any of the four fundamental element (availability; access; utilization; and stability) of food security which are—characterized by food inadequacy: to lack of resources to acquire food; utilization; improper use or consumption of food in the body; and unstable supply and consumption of nutritious food, respectively. As a complex process, food insecurity may occur in the form of, chronic or persistent food insecurity that manifests when a household or an individual is unable to meet basic food consumption requirements over a sustained period [16]. A report by the World Food Programme [23] shows that individuals who experience chronic food insecurity are unable to meet basic food necessities due to lack of sufficient economic power to acquire income, land or productive assets, or they experience high dependency ratios, acute sickness or social barriers. Such households or individuals are constantly at risk of being unable to afford or acquire adequate nutrition food over a sustained period [12, 13]. It is reasoned that chronic food insecurity could be sustainably overcome with deliberate measures used to address abject poverty and enhanced development such as education, employment, or access to productive or financial resources in the form of credits or loans. Furthermore, households affected by chronic food insecurity need more direct access to adequate food supply to enable them raise their productive capacity [22]. The importance of analyzing the notion of food security and insecurity is that it helps in fostering improved food security responses both at macro and micro levels in addition to influencing emergency interventions such as food aid programmes and projects, and action-oriented food security policies.

4. Malnutrition versus overnutrition: dietary intake

Malnutrition is a public health concern that is occasioned by deficiencies, excess or imbalances in macro and/or micronutrients in humans [22]. These deficiencies could result from chronic food insecurity, hunger, and poverty [13]. Other non-food factors that influence malnutrition are inadequate care practices, lack of health services, unhealthy environment, and ignorance. This implies that malnourished people in resource-poor communities, are at high risk of suffering from deficiencies of micronutrients caused by poverty and hunger. Hunger simply means food deprivation. Within this context, hunger and malnutrition are not only a threat to public health but are also among the leading cause of death in the middle and low income countries where the population is largely impoverished. On the other hand, nutrition refers to the quality and the quantity of food consumed for a healthy living. A healthy diet consists of four basic nutrients which are, proteins, carbohydrates, minerals and vitamins (meat, dairy, starch vegetable, and fruits). Other essential nutrients recommended for quality health lifestyle include fiber and lipids. Consequently, nutritional complications not only emerge from compromised-dietary intake but have adverse effects on human health resulting in death. On the other hand, when good eating habits are practiced, nutrition is one of the fundamental factors that enables people to stay healthy. Children especially those below the age of 10 have high nutritional requirements for their growth. However, in developing countries where poverty and food insecurity are high, undernutrition and lack of adequate dietary diversity is a major contributor to child mortality [24]. Research on *Maternal and child malnutrition in low-income and middle-income countries* [25] shows that in 2011, undernutrition contributed to 45% of child mortality in the low income and middle income countries.

It is also worth noting that dietary intake refers to the daily absorption or consumption of nutrients such as protein, carbohydrate, fats and vitamins and other food components such as fiber as recommended daily allowances for a healthy living. This also implies taking sufficient amount of calories (units of energy) from the food that is consumed. Hence, good dietary intake will mean that an individual should take at least a minimum required calories per day. Dietary measurements area also keys to assessing food, and nutrient intake of households or individuals. For example, the recent global report by the World Health Organization [26] echoed that healthy diet practices means calories intake should resonate with the energy expenditure. Conversely, to avoid unhealthy weight gain, total lipid should not exceed 30% of total energy intake; while consumption of saturated fat should not be more than 10% of total energy intake. Further, free sugars intake should be less than 10% of the total energy consumption [26]. Meanwhile, public health problems such as cardiovascular diseases have been on the rise. Most recent estimates by the World Health Organization [26] also shows that cardiovascular diseases mostly originate from compromised dietary intake and lack of physical activities and that, they are a primary cause of death globally. The WHO echoed that cardiovascular diseases claim about 31% or 17.9 million lives annually, and that the diseases are characterized by high levels of blood pressure, glucose, and lipids. Other symptoms include obesity and overweight and these result in some cancers, type-2 diabetes, stroke, heart attack, and cardiac arrest [26]. The problem of obesity and overweight is also on the rise in middle-income countries such as South Africa.

To enhance nutritional health, in 2003 South Africa launched its Food-Based Dietary (FBNGs), which it revised in 2013 using a multi sectorial approach comprising the National Department of Health- Directorate of Nutrition, the medical research council, Nutritional Society of South Africa, food producer organizations, academics and the United Nations organizations such as the FAO, as the national working group. The 2003 South African FBNGs had the following items (mostly local and affordable foods) to be consumed regularly by individuals who are ≥7 years as necessity for health eating which lowers the risk of noncommunicable diseases [27]:

- Enjoy a variety of foods.
- Be active.
- Make starchy foods the basis of most meals.
- Eat dry beans, peas, lentils and soy regularly.

- Chicken, fish, meat or eggs can be eaten daily.
- Drink lots of clean, safe water.
- Eat plenty of vegetables and fruit every day.
- Eat fats sparingly.
- Use salt sparingly.
- If you drink alcohol, drink sensibly.

Use foods and drinks containing sugar sparingly, and not between meals.

The limitation in the first (2003) guide was that while it recommended the consumption of food groups it neither specified the items (such as highly processed foods, energy dense food, fat and salt) whose consumption should be limited nor provided the absolute values for the recommended daily allowance or calories. The implication is that the supposed evidence based guideline to comprehensive dietary patterns and healthy lifestyles overlooked the issue of overnutrition, an emerging public health concern in high income and middle income countries including South Africa [27].

Overnutrition is the overconsumption of any food or nutrients regardless of the food group (source) such that one's health is compromised. Overnutrition can result in obesity and overweight which in turn increases the risk of metabolic syndrome, noncommunicable diseases and/or cardiovascular diseases. Additionally, studies [27–31] conducted in South Africa and around the world have shown that overnutrition is among the leading cause of metabolic syndrome in children and adolescents (conditions such as increased blood pressure, high blood sugar, excess body fat around the waist, and abnormal cholesterol or triglyceride levels) and that it increases among others, the risk of heart disease and type-2 diabetes.

The 2012-reviewed revised general FBDGs for South Africans had the following items [27]:

- Enjoy a variety of foods.
- Be active!
- Make starchy foods part of most meals.
- Eat plenty of vegetables and fruit every day.
- Eat dry beans, split peas, lentils and soya regularly.
- Have milk, maas (sour milk) or yoghurt every day.
- Fish, chicken, lean meat or eggs can be eaten daily.
- Drink lots of clean, safe water.
- Use fats sparingly. Choose vegetable oils, rather than hard fats.
- Use sugar and foods and drinks high in sugar sparingly.
- Use salt and food high in salt sparingly.

5. South African inequalities, poverty and compromised dietary-intake: implications on public health

Africa is the most unequal society in the world of which South Africa is the leading unequal country, mainly due to the nation's historical injustices that were driven by colonial and the apartheid regimes. In fact, poverty and food insecurity related problems are not new in South Africa. The nation's socio-economic inequalities can be traced back to the arrival of the Europeans in the present day Western Cape province and the subsequent apartheid governance whose racialized policies disadvantaged and left the majority (black population) in chronic poverty. This increased their vulnerability to hunger and malnutrition related conditions evidenced by the 1994 demographic records which revealed that at the end of the apartheid government, about 41% of children from South Africa's impoverished households were chronically hungry and undernourished [32]. Of note is that, that during the apartheid regime, South Africa was food secure in terms of food availability. This was due to increased food production by commercial farming—a white dominated industry. However, cheap labour was sourced from the black population whose wage could not sustain their basic human needs including household food security.

Consequently, the issue of food insecurity and poverty was worsened by unjust and racialized policies that deprived the majority socially and economically [33]. More evidence of the existing inequalities such as high poverty levels among the black population is reported in several studies that were conducted during the first decade of post-apartheid South Africa. Likewise, a study [34] recounts that in 1995, in terms of annual income quantile by race, South Africans of African ancestry constituted the poorest households in terms of annual income such that an estimated 26% of them had incomes between R0. 00 and R6 839.00 per annum. This was followed by the mixed race ancestry households who constituted 12%, and only 2% of both Indian, and white households.

Additionally, in 1994, South Africa conducted its first national survey on child malnutrition whose findings revealed that one out of four children aged between 6 months and six years were malnourished. Of these 10% were underweight [35]. Having a low Body Mass Index or being underweight compromises one's immunity system, and leads in poor health. Despite that these results only linked poverty to child malnutrition, they are significant to this research as they underscore the potential correlation between lack of dietary diversity and malnutrition, and poverty or the inability to afford a good diet for a healthy living.

Similarly, research by, Woolard [9] concluded that the Africa National Congress (ANC) government inherited extremely unequal economic opportunities which saw the black population accounting for 95% of the impoverished South Africa. The prioritization of the household food security as a basic human necessity by the ANC government is evident in section 27 of the Constitution, which stipulates that "Everyone has the right to have access to (a) health care services; (b) sufficient food and water; (c) social security' [36] and that; government should "take reasonable legislative and other similar measures within the context of its available resources to achieve the progressive realization of services such as sufficient food and water, and health care" [36]. Further recognition of the right to food is enshrined in the socio-economic policies such as the Reconstruction Development Programme (RDP) and the Broad Based Black Economic Empowerment (B-BBEE) programmes which seek to eradicate the nation's high levels of poverty and deprivation that have been compounded by relatively high level of disparities between the white population and the historically disadvantaged population. The former was favored during apartheid. The RDP is a government programme whose priority is to rectify the inequalities fabricated by the apartheid government to the majority of South Africans [37, 38]. As observed by Hendriks [39] the RDP identified household food security as a basic human necessity and food insecurity as a legacy of the oppressive apartheid laws which favored the minority white race.

Despite that the apartheid government collapsed in 1994, and that the new government ushered into new policies such as the RDP of 1994 and the B-BBEE of 2003, poverty levels are still high in the country and majority of those affected are the black population and the youth. These vast populations are not only impoverished but have also been found to be food insecure [40]. Evidence of the existing poverty and poor nutrition is the government social protection policies that have been implemented through social grant financial packages and the national nutritional programmes [such as the National School Nutrition Programmes (NSNP)] which are meant to easy household poverty and vulnerability to hunger.

The NSNP is a fundamental government initiative that directly addresses macro and micro nutritional needs among the historically disadvantaged children in South Africa. The program is part of the National Policy on Food and Nutrition Security that enhances a broad framework for the reorientation of household food security interventions such as the nutrition programs in the country [41]. One of the aim is to address nutritional needs among the most vulnerable groups such as the school age. Adequate nutrition is essential for keeping humans healthy across their lifespan. Thus, a healthy diet helps children grow and develop properly. It also reduces their risk of chronic diseases, including obesity. Adults who eat a healthy diet live longer and have a lower risk of obesity, heart disease, type 2 diabetes, and certain cancers. Healthy eating habits can help individuals with chronic diseases to manage these conditions and prevent complications.

Another strategy in which South African government addresses poverty and household food insecurity, and vulnerability is through social grants. Social grants are a government initiative that target household food insecurity in South Africa. In particular, the grants target sub-population groups such as the impoverished, including other vulnerable groups such as people with disabilities, children and older persons above the age of 60 years. The social financial grants are distributed in form of old age pension funds, foster care grants, disability grants, care dependency grants and child support grants [32]. In 2016, 30% of the vulnerable groups were beneficiaries of social grants that translated into 44% of all households in South Africa [32]. In the same year, the Child Support Grant benefited 11, 9 million children whereby each of them was paid R350.00 per month, making it the highest form of paid social grant. On the other hand, the Older Persons Grant benefitted from an estimated R3.2 million elderly people whereby those who were aged between 60 and 74 years received R1 505.00 each per month; while R1 525.00 was granted to each beneficiary aged >75-year-old [32, 42]. A disability grant beneficiary received R1 505.00 per month, a foster Care grant received R890.00 per month; while the Care Dependency Grant beneficiary received R1 505.00 per month.

These grants are shown to have improved household food access and other basic household needs among the beneficiaries. In 2012 the Statistics South Africa [39] reported that social grants contributed to 42% of household income in impoverished families and were their major source of income. Despite such a remarkable mile stone in public spending on improving the welfare of vulnerable people, the challenge is that not all the targeted beneficiaries have access to the grants arguably due to bureaucracy in selecting those who qualify to be beneficiaries among the millions who are impoverished in the country. As a result, about 20% [43, 44] of the economically disadvantaged South Africans lack financial support from the state and are thus malnourished and live in abject poverty.

Some empirical studies [45] have reported about caregivers of child support grants citing forgery of more birth certificates including having multiple children so that they could secure more grants as safety nets. Similarly, there are also reports of increased teenage pregnancy in households particularly in rural areas as strategy to secure more child grant support. In turn, this increases poverty and unemployment among such households because the young mothers are likely to drop out of school and stay unemployed; in cases where they fail to secure their child support grants, such families find it difficult to cope with the cost of maintaining large households. Alcohol abuse is another identified risk factor for poverty and compromised healthy lifestyle in South Africa. Some studies revealed that some grant caregivers do not utilize the money for the intended purposes but divert a portion of it on alcohol consumption [46].

Furthermore, it is reasoned that poverty levels in South Africa are also escalated by undocumented immigrants in the country. For instance, given that the grants are exclusive to documented persons or citizens (vulnerable groups) of South Africa, this leaves the resource-poor undocumented or illegal immigrants in the country to fend for themselves. Of note is that, South Africa has the highest number (>4 million) of immigrants legal and undocumented (mostly from low income countries), in Africa [47] most of whom are highly vulnerable to poverty and hunger.

In 2010–2011, South Africa drafted a National Development Plan-2030 (NDP-2030) as a broad strategic framework for a more prosperous and equitable South Africa, where poverty and its related conditions such as individual food insecurity and non-communicable diseases will be adequately addressed by enhancing social-economic opportunities such as health care, education, social security and safety nets [48]. The implementation and success of the plan would depend on every South African taking responsibility for the NDP, led by the head of state and the Cabinet. However, several years after the implementation of the program whereby, less than a decade is remaining to reach the year 2030, the problem of social-economic inequalities persistent common in South Africa. Likewise, a report on South African household poverty as proxy for household food insecurity revealed that in 2015, some 13,8 million individuals were vulnerable to hunger because they lived below the national food poverty line of R441.00 per person per month [49]. This was an increase from 11 million people in 2011. The most affected were the historically disadvantaged, single-parent households, and the rural households.

Consequently, most recent research shows that poverty, vulnerability to hunger, and compromised health lifestyle are still common in South Africa. Accordingly, the 2019 Statistics South Africa report showed that, 11.3% or 6.5 million people by head count experienced hunger while vulnerability to hunger by households was 9.7%. In terms of food access inadequacy, 15.7% of the households that lived in metropolitan areas had experienced inadequate or severely inadequate access to food during the preceding year [50]. At the same time, severe inadequate food access affected 5.2% of the households. Moderate food access inadequate stood at 15.0%. In the same study, it was reported that inadequate food access was influenced by rising economic challenges or poverty in the country. More so, rural poverty areas remained much poorer, despite that the urban–rural economic gap has narrowed.

Another research [51] revealed that in South Africa, chronic malnutrition coexisted in increasing cases of obesity and overweight whereby compromised diet often caused high levels of malnutrition. As such, high food prices, high poverty levels and socio-economic inequalities meant that many households were unable to consume a diverse diet. In the same study, socio-economic status was measured using income and relative asset index. The study concluded that a consistence of pro-rich Socio Economic Status (SES) influenced dietary intake among high income households. Of note is that, although, consumption of starch and energy dense food (high sugar) was common in both categories of the surveyed, low income households had a low intake of fruit, vegetable, and meat than their high SES counterparts whose households also consumed food rich in vitamins, minerals and protein. The findings also concluded that inequality in both dietary diversity and the frequency of consuming all food categories favored high income households whose dietary intake resonated with both the South African national and the WHO. On the same subject, a different research [27] shows that an intake of fruits and vegetables reduces the risk of non-communicable diseases such as diabetes, obesity, cancer and cardiovascular mortality and all cause of mortality among resource-poor communities.

6. Conclusions and recommendations

This chapter concludes that in a developing country like South Africa, poverty is one of the influencers of compromised-dietary intake and vulnerability not only to cardiovascular diseases such as stroke, heart attack and heart failure, but also to other non-communicable diseases, malnutrition and undernutrition, and type 2 diabetes. This is evident in the majority of the historically disadvantaged group in South Africa.

A comprehensive public health approach is needed to curb the inequality and ignorance which are the main source of compromised dietary intake among vulnerable groups. The problem associated with malnutrition related diseases cannot be left in the hands of government alone. It requires multi sectorial approach from civil society actors, researchers and the public itself; the approach that requires public awareness.

As the world continues to nurse its latest public health disaster—COVID-19 pandemic which infected >62 million people and claimed >1.5 million lives in 2020 [52, 53], individuals with pre-existing unhealthy conditions such as malnutrition, cardiovascular disease, and diabetes are highly vulnerable to succumbing to the virus. Deliberate policies that promote household food security are critical in fostering dietary diversity, and health lifestyle such as physical exercises.

Furthermore, global extreme poverty is expected to rise in 2020/2021 for the first time in over two decades. This is due to the disruption of the COVID-19 pandemic that has worsened the pressures of conflict and climate change, which were already slowing poverty reduction progress in Sub-Saharan Africa. As a result of the COVID 19 pandemic, Sub-Sahara Africa's fragile economy, will negatively affect the vulnerable groups who are dependent on government handouts for their livelihood as is the case in South Africa.

Author details

Stella Chewe Sabi
Researcher of Food Security and Consumer Sciences, Department Consumer Science, University of Zululand, Richards Bay, South Africa

*Address all correspondence to: stellasabi@yahoo.co.uk; stellas@uj.ac.za

References

[1] World Bank. Poverty and Shared Prosperity 2020: Reversals of FortuneWashington DC: The World Bank; 2020.

[2] Simon GA. Food Security: Definition Four Dimensions History Basic Readings as an Introduction to Food Security for Students from the IPAD Master SupAgro Montpellier Attending a Joint Training Programme in Rome from 19th to 24th Marc. Rome: FAO; 2012. pp. 1-28.

[3] United Nations General Assembly. Report of the World Food Conference, Rome, 5-16 November 1974. New York: United Nations; 1975.

[4] World Bank. The 1990 World Development Report: Poverty— World Development Indicators. Oxford: Oxford University Press; 1990.

[5] Food and Agriculture Organization. Globally Almost 870 Million Chronically Undernourished - New Hunger Report. Rome: FAO Publications; 2012.

[6] United Nations General Assembly. Resolution Adopted by the General Assembly on 25 September 2015, A/RES 70/1. Transforming our World: the 2030 Agenda for Sustainable Development. New York: UN General Assembly; 2015.

[7] FAO, IFAD, WFP. The State of Food Security in the World, 2015. Meeting the 2015 International Hunger Targets: Taking Stock of Uneven Progress. Rome: FAO Publications; 2015.

[8] World Bank. No poverty: End poverty in all its Forms Everywhere. 2017. Available from: https://datatopics.worldbank.org/sdgatlas/archive/2017/SDG-01-no-poverty.html [Accessed 2/11/2020].

[9] Woolard I. An overview of Poverty and Inequality in South Africa. Unpublished briefing paper. Pretoria: HSRC; 2002.

[10] Republic of South Africa. Government Gazette. Vol 621. (No. 40759). Pretoria: Government Printers; 2017.

[11] Food and Agriculture Organization, Rome Declaration on World Food Security and World Food Summit Plan of Action. In: World Food Summit. Rome: FAO; 1996.

[12] Maxwell D, Ahiadeke C, Levin C, Armar-Klemesu M, Zakariah S, Lamptey G M. Alternative food-security indicators: revisiting the frequency and severity ofcoping strategies. Food Policy. 1999; **24**(4):411-429.

[13] Chung K, Haddad L, Ramakrishna J, Riely F. Identifying the Food Insecure: The Application of Mixed-Method Approaches in India. Washington, DC: International Food Policy Research Institute; 1997.

[14] Maxwell S, M. Smith. Household food security: a conceptual review. In: Maxwell, S., Frankenberger, T. (Eds.). Household Food Security: Concepts, Indicators, Measurements. Rome: IFAD. 1992 (1):1-72.

[15] FAO, IFAD, WFP. The State of Food Insecurity in The World: How does International Price Volatility Affect Domestic Economies and Food Security. Rome: FAO; 2011.

[16] Devereux S, Distinguishing Between Chronic and Transitory Food Insecurity in Emergency Needs Assessments. World Food Program, Emmergency Needs Assessment Branch. Rome: WFP; 2006.

[17] Organisation for Economic Co-operation and Development. The DAC guidelines: Poverty Reduction. Paris: OECD Publishing; 2001.

[18] Barrett C, Lentz EC. Hunger and food insecurity. In: The Oxford

Handbook of the Social Science of Poverty. (Eds). Brady D, Burton LM. Oxford: OUP; 2013.

[19] Booth S, Smith A. Food security and poverty in Australia-challenges for dietitians. Australian Journal of Nutrition and Dietetics. 2001; **58**(3):150-156.

[20] Sorsdahl K, Slopen N, Siefert K, Seedat S, Stein D, Williams D. Household food insufficiency and mental health in South Africa. Journal of Epidemiology & Community Health.2011; **65**(5): 426-431.

[21] Dixon LB, Winkleby MA, Radimer KL. Dietary intakes and serum nutrients differ between adults from food-insufficient and food-sufficient families: Third National Health and Nutrition Examination Survey, 1988-1994. The Journal of Nutrition. 2001; **131**(4):1232-1246.

[22] Food and Agricultural Organisation. Food Security Information for Action Practical Guides. Rome: FAO; 2008.

[23] World Food Programme. Emmergency Needs Assessment. Rome: World Food Programme Rome; 2004.

[24] World Health Organization. Infant and young child nutrition: Technical consultation on infant and young child feeding. Fifty-third World Health Assembly. Geneva: WHO; 2000.

[25] Black RE, Victora CG, Walker SP, Bhutta ZA, Christian P, De Onis M, Ezzati M, Grantham-McGregor S, Katz J, Martorell R, Uauy R, Maternal and child undernutrition and overweight in low-income and middle-income countries. The Lancet. 2013; **382**(9890)427-451.

[26] World Health Organisation. Healthy Diet. 2020a. Available from: https://www.who.int/news-room/fact-sheets/detail/healthy-diet [Accessed 2/11/2020].

[27] Jinabhai CC, Taylor M, Sullivan KR. Implications of the prevalence of stunting, overweight and obesity amongst South African primary school children: a possible nutritional transition?. European Journal of Clinical Nutrition. 2003; **57**(2):358-365.

[28] Stabouli S. Papakatsika S, Kotsis V. The role of obesity, salt and exercise on blood pressure in children and adolescents. Expert review of cardiovascular therapy. 2011; **9**(6): 753-761.

[29] Kimani-Murage EW, Kahn K, Pettifor JM, Tollman SM, Dunger DB, Gómez-Olivé XF, Norris SA. The prevalence of stunting, overweight and obesity, and metabolic disease risk in rural South African children. BMC Public Health. 2010; **10**(1);1-13.

[30] Danquah FI, Ansu-Mensah M, Bawontuo V, Yeboah M, Udoh RH, Tahiru M, Kuupiel D. Risk factors and morbidities associated with childhood obesity in sub-Saharan Africa: a systematic scoping review. BMC Nutrition. 2020; **6**(1);1-14.

[31] Tathiah N, Moodley I, Mubaiwa V, Denny L, Taylor M. South Africa's nutritional transition: Overweight, obesity, underweight and stunting in female primary school learners in rural KwaZulu-Natal, South Africa. South African Medical Journal. 2013; **103**(10);718-722.

[32] Devereux S, Waidler J. Why does Malnutrition Persist in South Africa Despite Social Grants, in Centre of Excellence in Food Security. Working paper 1; 2017.

[33] Seekings J. South Africa: Democracy, poverty and inclusive growth since 1994. In Democracy Works–Conference Paper.

Centre for Development and Enterprise (CDE); 2014.

[34] Hirschowitz R. Living in South Africa: Selected findings of the 1995 October household survey. (ISBN 0-621 17597 8). Pretoria: Central Statistical Service; 1996.

[35] Labadarios D, Van Middelkoop A, Coutsoudis. South African Vitamin A Consultative Group (SAVACG). Anthropometric, vitamin A, iron and immunisation coverage status in children aged 6-71 months in South Africa. South African Medical Journal. 1994;(86):354-357.

[36] Republic of South Africa. The Bill of Rights of the Constitution. Government Gazette. (No. 17678). Pretoria: Government Printer; 1996.

[37] Republic of South Africa. Broad-based Black Economic Empowerment Act, No. 53 of 2003, 2004. Pretoria: Government Printer; 2004.

[38] Republic of South Africa, Department of Agriculture. The Integrated Food Security Strategy For South Africa. Pretoria: Government printers; 2002.

[39] Hendriks S. Food security in South Africa: Status quo and policy imperatives. Agrekon. 2014; **53**(2):1-24.

[40] Statistics South Africa. Poverty trends in South Africa: An examination of absolute poverty between 2006 and 2015. Pretoria: Statistics South Africa; 2017.

[41] Department of Agriculture, Forestry and Fisheries. Food Security. Pretoria: Directorate Economic Services: Production Economics Unit; 2011.

[42] Statistics South Africa. General Household Survey Series Volume IV: Food security and agriculture 2002-2011. Depth analysis of the General Household Survey data. GHS Series Volume IV. (Report No.0318-03 (2002-2011). Pretoria: Statistics South Africa; 2012.

[43] Devereux S, Waidler J. Why does malnutrition persist in South Africa despite social grants. Food Security South Africa Working Paper Series (001). Pretoria: DST-NRF Centre of Excellence in Food Security; 2017.

[44] Statistics South Africa. Consumer Price Index: Statistical release P0141. Pretoria: Statistics South Africa; 2016.

[45] Ndlovu BN. Challenges facing the recipients of the child support grant in the Umhlathuze Municipality (Unpublished Doctoral dissertation, University of Zululand); 2009.

[46] Khosa P, Kaseke E. The utilisation of the child support grant by caregivers: the case of Ba-Phalaborwa municipality in Limpopo Province. Social work. 2017; **53**(3): 356-367.

[47] United Nations Department of Economic and Social Affairs. International Migration Report: 2017 Highlights. New York: United Nations; 2017.

[48] Republic of South Africa, National, National Planning Commission. 2013. National Development Plan vision 2030: Our future, make it work, Pretoria: Government Printers; 2013.

[49] Statistics South Africa. General Household Survey Statistical Release P0318. Pretoria: Statistics South Africa; 2019.

[50] Jonah CMP, JD. Evidence of the existence of socioeconomic-related inequality South African diets: A quantitative analysis of the 2017 General Household Survey. World Nutrition, 2019; **10**(4): 27-42.

[51] Okop KJ, Ndayi K, Tsolekile L, Sanders D, Puoane. Low intake of commonly available fruits and vegetables in socio-economically disadvantaged communities of South Africa: influence of affordability and sugary drinks intake. BMC Public Health; 2019. **19**(1): 1-14.

[52] World Health Organisation. WHO Reveals Leading Causes Of Death And Disability Worldwide: 2000-2019. 2020b. Available from: https://www.who.int/news/item/09-12-2020-who-reveals-leading-causes-of-death-and-disability-worldwide-2000-2019 [Accessed 2021/1/6].

[53] World Health Organisation. Cardiovascular Diseases. 2020c. Available from: https://www.who.int/health-topics/cardiovascular-diseases#tab=tab1 [Accessed 2021/1/7].

Chapter 4

Double Burden of Poverty and Cardiovascular Disease Risk among Low-Resource Communities in South Africa

Wilna Oldewage-Theron and Christa Grobler

Abstract

Limited studies evaluating the prevalence of cardiovascular risk (CVR) in resource-poor black communities in South Africa (SA), exist. The objective of this chapter is to evaluate the prevalence of CVR in a cross-sectional studies in randomly selected low income children, adults and elderly in Gauteng, Free State and Eastern Cape, SA. The test panel of CVR markers included: anthropometry, lipid profile, blood pressure, fibrinogen, high sensitive–C–reactive protein (HS–CRP), homocysteine, vitamin B12, folate, glucose and dietary intakes. The main findings indicated high CVR with prevalence of overweight/obesity, Hypertension, hyperhomocysteinaemia, increased fibrinogen and HS-CRP, as well as low intakes of dietary fibre, vitamins B6 and B12, folate and polyunsaturated- and monounsaturated fatty acids, and high intakes of dietary sodium, saturated and trans fatty acids, and added sugars. Multiple CVR factors are present among all the communities. It can thus be concluded that a double burden of poverty and risk of CVD exists across the different age groups and geographical locations in these resource-poor communities.

Keywords: cardiovascular risk, poverty, South Africa, children, adults, elderly

1. Introduction

South Africa (SA) is a middle-income country that is characterised by contrasting living conditions ranging from wealthy urban suburbs to lower-income, underdeveloped areas. [1] SA has faced many socio-economic challenges such as high levels of poverty, inequality and unemployment [1, 2] despite having the second largest economy on the African continent. Since the country's transition to democracy in 1994, progress has been made, but unemployment rates and poverty levels remain high. [1] Poverty is the main underlying factor contributing to food insecurity. [3, 4] The food insecure often use strategies to cope with the inability to access food. One of these include reducing the quality and quantity of food consumed, thus consuming poor diversity diets which can have detrimental consequences such as hunger, malnutrition [5, 6] and increased prevalence of metabolic and cardiovascular diseases (CVDs) [7] due to it hindering individuals' ability to choose the most appropriate foods and beverages for an adequate diet. [8] A disadvantage of food insecurity is thus monotonous diets with consumption of more affordable energy-dense staples and foods that may have detrimental health outcomes such as obesity and its chronic disease comorbidities. [9] Food insecurity thus does not only cause under-nutrition, but also in over-nutrition such as obesity and its comorbidities, especially in low-income communities. [10] SA is a country in health transition and suffers from a quadruple burden of (a) poverty and nutrition-related chronic diseases of lifestyle [CDL], (b) communicable diseases, (c) peri-natal, maternal and injury-related disorders, [11] and (d) a nutrition transition. A recent study has found that this quadruple burden of disease is predominantly present in the black African population. [1] Urbanisation and westernisation of the Black African population of SA is marked not only by demographic transition, but also by increased animal protein, total dietary fat and added sugar intakes [11] and a health transition resulting in an increased prevalence of obesity [6] and CDL such as CVD. [11, 12]

2. Double burden of poverty and cardiovascular disease among black south Africans

The South African population of approximately 59 million people consists of 81% black Africans. [13] In 2017, it was reported that 56% of the SA population lived in poverty [14] with 28% living in extreme poverty, thus not having enough money to purchase enough food to consume around 2,100 calories per day for a month (food poverty). The most vulnerable to food poverty are women, children (66.8%), those with low education (79.2%) and people from the black population group (64.2%). [15, 16]

CVD incidence is increasing rapidly among all population groups in SA. [11] CDLs contribute 51% to the mortality rate, with CVD and diabetes accounting for 19% and 8% of the total deaths. Many people in SA have poor living conditions and limited resources to maintain health and well-being. [15] In spite of cultural background, people that has been subjected to urbanisation, has adopted a more Western lifestyle with lower dietary fibre and higher dietary fat and added sugar intakes, as well as lower physical activity levels. These dietary changes have led to higher prevalence of CDL, [17] specifically an increased risk and susceptibility of CVD among the black population, [18] and not only in adults, but also among children. [19] The face of CVD has thus changed in recent years. Initially it was a disease of the white population group, the affluent and older generations, but since the 2000s, it was also observed that the prevalence of CVD risk factors, such as dyslipidaemia and obesity, has increased among black Africans [20] as well as children and adolescents. [21–24]

The aim of this chapter was thus to investigate the prevalence of the various cardiovascular risk factors, specifically those that are irreversible, among children (6–18 years old) in peri-urban Free State (FS), [25] rural Eastern Cape (EC), [24, 26–28] peri-urban [29] and urban [30–33] Gauteng; adults (19–59 years old) in urban Gauteng [30, 31, 34–37] and peri-urban FS; [38–40] and elderly (≥60 years) in urban Gauteng, [41–43] including both genders, living in poverty in SA. Gauteng was chosen as the authors both resided in Gauteng and it was the focus of the university for funding. No data had been available for the cardiovascular risk factors in the above-mentioned communities and a valuable research opportunity was created to address the paucity of information in these communities. For this reason, the FS and EC provinces were chosen because of funding opportunities and gap in the knowledge base on the areas included in these studies.

3. Methodology

A search of electronic databases focusing on poverty, food insecurity and cardiovascular risk factors was carried out between 2010 and 2020. Databases used included: MEDLINE (PubMed), Web of Science, ScienceDirect, Scopus, EBSCOHost, Springer Link, and Sabinet. The keywords used included: "poverty", "food security", "nutrition security", "food and nutrition security", "cardiovascular disease", "CVD", "cardiovascular risk", "CVR", "cholesterol", "triglycerides", "HDL", "LDL", "C-reactive protein", "CRP", "fibrinogen", "homocysteiene", "vitamin B6", "vitamin B9", "folate", "folic acid", "vitamin B12", "glucose", "insulin", "obesity", "overweight", "nutritional status", "hypertension", "high blood pressure", "dietary diversity", "dietary intake", "children", "adults", "elderly", "older people", "aged", "double burden", and "South Africa".

The data used for this chapter included all the databases and articles published for the various studies undertaken by the authors between 2000 and 2020 among black children in the EC, FS and Gauteng, [24–28, 30–32, 36] adults in Gauteng and the FS [25, 30, 35, 37, 40] and the elderly in Gauteng [37, 41, 43] in various urban, peri-urban and rural areas of SA. For the purpose of this book chapter, urban areas include cities and towns that are developed, thus having a density of human structures such as houses, commercial buildings, roads, and public transport. Peri-urban areas are underdeveloped areas on the outskirts of the towns and cities where people live, but no public transportation or commercial buildings are present. Rural areas refer to areas with low population density and large areas of undeveloped land where people mainly live far apart from their neighbours.

Comparative tables were drawn up using the published articles and, where data were not published, descriptive statistical analyses (frequencies) were calculated using IBM SPSS Statistics, version 26, from the study databases that had not been destroyed. The ethical and scientific procedures for the sampling strategy and data collection methods were the same for the published and unpublished data.

4. Poverty and food insecurity

Poverty and food insecurity were observed in all seven study communities. A large majority of the adults (75.7%–78.0%) [35, 44] and child caregivers (53.0%–94.0%) [27, 29, 30, 44] were unemployed, had either no or only primary education (39.9%–78.8%), [27, 29, 30, 34, 36, 43, 44] and lived in poverty (67.7–100%). [27, 29, 35, 36, 44] The poverty rates of all the communities were more than double the 25.2% national food poverty rate. [15] This may have been due to the high unemployment rate and low education levels found among the adults in all the communities. A chronic money shortage to buy food was also reported in large percentages of the study population.

5. Cardiovascular risk factors

Many risk factors for CVD have been identified in the scientific literature and can be reversible or irreversible (**Table 1**). In 2016, 20% of the South African adults (15+ years) were smoking. [45] Risk factors present in the South African adult (18+ years) population are obesity (68% women; 31% men) hypertension (46% in women and 44% in men), [46] physical inactivity (37%), high blood pressure (24%) and hyperglycaemia (10%). [45] There is a paucity of national data for other CVD risk factors in adults, and very little CVD national data are available for children, except for the prevalence of overweight and obesity.

Irreversible	Gender (male)
	Ageing
	Genetically inherited factors
Potentially reversible factors	Cigarette smoking
	Obesity
	Hypertension Physical activity
	Hyperglycaemia, diabetes
	Increased haemostatic factors, decreased fibrinolysis, increased platelet aggregration
	Increased levels of homocysteine
	Increased inflammatory response (HS-CRP)
	Dyslipidaemia (increased cholestrol, LDL, Triglyseride, decreased LDL)
	Diet and dietary diversity
Psyschosocial	Low socio-economic class
	Stressful environment
	Personality types
Geographic	Climate and season (cold weather increased risk)
	Soft drinking water
	Environmental pollution

Table 1.
Reversible and irreversible cardiovascular risk factors.

5.1 Socio-demographic risk factors

The history of CVD of an individual is directly proportional to the risk of CVD (the earlier the age of onset and the more family members affected the greater is the risk of CVD). [47] It is known that men are at greater risk of developing CVD than women [47, 48] maybe because oestrogen has an inhibiting effect on low density lipoprotein-cholesterol (LDL-C) oxidation and increasing the production of large very low-density lipoproteins (VLDL) and therefore has a protective effect against atherogenesis. [50] Low levels of education in middle-income countries like SA had a significantly higher risk of major CVD events compared to those with high incomes. [49] The majority (>70%) of our communities showed low education (no or primary school education), [29, 31, 34, 35, 43] except for the peri-urban adults in the FS (44.2%); [44] and caregivers of the peri-urban children in Gauteng (39.9%), [29] however, these percentages are still high. High unemployment rates (53.0–94.0%) [29–31, 35, 44] for the majority of all the communities were also observed. The low education and high unemployment rates of the communities could be some of the main reasons for the high poverty rates in the study communities (67.7–100%). [26, 35, 36, 44] Research has found that people with low education may not have access to health care that may prevent detecting and treating disease and thus compromise their health even further. [50]

5.2 Cigarette smoking

Cigarette smoking doubles the risk of coronary artery disease and contributes seven-fold to the increase in risk for peripheral arterial disease. [51] Cigarette smoking and increases blood pressure and increases the heart's workload. It deprives the heart muscle of oxygen and damages the platelets that increase coagulation and clot formation. Toxins in cigarettes may also damage the blood vessels and increase atherosclerosis. [48, 52] In SA, the proportion of adult (15+ years) women that smoke (37%) daily is higher than in men (8%). [46] Smoking patterns among children were not measured in our studies, but we previously reported 11.7%, 15.2% and 23.6% smoking among urban elderly, [43] peri-urban adults in Gauteng [31] and rural adults in the FS. [37]

5.3 Obesity

Obesity is considered a multi-factorial condition [20, 53, 54] associated with an increased risk for comorbidities such as type 2 diabetes, insulin resistance, cancer, stroke, [53] hypertension, dyslipidaemia, [53, 55] and hypertriglyceridaemia. [55] Obesity is also considered an independent risk factor for CVD. [40] For every 1% increase above ideal body mass index (BMI), the cardiovascular risk (CVR) increases by 3.3% for females and 3.6% for males. [56] In our studies, the majority of the adults and elderly were overweight/obese. [44, 57] Although we did not report gender differences in this chapter, previous published results confirmed a higher prevalence among women in rural FS [37] and urban elderly [41] than in men. Our results further showed that the urban women in Gauteng had the highest prevalence (82.3%) of overweight/obesity, but cannot be compared to the peri-urban adults and urban elderly that included both men and women. However, the overweight/obesity prevalence among the urban elderly in Gauteng [57] and the peri-urban adults in the FS [44] was consistent with the national prevalence.

There is usually a higher prevalence of overweight/obesity in urban than rural. [20] We did not have any rural adult communities to compare our results, but the urban elderly in Gauteng (61.0%) [57] had lower prevalence of overweight/obesity than the peri-urban adults in the FS (67.9%). [44] This was inconsistent with research from sub-Saharan Africa (SSA) [54] and SA where it was found that age is positively correlated with overweight and obesity. [58, 59] In all three the adult communities, the prevalence of obesity was higher than the prevalence of overweight. (**Table 2**). The increasing prevalence of childhood overweight/obesity in SA [11] is presenting a major public health problem. Childhood overweight/obesity is associated with early onset of hypertension and hyperglycaemia, both risk factors for CVD, [71] as well as adult obesity, [54] premature death and disability. [54] Similar to adults, a higher prevalence of overweight/obesity among children is found in urban areas. [54, 72, 73] (**Table 3**) However, our results showed higher prevalence among the rural children (4.3%) [24] compared to the urban children (1.0%). [32] In addition, the rural [28] and urban [32] children had the lowest prevalence of overweight and no obesity prevalence. Both peri-urban areas showed a prevalence of 21.0% in the FS [25] and 18.3% in Gauteng. [32, 33] This was higher than the national prevalence. In our studies among resource-poor communities, the prevalence of obesity was much lower than the prevalence of overweight. Our studies have found significantly higher prevalence of overweight/obesity in girls when compared to the boys. [24, 26] These results were consistent with national data [77] and for SSA, [54] but inconsistent with a recent systematic review and meta-analysis investigating overweight/obesity among 5–19 year old children in 15 countries in Africa where the boys and girls were equally affected by overweight/obesity. [71].

To summarise, overweight/obesity is common among the poor-resource adults and elderly in our study population. The high prevalence observed among the adults, specifically women, and elderly may be due to poor nutrition (**Table 2**). Although the prevalence of obesity is not yet high among the children in our study

Variable	Reference values	Urban women Gauteng (n = 628) %	Peri-urban adults Free State (n = 271) %	Urban elderly Gauteng (n = 170) %
Overweight	BMI ≥ 25 < 30 [60]	39.3 [37]	26.0 [44]	29.5 [57]
Obese	BMI ≥ 30 [60]	43.0 [37]	41.9 [44]	31.5 [57]
High serum TC levels	≥6.2 mmol/L [61]	0.5 [37]	16.7	22.3 [57]
Low HDL-C levels	<1 mmol/L (adult men) <1.3 mmol/L (adult women) [61, 62]	43.0 [37]	62.7 [39]	76.2 [57]
High LDL-C levels	>4.1 mmol/L [60, 63]	0.5 [37]	16.7	14.6 [57]
Hypertriglyceridaemia (High TRG levels)	≥2.3 mmol/L [60, 63]	24.7 [37]	12.7 [39]	13.8 [57]
High normal BP	130–139 mm Hg/85–89 mm Hg (systolic/diastolic blood pressure) [64]	11.6 [37]	12.7	10.8 [57]
Hypertensive	≥140/≥90 mm Hg (systolic/ diastolic blood pressure) [64]	36.4 [37]	53.2 [39]	68.0 [57]
Hyperhomocysteienemia	>15 umol/L [61] (serum homocysteiene)	—	—	66.4 [57]
Fibrinogen	>3.5 g/L [65]	—	—	68.0 [57]
Inflammation (HS-CRP)	≥3 mg/dL [62]	—	56.9	68.3 [57]
Hyperglycaemia (serum glucose)	>5.5 mmol/L [66]	—	16.0 [39]	38.5 [57]
Serum vitamin B6	<8.6 mcg/L [67]	—	—	98.0 [57]
Serum vitamin B12	<156 pmol/L [68, 69]	—	—	4.8 [57]
Serum folate	<5.9 nmol/dL [70]	—	—	9.6 [57]

Table 2.
Cardiovascular risk factors in adults and elderly.

communities, the results highlight the increasing burden of overweight among children (**Table 3**). The high prevalence of overweight and obesity in our study communities is a concern as the comorbidities associated with overweight/obesity have negative effects on health across the life cycle. [71]

5.4 Hypertension

Hypertension (blood pressure ≥ 140/90 mm Hg) [64] is considered one of the most important risk factors for developing CVD [50, 78] due to organ injury to the heart and kidneys. [79] Sharp increases in childhood hypertension have been reported in SA recently. [11] In childhood, hypertension treatment does not reverse the target organ injury and although hypertension treatment will significantly reduce event rates, the burden of CVD event rates will remain high though adulthood. [79] SA has a high hypertension burden with 44% and 41% of adult (≥15 years) black African women and men respectively. [46] In our adult populations the urban women in Gauteng had lower prevalence of 36.4% compared to the peri-urban adults in the FS (53.2%). [39] The elderly in urban Gauteng had the highest prevalence (68.%). [57] (**Table 2**) This was consistent with the national prevalence (84% among both genders aged ≥65 years), indicating that

Variable	Reference values	Rural children Eastern Cape (n = 232) %	Peri-urban children Free State (n = 98) %	Peri-urban children Gauteng (n = 203) %	Urban children Gauteng (n = 152) %
Overweight	BMI:A ≥ 2 < 3 [74]	4.3 [24]	17.0 [25]	15.8 [29]	1.0 [32]
Obese	BMI:A ≥ 3 [74]	0.0 [24]	4.0 [25]	2.5 [29]	0.0 [32]
High serum TC levels	≥5.18 mmol/L [75]	1.3 [24]	19.4	3.0	10.2 [32]
Low HDL-C levels	<1.04 mmol/L [75]	42.5 [24]	30.6	19.2	95.9 [32]
High LDL-C levels	≤3.37 mmol/L [75]	2.12 [24]	12.2	2.5	28.6 [32]
Hypertriglyceridaemia (High TRG levels)	≥1.12 mmol/L (0–9 years old) ≥1.47 mmol/L (10–19 years old) [75]	12.4 [24]	35.7	4.4	1.0 [32]
Hyperhomocysteienaemia	>15 umol/L [61]	1.6	—	—	—
Fibrinogen	>3.5 g/L [65]	14.8	—	—	—
Inflammation (HS-CRP)	≥3 mg/dL [62]	19.0 [24]	7.8	—	—
Hyperglycaemia (serum glucose)	>6.1 mmol/L [76]	10.3[24]	6.5	6.9	—
Serum vitamin B12	<156 pmol/L [69]	7.6	—	—	—
Serum folate	<5.9 nmol/dL [70]	4.6	—	—	—

Table 3.
Cardiovascular risk factors of children.

the hypertension burden increases with age. [46, 80] A recent national survey has found an overall prevalence of 43%, of which 58% were unaware of the condition and thus did not receive treatment. [80] Similar results were observed where only 36.8% of the hypertensive urban elderly in Gauteng used hypertensive medication. [43] No hypertension data were available for the children.

In summary, our results showed high levels of hypertension in adults and the elderly in both urban and peri-urban areas. A recent national survey has found older age, obesity and lower education levels as the main risk factors for hypertension in SA. [80] High prevalence of obesity and poor education levels have been identified in all our adult communities.

5.5 Hyperglycaemia, diabetes and metabolic syndrome

Diabetes mellitus is the most common, but also the most complex CDL. [81, 82] Hyperglycaemia affects multiple organs and can lead to arterial hypertension. [83] It is estimated that the cause of death in 80% of individuals suffering from type 2 diabetes will be due to thrombotic complications of which 75% will result from a cardiovascular event. [84] Data on the incident rates of children with diabetes are available for only 6% of African countries and may be due to lack of screening tests available in the poor and low income communities. [84] Results in **Tables 2** and **3** indicated that 38.5% urban elderly (Gauteng), [57] 16.0% peri-urban adults (FS), [39] 10.3% rural children

(EC), [24] 6.5% peri-urban children (FS), and 6.9% peri-urban children (Gauteng) had high serum glucose levels. An increased prevalence of diabetes was reported for developing countries, [85] and it can be concluded that the prevalence of hyperglycaemia in all age groups in urban, peri-urban and rural areas in SA is concerning.

5.6 Haemostasis

The development of coronary artery disease and myocardial infarction has both atheromatous and thrombotic components. Haemostasis is a finely balanced system of clot formation and fibrinolysis. [86–88] Fibrinogen is recognised as an independent risk marker of CVD. Fibrinogen, because of its mass, also has a direct effect on the blood viscosity and a physical functional effect on platelet aggregation. [65, 89] Studies have indicated an increased level of plasma fibrinogen in black South Africans. [12, 57, 90] An increase of one gram per litre in plasma fibrinogen doubles the risk of CVD. [89] The fibrinogen levels were measured in two of the communities. High fibrinogen levels were observed in 68.0% of the elderly [57] (**Table 2**) and 14.8% of the rural children (**Table 3**), indicating an increased risk for CVD.

5.7 Homocysteine metabolism

5.7.1 Homocysteine

Several mechanisms have been proposed to clarify the link between homocysteine and pro-thrombotic state. The oxidative damage to the endothelium, combined with inhibition of the vasculo-protective function of nitric oxide, enhances thrombogenecity. [91] Homocysteine is metabolised by (a) the trans-sulphuration pathway which results in the production of cystathionine - a process that requires vitamin B6 and the main route of metabolism is via a methionine-conserving pathway - a process that requires methyltetrahydrofolate (from folic acid) and vitamin B12 as co-factor or alternatively (b) by the remethylation pathway taking place in the kidney and liver (where betaine is utilised instead of folate). [92–95] An association between elevated plasma homocysteine and the development of atherosclerosis has been confirmed. [96] Studies in animal models have shown that elevated homocysteine promoted atherosclerosis by increased oxidative stress impaired endothelial function and increased thrombogenecity. [92, 93, 95–99] Epidemiological retrospective and prospective clinical studies established homocysteine as a potent independent risk factor for atherothrombotic vascular disease. [91, 92, 100] Additionally, homocysteine increase superoxide (O_2^{-}) levels resulting in increased oxidative stress, causing an inflammatory state and increased atherosclerosis and ischemia reperfusion. Oxidative stress in return inhibits the cobalamine metabolism and enhances the cycle. [101, 102] The frequency of hyperhomocysteienaemia as an independent risk factor for atherothrombotic vascular disease [91, 92, 100] was found in 66.4% and 1.6% of the urban elderly [57] and rural children respectively. Thus, although homocysteine measurement did not form part of the objectives in all our communities, prevalence of hyperhomocysteienaemia in the urban elderly (Gauteng) (**Table 2**) and the rural children (EC) (**Table 3**) is an additional confirmation of an increased risk for CVD in the low income South African population.

5.7.2 Serum vitamin B6 levels

Vitamin B6 acts as coenzyme in the irreversible trans-sulfuration of homocysteine to cysteine. Higher vitamin B6 level are associated with lower homocysteine levels. Fat metabolism requires carnitine, obtained either directly [103] through diet or via synthesis requiring lysine and vitamin B6. Vitamin B6 deficiency was also found to be associated with decreased plasma PUFAs (n-6 and n-3) which may be associated with elevated cardiovascular risk and a contributing factor to the anti-inflammatory response. [104, 105] Low circulating vitamin B6 levels have been found inversely related to inflammatory markers (HS-CRP, fibrinogen, IL-6 and TNF-α) and are related to the incidence of inflammatory diseases (rheumatoid arthritis, CVD, and diabetes). [106, 107] Vitamin B6 levels were only available for the urban elderly and 98% of the respondents had low serum vitamin B6 levels (**Table 2**). Vitamin B6 levels were not available for any of the children, but pre-school children in Zambia indicated a suboptimal vitamin B6 in the studied group. [108] It would, therefore, be beneficial to include vitamin B6 serum levels in their analytical profile in future.

5.7.3 Serum folate levels

Low serum folate levels is a cardiovascular risk marker independently from homocysteine level. [109] Folate, as a donor of one-carbon units, is essential for methylation and affects numerous metabolisms involved in CVD [110] and accurate replication of deoxyribonucleic acid (DNA) and its repair. If DNA repair capacity of the cell is exceeded by the rate of damage to the genome, serious defects in cellular and tissue physiology occur, resulting in degenerative diseases including CVD. [111] The four mechanisms by which folate is involved in reducing atherosclerosis are: (1) Optimising methylation cycle and thereby directly reducing the homocysteine levels; (2) Acting directly as an antioxidant; (3) Interacting with enzyme endothelial nitric oxide synthase; (4) Affecting cofactor bioavailability of nitric oxide. Apart from being an independent cardiovascular risk marker, decreased serum folate levels also Indicate a decreased cell regeneration. [112] The serum folate levels were only available for two of the communities and 4.8% and 7.6% had low folate levels in the elderly [57] (**Table 2**) and rural children (EC) (**Table 3**) respectively. Study communities included in this study are therefore at risk for CVD and the general effect of ineffective cell recovery.

5.7.4 Serum vitamin B12 levels

The cofactor cobalamin is required for the optimal function of the enzymes methionine synthase and L-methylmalonyl-CoA. [113, 114] During methionine synthase, homocysteine is converted to methionine, when the methyl group is transferred from 5-methylene tetrahydrofolate to cobalamin to form methylcobalamin and tetrahydrofolate while methylcobalamin donates its methyl group that binds to homocysteine to form methionin (required for the synthesis of S-adenosylmethionine [SAM]). [87, 115] SAM is required in many cellular methylation reactions, including the methylation ribonucleic acid (RNA) and DNA. [116, 117] Reduced synthesis of methionine as a result of insufficient cobalamine results in increased homocysteine levels. [104] Vitamin B12 is also the coenzyme required to remove the methyl group from folate, thereby activating folate. [117, 118] Serum vitamin B12 was only available for the elderly in Gauteng (**Table 2**) and the rural children (EC) (**Table 3**) and 4.8% [57] and 7.6% had low folate levels respectively, thus at risk of impaired homocysteine metabolism and CVD.

5.8 Inflammation

An inflammatory response is initiated by damage to the vascular cell lining resulting in a series of mechanisms (acute-phase response) including haemodynamic (vasodilatation) activation of endothelial cells (increased adhesion molecule expression), increased permeability (enhanced protein movement) and an increase in acute-phase proteins. [119, 120] Vessel injury can also be caused by high LDL-C, hypertension, cigarette toxins and elevated homocysteine levels. During the inflammatory response that aims to repair the damage to the artery wall, LDL-C becomes trapped in the lesion that is engulfed by the macrophages and the free radicals oxidise the LDL trapped in the macrophage and eventually become plaque. [48] CRP is a β-globulin which is bound strongly to phospholipids and increases twentyfold to thirtyfold during an infectious or inflammatory response and is, therefore, considered a credible marker for systemic inflammation. [47] The prevalence of systemic inflammation was found in 56.9% of the adult respondents (peri-urban FS) and in 68.3% of the elderly, [57] (**Table 2**) as well as 19% and 7.8% of the rural (EC) [26] and peri-urban children (FS) respectively. (**Table 3**) Elevated CRP is a strong independent predictor of risk of future cardiovascular events. [121, 122] Thus, the results from our studies indicate an increased risk for CVD.

5.9 Dyslipidaemia

The prevalence of dyslipidaemia varies across the regions in SSA due to increased urbanisation and change of lifestyle factors (epidemiological transition). [123] A similar variation was observed in SA where a significant difference in the prevalence of dyslipidaemia occurs in different ethnic groups. [124] Although, studies indicated that people from an African decent showed an athero-protective lipid profile (lower total cholesterol) compared to their white European or Indian fellow countrymen, widespread low High density Lipoprotein (HDL-C) was present. [125] The use of antiretroviral therapy (ARV) also leads to an increase in dyslipidaemia. With the high prevalence of HIV/AIDS in SA [45, 46], is ARV treatment (the largest health programme internationally) is considered as a contributing factor to dyslipidaemia in SA. [126]. Previous studies indicated that prevalence of dyslipidaemia among black South Africans (independent of rural or urban) varies between 30% and 63%. [125, 127, 128]

The high protein component of high-density lipoprotein-cholesterol (HDL-C) accounts for its metabolic function of removing cholesterol from tissue back to the liver, and is considered as an important anti-atherogenic pathway modulating inflammation. The inverse correlation between serum HDL-C and cardiovascular risk (CVR) is well known and widely accepted. [129] Studies showed that improving poor lifestyle habits to have a positive effect on the HDL-C levels. [130]

With reference to the reported results in **Tables 2** and **3**, the prevalence of increased total serum cholesterol (TC) with the lowest in the urban adult women in Gauteng where 0.5% of participants had an increased TC. The highest prevalence was observed among the urban elderly population of Gauteng, where 22.3% of participants had an increased TC. The prevalence of low serum HDL-C levels was significantly decreased in all the study communities with the lowest prevalence in the peri-urban children where 19.2% had a HDL-C of less than 130 mg/dl. The highest prevalence was in the urban children where 95.6% had a decreased HDL-C level. The percentage of participants with the highest prevalence of abnormal LDL-C levels was found in the urban children in Gauteng (28.6%) and the lowest prevalence was found in the urban women of Gauteng (0.5%). In contrast, the lowest prevalence of participants with increased serum triglyceride levels were found in the urban children of Gauteng and the highest prevalence was in the urban (Gauteng) women (24.7%). Results obtained from our studies are in line with results obtained from other studies in SA [125–128], confirming that prevalence of dyslipidaemia (mainly decreased HDL-C) is becoming an increasing concern that needs to be consciously addressed in planning for Health care interventions.

Dyslipidaemia is regarded as an independent CVR marker. [124] As indicated in **Figure 1**, a total of 4.1% Peri-urban children from the FS had four elevated lipid

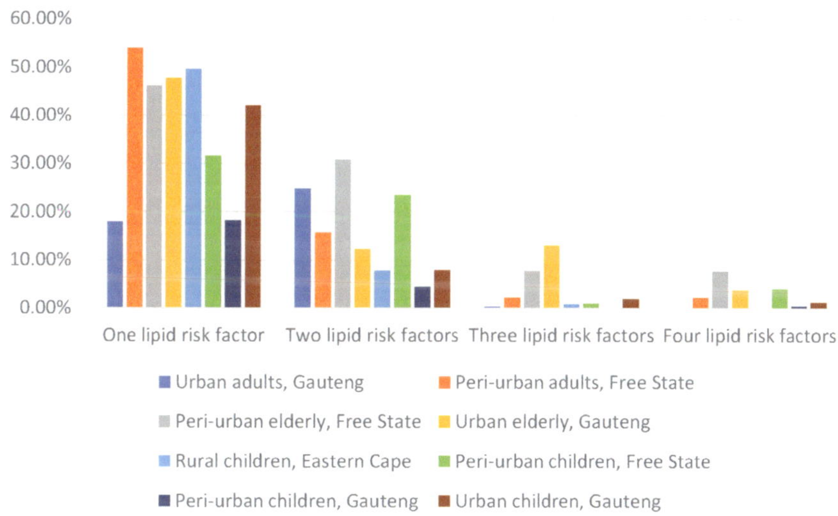

Figure 1.
Dyslipidaemic factors present in study groups.

risk factors, additionally, of the urban elderly from Gauteng 3.8% had four, 13.1% had three, 12.3% had two and 47.7% had one elevated lipid parameter. Interestingly, more than one lipid risk factor were present in almost all the communities (>10% of adults and elderly), even in the children (>5%).

5.10 Dietary intake factors

Dietary diversity has a significant positive association with health. [34] An inverse relationship between dietary diversity and CVD risk factors, namely hypertension, hypercholesterolaemia and high HDL-C has been observed. [131] Although we did not measure dietary diversity in all the communities, poor to moderate dietary diversity were observed in all of the communities. [26, 29, 33, 35, 38, 57]. This may have been due to their socio-economic status and food insecurity and may be a risk factor for CVD.

5.10.1 Added sugar intakes

An association between higher dietary sugar intakes and overweight/obesity and CDLs such as CVD exists. Increased dietary glycaemic load, caused by high sugar consumption, results in increased hepatic lipogenesis, dyslipidaemia,[132] and CVD. [133] Childhood overweight/obesity risk and morbidity were associated with consumption of sugar-sweetened beverages (SSBs) and highly processed foods and snacks. [54] The World Health Organisation recommends the intake of added sugar to be <10% of total energy intake. [134] More than 20% of the adults, elderly [57] and children in rural EC had high added sugar intakes whereas the children in peri-urban FS and urban Gauteng [33] had no added sugar intakes. Although SSB consumption has not been investigated in our studies, during the past 50 years, SBB consumption has increased [132] and SA is in the top 10 countries with the highest consumption of SSBs globally. [135]

5.10.2 Dietary fibre

Vegetables, legumes, whole grains and fruit all contribute to dietary fibre intake. Dietary fibre is differentiated as soluble (dissolves in water and forms a gel) and insoluble fibres. Good sources of soluble fibre are oats, citrus fruit, barley and legumes. It lowers LDL-C and glucose levels and, therefore, has a protective effect against CVD. [136] Lowering of cholesterol is achieved by the binding of fibre to bile acids, thereby escalating its excretion. This inhibits the production of cholesterol by the liver, resulting in lower blood cholesterol. [137] Food sources of insoluble dietary fibre include whole grains and vegetables. It cannot be fermented and promotes bowel movement and alleviates constipation. [138] A large majority (0–100%) of the children and adults in all our communities had low dietary fibre intakes. [24, 26, 29, 33–35, 38, 43, 44, 57] This may be due to the mainly refined carbohydrate-rich diet consumed by all these communities.

5.10.3 Dietary fats and fatty acids

Dietary fats consist mainly of cholesterol and fatty acids. Total dietary fat (% of total energy [TE]) intakes were higher than recommended for all the communities, ranging from 13.7% to 32.7% in urban Gauteng women and elderly respectively. [24, 26, 29, 32, 35, 36, 38, 39, 42–44, 57] High-fat diets cause an increase in postprandial triglyceride levels that are associated with risk of coronary heart disease (CHD). [139, 140] Fatty acids can be either protective against the development of CVD or can be risk factors for CVD. Saturated fatty acids (SFAs) and trans fatty acids (TFAs) have the greatest adverse effect on atherogenic cholesterol levels and are both associated with risk of CVD. [136, 141] Increased SFA intakes increase LDL-C levels. [142] TFAs have a HDL-C lowering effect and also increase LDL-C levels and, therefore, increase the risk of CVD.[47]. The contribution of TFA to CVD is a multiple pathway mechanism affecting lipid metabolism, increased inflammatory response and adiposity, and decreased endothelial function and insulin sensitivity. [143]

Dietary SFA intakes of <10% and TFAs of <1% of total energy intakes are recommended. [144] High TFA intakes were observed in less than 10% of our communities, except for the children in rural EC where the proportion of respondents with high intakes of TFAs was 36.7%. The proportion of the respondents that had high SFA intakes ranged from 18.6% to 42.9%. [24, 26, 32, 34, 37, 38, 42] The elderly (40.0%) [57] and peri-urban children (41.6% in Gauteng and 42.9% in the FS) [25, 29] had the highest prevalence of high TFA intakes (40.0%). Low-cost processed meats such as polony and Russians as well as chicken feet and heads were frequently consumed by our communities and may have contributed to the large intakes. Although there has been controversy about SFA intake and CVD risk, sufficient evidence exists that high SFA intakes cause increased LDL-C level by downregulating LDL receptors. [136]

PUFAs have a protective effect against CVD, specifically omega-6 PUFAs that significantly reduces total cholesterol and LDL-C levels as well as inflammatory markers. [145] High intakes of omega-3 PUFAs lowers the risk for myocardial infarction, CHD and CVD mortality and CVD events. [136] In addition, a diet rich in PUFA reduces the TC:HDL-C ratio and CHD incidence. [146] Linolenic acid (omega-3 fatty acid) and linoleic acid (omega-6 fatty acid) are essential fatty acids that cannot be physiologically produced and, therefore, need to be supplied by food sources. [147] Omega-3 decreases the risk of CVD by preventing thrombus formation, lowering blood pressure and protecting against irregular heart beat. [142] Replacing dietary carbohydrates and SFAs by an increased intake of omega-6 PUFAs lower LDL-C and increase HDL-C levels [148]. A large proportion of all of our communities had low PUFA intakes (33.0–100%), particularly for both omega-3 (93.1–100%) and omega-6 (2.4–29.7%) fatty acids. MUFA intakes were low in a large proportion of the participants (29.0–77.6%), except for the peri-urban children in Gauteng where only 4.8% of the children had low MUFA intakes. The majority of these children also showed high dietary cholesterol intakes (57.6%) whereas the rest of the study communities had relatively low prevalence (<20%) of high dietary cholesterol intakes. Because most of our communities live in poverty, it is questionable if they can afford oily fish, olive oil and the other MUFA and PUFA dietary sources, however, they do consume mostly sunflower oil, but in small quantities. [26, 29, 33, 34, 38, 57]

5.10.4 Dietary vitamin B6, B12 and folate intakes

Dietary sources of vitamin B6 include meat, fish, potatoes and bananas which are good sources. However, it is also present in nuts, whole grain, fortified cereal and leafy vegetables, chicken, legumes, non-citrus fruit, liver and soy products. [149–152] The bioavailability differs according to food type, with pyridoxine glycoside as the least bioavailable. Vitamin B6 (5–75%) obtained from plant sources is in the form of glycosylated pyridoxine. [153, 154] Owing to the abundance of vitamin B6 in a variety of food sources, deficiency is not very common, however, in our communities, large proportions of the adults (79.1% in peri-urban FS Province and 85.7% urban women in Gauteng) and elderly (91.0%) [57] had low vitamin B6 intakes. Among the children, 36.7% of the rural and 24.8% of the peri-urban children in Gauteng showed low intakes of vitamin B6. Vitamin B6 deficiency often occurs in conjunction with other nutritional disorders and is associated with an increased risk of CVD. [155] Vitamin B6 not only has a homocysteine lowering effect, but is also needed for the metabolism of omega-3 PUFAs. [96]

Folate is the major determinant of homocysteiene [96] and thus has homocysteiene lowering effect. A recent meta-analysis showed that folic acid supplementation resulted in a 4% reduced risk for CVD events and the benefit was even greater among participants without pre-existing CVD or low folate levels. [156] Because folate cannot be physiologically synthesised, concentration depends on consumption. [65] All of our communities showed large proportions of participants (>40.0% ≤ 95.0%) with low dietary folate intakes. Green leafy vegetables, citrus fruit, legumes, yeast, liver and organ meats contain the highest concentration of folate. [155] Low intakes of these food items have been found in our studies. [25, 26, 29–31, 33, 35, 38, 43, 44, 57] Folate is omnipresent in nature, but heat and oxidation during food preparation and storage have a destructive effect and can destroy up to 50% of the original concentration. [157]

Vitamin B12, together with folate, plays a key role for the enzyme methionine synthase needed for the re-methylation of homocysteine to methionine. [96] Dietary sources of vitamin B12 are animal products (meat, fish, chicken, milk and cheese) and rarely found in plants or yeast. [158] Vitamin B12 is stored in large quantities in the liver and a deficiency is developed over years. [65] The majority of our communities showed large proportions of participants (≥60% ≤ 95.2%) with low intakes of vitamin B12, except for the peri-urban children in Gauteng where 14.4% of the participants had low vitamin B12 intakes. This may be mainly due to the mainly carbohydrate-based diet with low meat and cheese intakes.

5.10.5 Dietary sodium intakes

Sodium is an essential nutrient that is required for many physiological functions. [146] The daily physiological requirement for sodium is estimated at 0.1–1.0 gram. [159] High sodium intakes have been established as the major cause of hypertension in many epidemiological, experimental, controlled clinical and population trials. [160, 161] Sodium is mainly consumed as (a) salt (sodium-chloride) which is added during food preparation and cooking or at meal time, and (b) from sodium used in processed foods in SA. [162] Unfortunately we did not measure dietary sodium intakes in all our communities. Bread was identified as the largest contributor to salt intakes and that 41.0% of the South African population has a high salt intake. [162] Bread also consistently appeared in the top 20 most commonly consumed foods among our study communities [26, 29–31, 33, 34, 38, 43, 44, 57]. Another contributor to sodium intake in SA is sodium glutamate that is used as a condiment, [163] as well as salt in soup, gravy and spice mixes and powders, margarine and atchar, a spicy condiment, [163] biscuits/cookies, and breakfast cereals [164]. Stock cubes are regularly used for flavouring meat and vegetable dishes in SA [165, 166]. High stock cube consumption has also been observed in these communities by the authors.

6. Conclusions

In the studies reported among various communities, low education and employment status were observed as well as poverty in a large majority of the respondents. The scientific literature shows a strong association between poverty and CVD [163]. Poverty is an underlying factor of food insecurity that often results in poor dietary intakes that were observed in our communities. Many of the dietary CVD risk factors were present in large proportions of the communities. The literature is clear

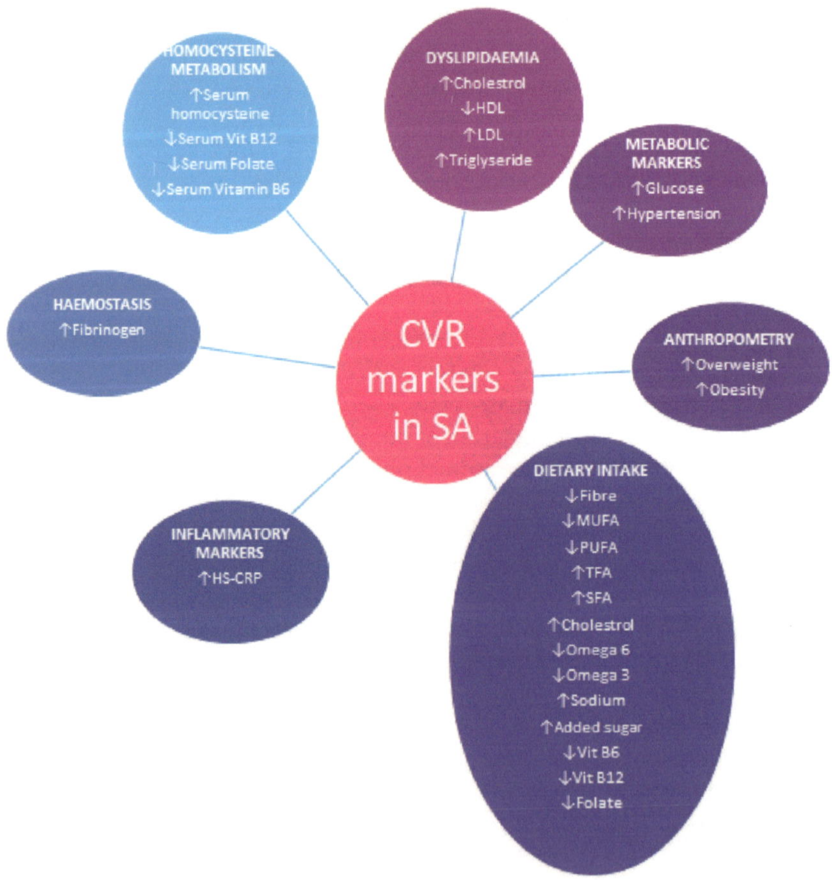

Figure 2.
Cardiovascular risk factors prevalent among children, adults and the elderly.

that these dietary factors may be associated with some of the risk factors for CVD, such as obesity, hypertension and the biochemical risk factors for CVD. Irreversible and potentially reversible and physiological (low income) risk markers were found to prevail. A summary of the elevated cardiovascular risk markers in our study is schematically presented in **Figure 2**. Multiple preventable CVR markers were present among the children, adults and elderly in rural, peri-urban and urban areas. It can thus be concluded that a double burden of poverty and risk of CVD exists across the different age groups and geographical locations in these resource-poor communities. Prevention of CVD can be achieved through nutrition education and awareness programs. It is recommended that policy makers give serious attention to CVR and screening should be done from an early age to identify those at risk and implement appropriate interventions.

Acknowledgements

We thank the National Research Foundation (NRF) and Vaal University of Technology (VUT) for financial support. Replamed (Cornel Pretorius) provided technical support, Prof A Egal, Centre of Sustainable Livelihoods (VUT) staff member and team members from the CARE research group for their operational support.

Conflict of interest

The authors have no conflict of interest to declare.

Author details

Wilna Oldewage-Theron[1] and Christa Grobler[2]*

1 Texas Tech University, Lubbock, United States of America and University of Free State, Bloemfontein, South Africa

2 Vaal University of Technology, Vanderbijlpark, South Africa

*Address all correspondence to: christa@vut.ac.za

References

[1] Bradshaw D, Nanna N, Pillay-van Wyk V, Laubscher R, Groenewald P, Dorrington RE. Burden of disease in South Africa: Protracted transitions driven by social pathologies. South African Medical Journal. 2019;109(11 Suppl 1):69-76. DOI: 10.7196/SAMJ.2019.v109i11b.14273

[2] Statistics South Africa (Stats SA). Towards measuring the extent of food security in South Africa: an examination of hunger and food adequacy. 2019. Pretoria: Stats SA.

[3] Koch J. The food security policy context in South Africa. International Policy Centre for Inclusive Growth. 2019. Available from: https://ipcig.org/pub/IPCCountryStudy21.pdf [Accessed 2020-12-10]

[4] Wight V, Kaushal N, Waldfoge, J, Garfinkel I. Understanding the link between poverty and food insecurity among children: Does the definition of poverty matter? Journal of Children and Poverty. 2014;20(1), 1-20. DOI: 10.1080/10796126.2014.891973

[5] Walsh CM, van Rooyen FC. Household FS and Hunger in Rural and Urban Communities in the Free State Province, South Africa. Ecology of Food and Nutrition. 2015;54(2):118-137. DOI: 10.1080/03670244.2014.964230

[6] Tacoli C. Food (in) security in rapidly urbanizing, low-income contexts. International Journal of Environmental Research and Public Health. 2017;14:1554. 8 pages.

[7] United Nation's Children's Fund (UNICEF). Improving child nutrition: the achievable imperative for global progress. 2013. Available from: https://www.unicef.org/publications/index_68661.html [Accessed 2020-12-14]

[8] Vorster HH, Badham JB, Venter CS. An introduction to the revised food-based dietary guidelines for South Africa. South African Journal of Clinical Nutrition. 2013;26(3)(Suppl):S5-S12.

[9] Naicker N, Mathee A, Teare J. Food insecurity in households in informal settlements in urban South Africa. Issues in public health. 2015;105(4). Available from: https://www.researchgate.net/publication/276102768_Food_insecurity_in_households_in_informal_settlements_in_urban_South_Africa [Accessed 2020-12-08]

[10] Global Nutrition Report 2020. Available from: file:///C:/Users/Dr.%20Oldewage/Downloads/Executive_Summary_2020_Global_Nutrition_Report.pdf. [Accessed 2020-12-16]

[11] Wentzel-Viljoen E, Lee S, Laubscher R, Vorster HH. Accelerated nutrition transition in the North West Province of South Africa: results from the Prospective Urban and Rural Epidemiology (PURE-NWP_SA) cohort study, 2005-2010. Public Health Nutrition. 2018;21(14):2630-2641. DOI: 10.1017/S1368980018001118

[12] Hills AP. Exercise: an integral and non-negotiable component of a healthy lifestyle. European Journal of Clinical Nutrition. 2018;72:1320-1322

[13] Republic of South Africa. South African year book 2018-2019. Available from: https://www.gcis.gov.za/sites/default/files/docs/resourcecentre/yearbook/yb1919-1-Land-and-its-People.pdf [Accessed 2020-12-11]

[14] The World Bank. Poverty. Available from: https://www.worldbank.org/en/topic/poverty#:~:text=Based%20on%20information%20about%20basic,poverty%20lines%20have%20been%20introduced [Accessed 2020-12-16]

[15] Gooding HC, Gidding SS, Moran AE, Redmond N, Allen NB, Bacha F, Burns TL, Catov JM, Grandner MA, Harris KM, Johnson HM, Kiernan M, Lewis TT, Matthews KA, Monaghan, Robinson JG,Tate D, Bibbins-Domingo K, Spring B. Challenges and Opportunities for the Prevention and Treatment of Cardiovascular Disease Among Young Adults: Report From a National Heart, Lung, and Blood Institute Working Group. Journal of American Heart Association. 2020. DOI: https://doi.org/10.1161/JAHA.120.016115

[16] Grimaccacia E, Naccarato A. Food insecurity individual experience: A comparison of economic and social characteristics of the most vulnerable groups in the world. Social Indicators Research.02019; 143: 391-410. DOI: https://doi.org/10.1007/s11205-018-1975-3

[17] Goryakin Y, Rocco L, Suhrcke M. The contribution of urbanization to non-communicable diseases: Evidence from 173 countries from 1980 to 2008. Economics & Human Biology. 2017; 26:151-163. https://doi.org/10.1016/j.ehb.2017.03.004

[18] Burger A, Pretorius R, Fourie CMT, Schutte AE. The relationship between cardiovascular risk factors and knowledge of cardiovascular disease in African men in North-West Province. Health SA Gesondheid. 2016; 21. https://doi.org/10.1016/j.hsag.2016.07.003

[19] Müller I, Walter C, Du Randt R, *et al.* Association between physical activity, cardiorespiratory fitness and clustered cardiovascular risk in South African children from disadvantaged communities: results from a cross-sectional study. British Medical Journal Open Sport & Exercise Medicine. 2020; 6:e000823. DOI: 10.1136/bmjsem-2020-000823

[20] Adeboye B, Bermano G, Rolland C. Obesity and its health impact in Africa: a systematic review. Cardiovascular journal of Africa. 2012;22(9):512-521.

[21] Kelishadi R, Pour MH, Zadegan NS, Kahbazi M, Sadry G, Amani A, Ansari R, Alikhassy H, Bashardoust N. Dietary fat intakc and lipid profiles of Iranian adolescents: Isfahan Healthy Heart Program – heart health promotion from childhood. Preventive Medicine. 2004;39 760-766.

[22] Boodai SA, Cherry LM, Sattar N & Reilly JJ. Prevalence of cardiometabolic risk factors and metabolic syndrome in obese Kuwaiti adolescents. Diabetes, Metabolic Syndrome and Obesity: targets and therapy. 2014;7:505-511.

[23] Martin L, Oepen J, Reinehr T, Wabitsch M, Glaussnitzer G, Waldeck E, Ingrisch S, Stachow R, Oelert M, Wiegand S & Holle R. Ethnicity and cardiovascular risk factors: evaluation of 40 921 normal-weight, overweight or obese children and adolescents living in Central Europe. International Journal of Obesity. 2015;39:5-51.

[24] Oldewage-Theron, Egal AA, Grobler C. Lipid profile, hyperglycaemia, systemic inflammation and anthropometry as cardiovascular risk factors and their association with dietary intakes in children from rural Cofimvaba, Eastern Cape, South Africa. Journal of Consumer Sciences. 2017;2:1-15.

[25] Egal A, Oldewage-Theron W. Association of micronutrients and child growth in children aged 7-15 years from Qwa-Qwa, South Africa. South African Journal of Clinical Nutrition.2017;4(1):1-5. DOI: 10.1080/16070658.2017.1392743.

[26] Oldewage-Theron W, Kruger R. The association between diet quality and subclinical inflammation among children aged 6-18 years in the Eastern Cape, South Africa. Public Health

Nutrition. 2016; 10 pages. DOI: 10.1017/S1368980016001956

[27] Oldewage-Theron WH, Egal AA, Moroka T. Socio-economic factors as determinants of nutrition knowledge of adolescents in Cofimvaba, Eastern Cape of South Africa. African Journal of Physical, Health Education, Recreation and Dance. 2014; 20(3:1):858-869.

[28] Otitoola O, Oldewage-Theron W, Egal A. Prevalence of overweight and obesity among selected schoolchildren and adolescents in Cofimvaba, South Africa. South African Journal of Clinical Nutrition. 2020:6 pages. https://doi.org/10.1080/16070658.2020/1733305

[29] Nyathela T. Impact of a school feeding programme on the nutritional status of primary school children in Orange Farms. 2009. MTech dissertation. Vanderbijlpark: Vaal University of Technology (VUT), SA.

[30] Oldewage-Theron WH, Dicks EG, Napier CE. Poverty, household food insecurity and nutrition: Coping strategies in an informal settlement in the Vaal Triangle, South Africa. Public Health. 2006:120:795-804.

[31] Oldewage-Theron WH, Dicks EG, Napier CE, Rutengwe R. Situation analysis of an informal settlement in the Vaal Triangle. Development South Africa. 2005;22(1):13-26.

[32] Oldewage-Theron W, Napier C, Egal A. Dietary fat intake and nutritional status indicators of primary school children in a low-income informal settlement in the Vaal region. South African Journal of Clinical Nutrition. 2011;24(2):99-104.

[33] Napier C. Evaluation of a school feeding programme for primary school children in an informal settlement. 2006. DTech thesis. Vanderbijlpark: Vaal University of Technology (VUT), SA.

[34] Oldewage-Theron WH, Egal AA. A cross-sectional baseline survey investigating the relationship between dietary diversity and cardiovascular risk factors in women from the Vaal Region, South Africa. Journal of Nursing Education and Practice. 2014; 4(1):50-62.

[35] Oldewage-Theron WH, Kruger R, Egal AA. Socio-economic variables and nutrient adequacy of women in the Vaal Region of South Africa. Ecology of Food and Nutrition. 2014;53:514-527. DOI: 10.1080/03670244.2013.873423

[36] Oldewage-Theron W, Slabbert TJC. Depth of poverty in an informal settlement in the Vaal Region, South Africa. Health SA Gesondheid. 2010;15(1):6 pages. DOI: 10.4102/hsag.v15I.456

[37] Oldewage-Theron WH, Egal AA. Prevalence of and contributing factors to dyslipidaemia in low-income women aged 18-90 years in the peri-urban Vaal region. South African Journal of Clinical Nutrition. 2013;26(1):23-28.

[38] Oldewage-Theron W, Kruger R, Egal A. Diet quality in peri-urban settlements: South Africa. In: Preedy VR, Hunter LA, Patel VB, editors. Diet quality. Vol 2. New York: Springer Science + Business Media; 2013. p. 281-297. DOI: 10.1007/978-1-4614-7315-2_20

[39] Oldewage-Theron W, Egal. The effect of consumption of soy foods on metabolic syndrome in women: a case study from peri-urban Qwa-Qwa, South Africa. South African Journal of Clinical Nutrition. 2018;1(1):1-6. DOI: 10.1080/16070658.2018.1438340

[40] Oldewage-Theron W, Egal AA, Grobler C. Is overweight and obesity associated with iron status in low-income men and women? A case study from Qwa-Qwa, South Africa. Integrated Food, Nutrition and

Metabolism. 2014;4 pages. DOI: 10.15761/IFNM.1000110

[41] Otitoola O, Oldewage-Theron W, Egal A. Trends in the development of obesity in elderly day care attendees in Sharpeville, South Africa, from 2007-2011. South African Journal of Clinical Nutrition. 2015;28(1):12-17.

[42] Oldewage-Theron WH, Egal AA, Grobler C. Metabolic syndrome of free-living elderly from Sharpeville, South Africa: A prospective cohort study with 10-year follow-up. Journal of Aging Research and Clinical Practice. 2018;7:100-106. DOI: 10.14283/jarcp.2018.18

[43] Oldewage-Theron WH, Salami L, Zotor FB, Venter C. Health status of an elderly population in Sharpeville, South Africa. Health SA Gesondheid. 2008;13(3):3-17.

[44] Oldewage-Theron WH, Duvenage SS, Egal AA. Situation analysis as indicator of food security in low-income rural communities. Journal of Family Ecology and Consumer Sciences. 2012;40:38-58.

[45] World Health Organization (WHO). Country profile: South Africa. 2016. Available from: https://www.who.int/nmh/countries/zaf_en.pdf?ua=1 [Accessed 2020-12-11]

[46] National Department of Health (NDoH), Statistics South Africa (Stats SA), South African Medical Research Council (SAMRC), and ICF. South Africa Demographic and Health Survey 2016. Pretoria: NDoH.

[47] Walli-Attaei M, Joseph P, Rosengren A, Chow CK, Rangorjan S, Lear SA, Habib KFA, Davletov K, Dans A, Lanas F, Yeates K, Poirier P, Teo KK, Bahonar A, Camilo F, Chifamba J, Diaz R, Diolkowska JA, Irazola V, Ismail R, Kour M, Khatib R, Liu X, Mańczuk M, MirandaJJ, OguzA, Perez-MmayorgaM, zuba A, Tsolekile LP, Varma RP, Yusufali A, Yusuf R, Wei L, Anand SS, Ysug F. Variations between women and men in risk factors, treatments, cardiovascular disease incidence and death in 27 high-income, middle income and low0income countries (PURE): a prospective cohort study. The Lancet. 2020; 396(0244):97-109. https://doi.org/10.1016/S0140-6736(20)30543-2

[48] Kristian Thygesen, Joseph S. Alpert, Allan S. Jaffe, Maarten L. Simoons, Bernard R. Chaitman and Harvey D. White. Third Universal Definition of Myocardial Infarction. Circulation. 2012. http://circ.ahajournals.org/content/early/2012/08/23/CIR.0b013e31826e1058.citation

[49] Novella S, Laguna-Fernández A, Lázaro-Franco M, Sobrino A, Bueno-Beti C, Tarin JJ, Monsalve E, Sanchis J, Hermenegildo C. Estradiol Acting through estrogen receptor alpha, restores dimethylaminohydrolase activity and nitric oxide production in oxLDL-treated human arterial endothelial cells. Molecular and Cellular Endrocrinology. 2013; 365(1):11-16 DOI:https://doi.org/10.1016/j.mce.2012.08.020

[50] Rosengren A, Smyth A, Rangarajan S, Ramasundarahettige C, Bangdiwala SI, AlHabib KF, Avezum A, Boström KB, Chifamba J, Hulec S, Gupta R, Igumbor EU, Iqbal R, Ismail N, Joseph P, Kaur M, Khatib R, Kruger IM, Lamelas P, Lanas F, Lear SA, Li W, Wang C, Quiang D, Wang Y, Lopez-Jaramillo, Mohammadifard N, Mohan V, Mony PK, Poirier P, Srilatha S, Szuba A, Tea K, Wielgosz A, Yeates KE, Yusoff K, Yusuf R, Yusufali AH, Attqei MW, McKee M, Yusuf S. Socioeconomic status and risk of cardiovascular disease in 20 low-income, middle-income, and high-income countries: the Prospective Urban Rural Epidemiology (PURE) study. The Lancet. 2019;7:e748-3760.

[51] Egidija Rinkūnienė ,Petrulioniene Z, Dzenkeviciute V, Gimzauskaite S, Mainelis A, Puronaite R, Juceviciene A, Gargalskaite U, Laucevicius A. Trends in Cigarette Smoking among Middle-Aged Lithuanian Subjects Participating in the Primary Prevention Program between 2009 and 2016. Medcina. 2019; 55(5):130. DOI: https://doi.org/10.3390/medicina55050130

[52] Mudau M, Genis M, Lochner A, Strijdom H. Endothelial dysfunction: the early predictor of atherosclerosis. Cardiovascular Journal of Africa. 2012; 23(4): 222-231. DOI: doi: 10.5830/CVJA-2011-068

[53] Otang-Mbeng W, Otunola GA, Afolayan AJ. Lifestyle factors and co-morbidities associated with obesity and overweight in Nkonkobe Municipality of the Eastern Cape, South Africa. Journal of Health, Population ad Nutrition. 2017;36:22. DOI: 10.1186/s41043-017-0098-9

[54] Danquah FI, Ansu-Mensah M, Bawontu V, Yeboah M, Udoh RH, Tahiru M, Kuupiel D. Risk factors and morbidities associated with childhood obesity in sub-Saharan Africa: a systematic scoping review. BMC Nutrition. 2020;6:37. DOI: 10.1186/s40795-020-00364-5

[55] Norris T, Cole TJ, Bann D, Hamer M, Hardy R, Li L, Ong KK, Ploubidis GB, Viner R, Johnson W. Duration of obesity exposure between ages 10 and 0 years and its relationship with cardiometabolic disease risk factors: A cohort study. PLOS Medicine. 2020;17(12):e1003387. DOI: 10.1371/journal.pmed.1003387

[56] Kastorini, C.M., Milionis, H.J., Goudevenos, J.A. and Panagiotakos, D.B. Mediterranean diet and coronary heart disease: Is obesity a link? - A systemic review. Nutrition, Metabolism & Cardiovascular Diseases. 2010. 20: 536-551.

[57] CJ Grobler. Impact of vitamins B12, B6 and folate supplementation on the cardiovascular risk markers in an elderly community of Sharpeville. 2016. D Tech thesis. Durban: Durban University of Technology (DUT), SA.

[58] Craig E, Reilly JJ, Bland R. Risk factors for overweight and overfatness in rural South African children and adolescents. Journal of Public Health. 2016;38(1):24-33. DOI: 10.1093/pubmed/fdv016

[59] Kimani-Murage EW, Kahn K, Pettifor JM, Tollman SM, Klipstein-Grobusch K, Norris SA. Predictors of adolescent weight status and central obesity in rural South Africa. Public Health Nutrition. 2011;14(6):1114-1122.

[60] World Health Organization. Body mass index. Available from: https://www.euro.who.int/en/health-topics/disease-prevention/nutrition/a-healthy-lifestyle/body-mass-index-bmi [Accessed 2020-12-16]

[61] NCEP (National Cholesterol Education Program. Expert panel on Detection, Evaluation and Treatment of High blood Cholesterol in Adults. Executive Summary of the Third Report of the National Cholesterol Education Program (NCEP) Adult Treatment Panel (ATP III). 2002

[62] Tahmasebi H, Trajcevski K, Higgins V, Adeli K. Influence of ethnicity on population referencevalues for biochemical markers. Critical Reviews in Clinical Laboratory Science. 2018; 55(5). DOI: https://doi.org/10.1080/10408363.2018.1476455

[63] Rouvre, M., Vol, S., Gusto, G., Born, C., Lantieri, O., Tichet, J. and Lecomte, P. Low high density lipoprotein cholesterol: Prevalence and associated risk-factors in a large French population. Annals of Epidemiology. 2011; 21(2): 118-127.

[64] Seedat YK, Rayner BL, Veriava Y. South African hypertension practice guideline 2014. Cardiovascular Journal of South Africa. 2014;25(6):288-294. DOI: 10.5830/CVJA-2014-062

[65] Hoffbrand AV, Moss, PAH. Essential Haematology. 6th ed. Oxford: Blackwell publishing Ltd. 2011.

[66] Ichihara K, Ozarda Y, Barth JH, Klee G, Shimizu Y, Xia L, Hoffman M, Shah S, Matsha T, Wassung J, Smit F, Ruzhanskaya A, Straseski J, Bustos DN, Kimura S, Takahashi A. A global multicenter study on reference values: Exploration of sources of variation across the countries. Clinica Chimica Acta. 2017; 467:83-97. DOI: https://doi.org/10.1016/j.cca.2016.09.015

[67] Wang Y, Chen W, Hu C, Wen X, Pan J, Xu F, Zhu Y, Shao X, Shangguan X, Fan L, Sha J, Wang Z, Cai Y, Liu Q, Dong B, Xue W. Albumin and Fibrinogen combined prognostic grade predicts prognosis of patients with prostate cancer. Journal of Cancer. 2017; 8(19):3992-4001. DOI: https://dx.doi.org/10.7150%2Fjca.21061

[68] Babic B, Tagkalos E, Gockel I, Corvinus F, Hadazijusufovic E, Hoppe-Lotichius M, Lang zh, vd Sluis PC, Grimminger PP. C-reactive protein levels after Esopagectomy are associated withincreased surgical trauma and complications. The Annals of Thoracic Surgery. 2020; 109(5): 1574-1583. DOI: https://doi.org/10.1016/j.athoracsur.2019.12.016

[69] Frithioff-Bojsoe C, Lund MAV, Kloppenborg JT, Nielsen TTH, Fonvig CE, Lausten-Thomsen U, Hedley PL, Hansen T, Pedersen OB, Christiansen M, Baker JL, Hansen T, Holm J-C. Glucose metabolism in children and adolescents: Population based reference values and comparisons to children and adolescents enrolled in obesity treatment. Pediatric Diabetes. 2019; https://doi.org/10.1111/pedi.12859

[70] Strohle A, Richter M, Gonzalez-Gross M, Neuhauser-Berthold M, Wagner K-H, Leschik-Bonnet E, Egert S, The revised D-A-CH-Reference values for the intake of vitaminB12: Preventionof deficiency and beyond. Molecular Nutrition & Food Research. 2019; DOI: https://doi.org/10.1002/mnfr.201801178

[71] Adom T, Kengne AP, de Villiers A, Puoane T. Prevalence of overweight and obesity among African primary school learners: A systematic review and meta-analysis. Obesity Science & Practice. 2019:487-502. DOI: 0.1002/osp4.355

[72] Pretorius SS, Neophytou N, Watson ED. Anthropometric profiles of 8-11 year old children from a low-income setting in South Africa. BMC Public Health. 2019;19(1):314. DOI: 10.1186/s12889-019-6530-x

[73] Reddy SP, Resnicow K, James S, Funani IN, Kambaran NS, Omardien RG, Masuka P, Sewpaul R, Vaughan RD, Mbewu A.Rapid increases in overweight and obesity among South African adolescents: comparison of data from the South Africa National Youth Risk Behaviour Survey in 2002 and 2008. American Journal of Public Health. 2012;102(2):262-268. DOI: 10.2105/AJPH.2011.300222

[74] Ganji V, Kafai MR. Population reference values for serum Methylmalonic Acid concentration and its relationship with age, sex, race, -ethnicity, supplement use, kidney function and serum vitamin B12 in the post- folic acid fortification period. Nutrients. 2018; 10(1), 74. DOI: https://doi.org/10.3390/nu10010074

[75] World Health Organization. Training course on child growth assessment. Interpreting growth indicators. 2008. Available from: https://www.who.int/childgrowth/training/module_c_interpreting_indicators.pdf [Accessed 2020-12-16]

[76] United States Department of Health and Human Services (DHHS), National Institutes of Health (NIH), National Heart, Lung and Blood Institute. Expert Panel on Integrated Guidelines for Cardiovascular Health and Risk Reduction in Children and Adolescents. "Expert panel on integrated guidelines for cardiovascular health and risk reduction in children and adolescents: summary report." 2012. NIH Publication No.12-7486. Washington DC: NIH.

[77] Shisana O, Labadarios D, Rehle T, Simbayi L, Zuma K, Dhansay A, Reddy P, Parker W, Hoosain E, Naidoo P, Hongoro C, Mchiza Z, Steyn NP, Dwane N, Makoae M, Maluleke T, Ramlagan, S, Zungu N, Evans MG, Jacobs L, Faber M, SANHANES-1 Team, The South African National Health and Nutrition Examination Survey, 2012: SANHANES-1: the health and nutritional status of the nation. 2014. Available from: http://www.hsrc.ac.za/en/research-outputs/view/6493 [Accessed 2020-12-13]

[78] Akpa OM, Made F, Ojo A, Ovbiagele, Adu D, Motala AA, Mayosi BM, Adebamowo SN, Engel ME, Tayo B, Rotimi C, Salako B, Akinyemi R, Gebregziabher M, sarfo F, Wahab K, Agongo G, Alberts M, Ali SA, Asiki G, Boua RP, Gómez-Olivé FX, Mashinya F, Micklesfield L, Mohamed SF, Nonterah EA, Norris SA, Sorgho H, Tollman S, Parekh RS, Chishala C, Ekoru K, Waddy SP, Peprah E, Mensah GA, Wiley K, Troyer J, Ramsay M, Owolabi MO as members of the CVD Working Group of the H3Africa Consortium. Regional patterns and association between obesity and hypertension in Africa. Evidence from the H3Africa CHAIR study. Hypertension. 2020;75:1167-1178. DOI: 10.1161/hypertensionaha.119.14147

[79] Gidding SS, Robinson J. It is now time to focus on risk before age 40. Journal of the American College of Cardiology. 2019;74(3). DOI:10.1016/j.jacc.2019.04.064

[80] Ware LJ, Chidumwa G, Charlton K, Schutte AE, Kowal P. Predictors of hypertension awareness, treatment and control in South Africa: results from the WHO-SAGE population survey (Wave 2). Journal of Human Hypertension. 2019;33:157-166.

[81] Georgiev AM, Krajnovi D, Kotur-Stevuljevi J, Ignjatovi S, Valentina Marinkovi V. Undiagnosed hyperglycaemia and hypertension as indicators of the various risk factors of future cardiovascular disease among population of Serbian students. Journal of Medical Biochemistry. 2018; 37: 289-298. DOI: http://dx.doi.org/10.1515/jomb-2017-0059

[82] Di Meo S, Lossa S, Venditti P. Improvement of obesity-linked skeletal muscle insulin resistance by strength and endurance training. Journal of Endocrinology. 2017; 234(3):R159-R181. DOI: 10.1530/JOE-17-0186

[83] Grinnan D, Farr G, Fox G, Sweeney. The role of Hyperglycemia and Insulin resistance in the development and progression of pulmonary arterial hypertension. Journal of diabetes research. 2016; DOI: https://doi.org/10.1155/2016/2481659

[84] Karachaliou F, Simatos G, Simatau A. The challenges in the development of diabetes prevention and Care models in low-income settings. Frontiers in Endocrinology. 2020; 11:518. DOI: https://dx.doi.org/10.3389%2Ffendo.2020.00518

[85] Kearney K, Tomlins D, Smith K, Ajjan R. Hypofibrinolysis in diabetes: a therapeutic for the reduction of cardiovascular risk. Cardiovascular Diabetology. 2017;34. DOI: 10.1186/s12933-017-0515-9

[86] Patterson CC, Karuranga S, Salpea P, Saeedi P, Dahlquist G, Soltesz G, Ogle GD. Worldwide estimates of incidence, prevalence and mortality of type 1 diabetes in children and adolescents: Results from the International Diabetes Federation Diabetes Atlas, 9th edition. Diabetes Research and Clinical Practice. 2019. https://doi.org/10.1016/j.diabres.2019.107842

[87] Animaw W, Seyoum Y. Increasing prevalence of diabetesmellitus in a developing country and its related factors. PLOS ONE. 2017. DOI:https://doi.org/10.1371/journal.pone.0187670

[88] Faxaly L. Imaging Methods for Haemostasis Research. Sweden: LiU-Tryck, Linköping. 2009

[89] Russo, I. The Prothrombotic Tendency in Metabolic Syndrome: Focus on the Potential Mechanisms Involved in Impaired Haemostasis and Fibrinolytic Balance. Scientifica. 2012. 525374:117.

[90] Kaptoge S, White IR, Thompson SG, Wood AM, Lewington S, Lowe GDO, Danesh J, Kostis JB, Wilson AC, Folsom AR, Chambless L, Benderly M, GoldbourtU,WilleitJ,KiechlS,YarnellJWG, Sweetnam PM, Elwood PC, Cushman M, Psatyr BM, Tracy P, Tybjærg-Hansen, Haverkate F, de Maat MPM, Fowkes FGR, Lee AJ, Smith FB, Salomaa V, Harald K, Rasi V, Vahtera E, Jousilahti P, Pekkanen D'Agostino JR, Kannel WB, Wilson PWF, Tofler G, Levy Marchioli DR, Valagussa F, Rosengren A, Wilhelmsen L, Lappas,. Eriksson H, Cremer P,Nagel D, Curb JB, Rodriguez B, Yano K, The Fibrinogen Studies Collaboration. Associations of plasma fibrinogen levels with established cardiovascular disease risk factors, inflammatory markers, and other characteristics: Individual participants' meta-analysis of 154 211 adults in 31 prospective studies. American Journal of Epidemiology. 2007. DOI: https://doi.org/10.1093/aje/kwm191

[91] Pieters M, Wolkberg AS. Fibrinogen and fibrin: An illustrated review. Research and practice in Thrombosis and Haemostasis. 2019 DOI: https://doi.org/10.1002/rth2.12191

[92] Cronje HT, Nienaber Rousseau C, Zandberg L, de Lange Z, Green FR, Pieters M. Fibrinogen and clot-related phenotypes determined by fibrinogen polymorphisms: Independent and IL-6 interactive associations. 2017. DOI:https://doi.org/10.1371/journal.pone.0187712

[93] Antoniades, C., Antonopoulos, A.S., Tousoulis, D., Marinou, K. and Stefanadis, C. 2009. Homocysteine and coronary atherosclerosis: from folate fortification to the recent clinical trials. European Heart Journal. 30: 6-15Kaul, S., Zadeh, A.A. and Shah, P.K. 2006. Homocysteine hypothesis for atherothrombotic cardiovascular disease. Journal of the American College of Cardiology. 48(5): 914-923.

[94] Aghayan SS, Farajzadeh A, Bagheri-Hosseinabadi Z, Fadaei H, Yarmohammadi M, Jasarisani M. Elevated homocysteine, as a biomarker of cardiac injury, in panic disorder patients due to oxidative stress. 2020; ODI: https://doi.org/10.1002/brb3.1851

[95] Chouksey D, Ishar HS, Jain R, Athale S, Sodani A. Association between Serum Homocysteine Levels and Methylene-Tetrahydrofolate-Reductase Gene Polymorphism in Patients with Stroke: A Study from a Tertiary Care Teaching Hospital from Central India. Journal of Medical Science. 2020; DOI: 10.4103/jmedsci.jmedsci_170_20

[96] Dobrynina LA, Kalashnikova LA, Shabalina AA, Kostyreva MV, Aleksandrova EV, Gafarova ME, Shamtieva KV. Indicators of homeostasis, inflammation, and homocysteine in ischemic stroke in the young age. 2017; 117(12.Vyp.2):25-33.

DOI: https://doi.org/10.17116/jnevro201711712225-33

[97] Esse R, Barroso M, de Almeida IT, Catro R, Contribution of Homocysteine metabolism disruption to endothelial dysfunction: State-of-the-Art. International Journal of Molecular Science. 2019; 20(4):867. DOI:https://doi.org/10.3390/ijms20040867

[98] McCully, K.S. 1969. Vascular pathology of homocysteinemia: implications for the pathogenesis of arteriosclerosis. The American Journal of Pathology. 56(1):111-128.

[99] Acampa M, Lazzerini PE, Martini G. Postoperative arterial fibrillation and ischemic stroke: The role of homocysteine. European stroke journal. 2017; DOI:https://doi.org/10.1177%2F2396987317732648

[100] Zhang X, Huang Z, Xie Z, Chien Y, Zheng Z, Wei X, Huang B, Shan Z, Liu J, Fan S, Chen J, Zhao F. Homocysteine induces oxidative stress and ferroptosis of nucleus pulposus via enhancing methylation of GPX4. Free radical Biology and Medicine. 2020; 160:552-565. DOI:https://doi.org/10.1016/j.freeradbiomed.2020.08.029

[101] Chen C, Yang W-C, Hsiao Y-H, Huang S-C, Huang Y-C, High homocysteine, low vitamin B-6, and increased oxidative stress are independently associated with the risk of chronic kidney disease. Nutrition. 2016; 32(2):236-241. DOI: https://doi.org/10.1016/j.nut.2015.08.016

[102] Wang W-M, Jin H-Z. Homocysteine: A potential common route for cardiovascular risk and DNA methylation in Psoriasis. Chinese Medicine Journal. 2017; Aug 20 130(16):1980-1986. DOI:10.4103/0366-6999.211895

[103] Moreira, E.S., Brasch, N.E. and Yun, J. Vitamin B12 protects against superoxide-induced cell injury in human aortic endothelial cells. Free Radical Biology & Medicine. 2011: 51: 876-883

[104] Bourgonje AR, Abdulle AE, Al-Rawas AM, Al-Maqbali M, Al-Saleh M, Enriquez MB, Al-Siyabi S, Al-Hashmi K, A-Lawati I, Bulthuis MLC, Mulder DJ, Gordijn SJ, van Goor H, Saleh J. Systemic oxidative stress is increased in postmenopausal women and independently associates with homocysteine levels. International Journal of Molecular Science. 2020; 21(1):314. DOI: https://doi.org/10.3390/ijms21010314

[105] Ye, X., Maras, J.E., Bakun, P.J. and Tucker, K.L. Dietary intake of vitamin B6, plasma Pyridoxal 5'-Phosphate, and homocysteine in Puerto Rican adults. Journal of American Dietetic Association. 2010; 110(11):1660-1668.

[106] Adekunle, A.S. and Adedeji, A.L. Anti-atherogenic effects of supplementation with vitamin B6 (Pyridoxine) in albino rats. African Journal of Biochemistry Research. 2011; 5(13):352355.

[107] Zhao, R., Diop-Bove, N., Visentin, M. and Goldman, I.D. Mechanisms of membrane transport of folates into cells and across epithelia. Annual review of nutrition. 2011: 31

[108] Huang, R. S., Hu, G. Q., Lin, B., Lin, Z. Y., and Sun, C.C. MicroRNA-155 silencing enhances inflammatory response and lipid uptake in oxidized low-density lipoprotein-stimulated human THP-1 macrophages. Journal of Investigative Medicine. 2010; 58(8):961-967.

[109] Lotto, V., Choi, S-W. and Friso, S. Vitamin B6: a challenging link between nutrition and inflammation in CVD. British Journal of Nutrition. 2011; 106:183-195.

[110] Titcomb TJ, Schmaelzle ST, Nuss ET, Gregory JF, Tanumihardjo SA. Suboptimal vitamin B intakes of Zambian Preschool children: Evaluation of 24-hour dietary recalls. Food and Nutrition Bulletin. DOI:https://doi.org/10.1177/0379572118760373

[111] Imamura, A., Murakami, R., Takahashi, R., Cheng, X.W., Numaguchi, Y., Murohara T. and Okumura, K. Low folate levels may be an atherogenic factor regardless of homocysteine levels in young health nonsmokers. Metabolism Clinical and Experimental. 2010; 59:728-733.

[112] Abbenhardt, C., Miller, J.W., Song, X., Brown, E.C., Cheng, T.Y., Wener, M.H., Zheng, Y., Toriola, A.T., Neuhouser, M.L., Beresford, S.A.A., Makar, K.W., Baily, L.B., Maneval, D.R., Green, R., Manson, J.E., Van Horn, L. and Ulrich, C.M. Biomarkers of one-carbon metabolism are associated with biomarkers of inflammation in women. The Journal of Nutritional Epidemiology. 2014; 144(5) :714-721

[113] Fenech, M. 2012. Folate (vitamin B9) and vitamin B12 and their function in the maintenance of nuclear and mitochondrial genome integrity. Mutation Research / Fundamentals and Molecular Mechanisms of Mutagenesis. 2012; 733:21-33

[114] Ganeshan, S., Kartihumar, B.A., Viswanath, A., Renjith, A. and Alin, B. Effect of folic acis on serum homocysteine levels in patients with Cardiovacular disease (CVD). Journal of Chemical and Pharmaceutical Research. 2014; 6(3):1141-1148

[115] Riedel, B. M., Molloy, A. M., Meyer, K., Fredriksen, Å., Ulvik, A., Schneede, J., Nexø, E., Hoff, G. and Ueland, P. M. Transcobalamin polymorphism 67A-> G, but not 776C-> G, affects serum holotranscobalamin in a cohort of healthy middle-aged men and women. The Journal of Nutrition. 2011.;141(10):1784-1790.

[116] Lieberman, M. & Marks, A.D. 2013. Marks' Basic Biochemistry: a Clinical Approach. 4th ed. Baltimore, Maryland: Lippincott Williams & Wilkins.

[117] Jelkmann, W. The disparate roles of cobalt in erythropoiesis, and doping relevance. Open Journal of Hematology. 2012; 3:2-9

[118] Scheitl CPM, Ghaem Maghami M, Lenz AK, et al. Site-specific RNA methylation by a methyltransferase ribozyme. Nature 2020; 587, 663-667. https://doi.org/10.1038/s41586-020-2854-z

[119] Pepper, M.R., Black, M.M. B12 in fetal development. Seminars in Cell & Developmental Biology. 2011; 22:619-623.

[120] Froese DS, Fowler B, Baumgartner MR. Vitamin B12, folate, and the methionine remethylation cycle- biochemistry, pathways, and regulation. Journal of Inherited Metabolic Disease. 2018; DOI: https://doi.org/10.1002/jimd.12009

[121] Sedding DG, Boyle EC, Demandt JAF, Sluimer JC, Dutzmann J, Haverich A, Bauersachs J. Vasa Vasorum Angiogenesis: Key player in the initiation and progression of Atherosclerosisand petential target for the treatment of cardiovascular disease. Immunology. 2018; DOI: https://doi.org/10.3389/fimmu.2018.00706

[122] Guzik TJ, Touyz RM, Oxidative stress, inflammation, and vascular aging in hypertension. Hypertension. 2017 70(4):660-667. DOI: https://doi.org/10.1161/HYPERTENSIONAHA.117.07802

[123] Eltoft A, Arntzen KA, Hansen J-B, Wilsgaard T, Mathiesen EB,

Johnsen SH. C-Reactive proetein in atherosclerosis- A risk marker but not a causal factor? A 13-year population-based longitudinal study: The Tromso study. Atheroscvlerosis. 2017;263:293-300. DOI: https://doi.org/10.1016/j.atherosclerosis.2017.07.001

[124] Elci E, Kaya C, Cim N, Yildizhan R, Elci GG. Evaluation of cardiac risk marker levels in obese and non-obese matients with polycystic ovaries. Gynecological Endocrinology. 2017; 33(1). DOI: https://doi.org/10.1080/09513590.2016.1203893

[125] Noubiap JJ, Bigna JJ, Nansseu JR, Nyaga UF, Balti EV, Echouffo-Tcheugui JB, Kengre AP. Prevalence of dyslipidaemia among adults in Africa: a systematic review and meta-analysis. The Lancet. 2018;6(9): E998-E1007. DOI: https://goi.org/10.10.1016/S2214-109X(18)30275-4.119.14147

[126] Reiger S, Jardim TV, Abrahams-Gessel S, Crowther NJ, Wade A, Gomez F.X, Salomon J, Tollman S, Gaziano TA. Awareness, treatment, and control of dyslipidaemia in South Africa: The HAALSI (Health and Aging in Africa: A Longitudinal Study of an INDEPTH Community in South Africa) study. Plos One. 2017. DOI: https://doi.org/10.1371/journal.pone.0187347

[127] Sliwa K, Lecour S, Carrington MJ, Stewart S, Lyons JG, Stewart S, Marais AD, Raal FJ. Different lipid profiles according to ethnicity in the Heart of Soweto study cohort of *de novo* presentations of heart disease. Cardiovascular Journal of Africa. 2012 Aug; 23(7): 389-395. DOI: https://dx.doi.org/10.5830%2FCVJA-2012-036

[128] Levitt, N.S., Steyn, K., Dave, J. and Bradshaw, D. Chronic noncommunicacle diseases and HIV-AIDS on a collision course: relevance for health care deliveray, particularly in lowresource settings-insight from South Africa. American Journal of Clinical Nutrition. 2011.; 94(suppl):1690S-1696S.

[129] Raal, F.J., Blom, D.J., Naidoo, S., Bramlage, P. and Brudi, P. Prevalence of dyslipidaemia in statin-treated patients in South Africa: results of the DYSlipidaemia International Study (DYSIS). Cardiovascular Journal of Africa. 2013; 24(8):330-338

[130] Navab, M., Reddy, S.T., Van Lenten, B.J. and Fogelman, A.M. HDL and cardiovascular disease: atherogenic and atheroprotective mechanisms. Nature Reviews Cardiology. 2011; 8(4):222232.

[131] Azadbakht L, Mirmiran P, Esmaillzadeh A, Azizi F. Dietary diversity score and cardiovascular risk factors in Tehranian adults. Public Health Nutrition. 2005:9(6):728-736. DOI: 10.1079/PHN2005887

[132] De Salvo KB, Olson R, Casavale KO. Dietary guidelines for Americans. Journal of the American Medical Association. 2016;315:457-458.

[133] Te Morenga LA, Howatson AJ, Jones RM, Mann J. Dietary sugars and cardiometabolic risk: systematic review and meta-analyses of randomized controlled trials of the effects on blood pressure and lipids. American Journal of Clinical Nutrition. 2014;100:65-79.

[134] World Health Organization. Guideline: sugar intakes for adults and children. 2015. Available from: https://apps.who.int/iris/handle/10665/149782 [Accessed 2020-12-10]

[135] Vorster HH, Kruger A, Wentzel-Viljoen E, Kruger, HS, Margetts, BM. Added sugar intake in South Africa: findings from the Adult Prospective Urban and Rural Epidemiology cohort study. American Journal of Clinical Nutrition. 2014;99:1479-1486.

[136] Sikand G, Severson T. Top 10 dietary strategies for atherosclerotic

cardiovascular risk reduction. American Journal of Preventive Cardiology. 2020;4:100106. DOI: 10.1016/j.ajpc.2020.100106

[137] Yanai, H., Katsuyama, H., Hamasaki, H., Abe, S., Tada, N. and Sako, A. Effects of Carbohydrate and Dietary Fiber Intake, Glycemic Index and Glycemic Load on HDL Metabolism in Asian Populations. Journal of Clinical Medicine Research. 2014; 6(5):321-326.

[138] Kurniawan, I. and Simadibrata, M. Management of chronic constipation in the elderly. The Elderly. 2011. 43(3):195-205

[139] Skeaff CM, Miller J. Dietary fat and coronary heart disease: Summary of evidence from prospective cohort and randomised controlled trials. Annals of Nutrition and Metabolism, 2009;55(1-3):173-201.

[140] Chowdhury R, Warnakula S, Kunutsor S, Crowe F, Ward HA, Johnson L, Franco OH, Butterworth AS, Forouhi NG, Thompson SG, Khaw KT, Mozaffarian D, Danesh J, Di Angelantonio E. Association of dietary, circulating, and supplement fatty acids with coronary risk: A systematic review and meta-analysis. Annals of Internal Medicine. 2014;160(6):398-406.

[141] Steyn N, Eksteen G, Senekal M. Assessment of the dietary intake of schoolchildren in South Africa: 15 years after the First National Study. Nutrients. 2016;8:509. DOI:10.3390/nu8080509

[142] Vannice, G. and Rasmussen, H. Position of the academy of nutrition and dietetics: dietary fatty acids for healthy adults. Journal of the Academy of Nutrition and Dietetics. 2014; 114(1):136-153.

[143] Drouin-Chartier J-P, Tremblay AJ, Lepine M-C, Lemelin V, Mamarche B, Couture P. Substitution of dietary ω-6 polyunsaturated fatty acids for saturated fatty acids decreases LDL apolipoprotein B-100 production rate in men with dyslipidaemia associated with insulin resistance: a randomised control trial. The American Journal of Clinical Nutrition. 2018; 107(1):26-34. DOI: https://doi.org/10.1093/ajcn/nqx013.

[144] Food and Agriculture Organization of the United Nations. Fats and fatty acids in human nutrition. FAO food and nutrition paper 91. Available from: http://www.fao.org/3/i1953e/i1953e00.pdf. [Accessed 2020-12-01]

[145] Saks FM, Campos H. Editorial: Polyunsaturated fatty acids, inflammation, and cardiovascular disease: Time to widen our view of the mechanisms. The Journal of Clinical Endocrinology and Metabolism. 2006;91(2):398-400. DOI: 10.1210/jc.2005-2459

[146] Anand SS, Hawkes C, de Souza RJ, Mente A, dehgan M, Nugent R, Zulyniak MA, Weis T, Bernstein AM, Krauss RM, Kromhout D, Jenkins DJA, Malik V, Martinez-Gonzalez MA, Mozaffarian D, Yussuf S, Willett WC, Popkin BM. Food consumption and its impact on cardiovascular disease: Importance of solutions focused on the globalized food system. Journal of the American College of Cardiology. 2015;66(14). DOI: 10.1016/j.jacc.2015.07.050

[147] Saini RK, Keum Y-S. Omega -3 and omega-6 polyunsaturated fatty acids: Dietary sources, metabolism, and significance-A review. Life Sciences. 2018; 203:255-267. DOI: https://doi.org/10.1016/j.lfs.2018.04.049

[148] DiNicolantonio JJ, J O'Keefe JH. Omega-6 vegetable oils as a driver of coronary heart disease: the oxidized linoleic acid hypothesis. Open Heart. 2018; DOI: http://dx.doi.org/10.1136/openhrt-2018-000898

[149] Dhalla, N.S., Takeda, S. and Elimbam, V. Mechanisms of the beneficial effects of vitamin B6 and pyridoxal 5-phosphate on cardiac performance in ischaemic heart disease. Clinical Chemistry Laboratory Medicine. 2013; 51(3):535-543.

[150] Cellini, B., Montioli, R., Oppici, E., Astegno, A. and Voltattorni, C.B. The chaperone role of the pyridoxal 5'-phosphate and its implications for rare diseases involving B6-dependent enzymes. Clinical Biochemistry. 2014; 47:158-165.

[151] Kim, Y.N. and Cho, Y.O. 2014. Evaluation of vitamin B6 intake and status of 20-to 64-year-old Koreans. Nutrition Research and Practice. 2014. 8(6):688-694.

[152] Friso S, Lotto V, Corrocher R, Choi SW. Vitamin B6 and cardiovascular disease. Subcellular Biochemistry. 2012;56:265-290. DOI: 10.1007/978-94-007-2199-9_14

[153] McNulty H, Pentieva K, Hoey L, Ward M. Homocysteine, B-vitamins and CVD. Proceedings of the Nutrition Society. 2008;67:232-237. DOI: 10.1017/S0029665108007076

[154] Bassett, M.N. and Sammán, N.C. Folate content and retention in selected raw and processed foods. Archivos Latinoamericanos De Nutricion. 2010; 60(3):298-305.

[155] Li Y, Huang T, Zheng Y, Muka T, Troup J, Hu FB. Folic acid supplementation and the risk of cardiovascular diseases: A meta-analysis of randomized controlled trials. Journal of the American Heart Association. 2016;5:e003768. DOI: 10.1161/JAHA.116.003768

[156] Koike, H., Hama, T., Kawagashira, Y., Hashimoto, R., Tomita, M., Lijima, M. and Sobue, G. The significance of folate deficiency in alcoholic and nutritional neuropathies: Analysis of a case. Nutrition. 2012; 28:821-824.

[157] Schwingshackl L, Schwedhelm C, Hoffmann G, Knüppel S, Iqbal K, Andriolo V, Bechthold A, Schlesinger S, Boeing H. Food gropus and risk of hypertension: A systematic review and dose-response meta-analysis of prospective studies. Advances in Nutrition. 2017;8:793-803. DOI: 10.3945/an.1171.017178

[158] Burtis, C.A. and Bruns, D.E. Tietz Fundamentals of Clinical Chemistry and Molecular Diagnostics. 7th ed. St. Louis, Missouri: Elsevier/Saunders. 2015.

[159] Oyebode O, Oti S, Chen YF, Lilford R. Salt intakes in sub-Saharan Africa: a systematic review and meta-regression. Population Health Metrics. 2016;14:1. Available from: https://doi.org/10.1186/s12963-015-0068-7 [Accessed 2020-09-18]

[160] Psaltopoulou T, Hatzis G, Papageorgiou N, Androulakis E, Briasoulis A, Tousoulis D. Socioeconomic status and risk factors for cardiovascular disease: Impact of dietary mediators. Hellenic Society of Cardiology. 2017;58:38-42. DOI: 10.1016/j.hjc.2017.01.022

[161] Charlton KE, Steyn K, Levitt NS, Zulu J, Jonathan D, Veldman F, Nel JH. Diet and blood pressure in South Africa: Intake of foods containing sodium, potassium, calcium, and magnesium in three ethnic groups. Nutrition. 2005;21(1):39-50.

[162] Charlton K, Ware LJ, Baumgartner J, Cockeran M, Schutte AE, Naidoo N, Kowal P. How will South Africa's mandatory salt reduction policy affect its salt iodisation programme? A cross-sectional analysis from the WHO-SAGE Wave 2 Salt & Tobacco study. BMJ Open. 2018;8(3):1-9.

[163] World Health Organization. Salt reduction. 2016. Available from: https://www.who.int/news-room/fact-sheets/detail/salt-reduction [Accessed 2019-09-18]

[164] Vorster HH, Badham JB, Venter CS. Food-based dietary guidelines for South Africa: an introduction. South African Journal of Clinical Nutrition, 2013;26(3):5-12.

[165] Soto-Ecageda JA, Estañol-vidal B, et al. Does salt addiction exist? Salud Ment. 2016;39(3):175-181.

[166] Chen Z, Oldewage-Theron WH. Household consumption of stock cubes and stock powder in the Vaal Triangle of SA. Nutrition and Food Science. 2004;34(4):174-178.

Section 2

Risk Factors for Cardiovascular Diseases

Chapter 5

Ambulatory Isolated Systolic Hypertension and Cardiovascular Target Organ Damage in People of African Ancestry

Muzi Maseko, Bongubuhle Mlambo, Edgar Phukubje and Thamsanqa Nyundu

Abstract

Isolated systolic hypertension (ISH) is a major contributor to cardiovascular disease morbidity and mortality worldwide, however, diagnosis of ISH is mainly dependent on conventional blood pressure (BP) techniques. Studies that have used ambulatory blood pressure monitoring (ABPM) were only limited to 24-hour BP. To date ambulatory isolated BP subtypes have never been identified. Therefore, the prevalence of ambulatory subtypes of ISH unknown. Conventional and ambulatory BP was measure in 549 participants and based on the results, they were stratified into ISH subtypes (Conventional, Daytime, Night-time and 24-hour ISH). Participants further underwent measurements of pulse wave velocity (PWV) and left ventricular mass index (LVMI) to determine the extent of arterial stiffness and left ventricular hypertrophy. We further assessed whether the target organ changes are associated with any ISH subtype. The prevalence of Conventional ISH (ISHC), 24-hour ISH (ISH24), Night-time ISH (ISHN) and Daytime ISH (ISHD) was 7.5%, 7.1%, 7.7% and 7.5% respectively. Compared to normotensives, all ISH subtypes had higher PWV and LVMI. These target organ changes were similar to those observed in hypertensives. Our results indicate that isolated systolic hypertension, whether conventional or ambulatory, is as detrimental as hypertension on cardiovascular target organs.

Keywords: hypertension, hypertrophy, ambulatory nocturnal, conventional, cardiovascular

1. Introduction

By definition, hypertension is a chronic condition characterised by persistent elevated blood pressure [1]. Traditionally, the term hypertension has been used to describe a condition in which systolic BP (SBP) is equal or above 140 mm Hg and/or a diastolic BP (DBP) is equal or above 90 mm Hg [2]. The term Systolic-diastolic hypertension (SDH) is slowly replacing 'hypertension' in this regard as the latter becomes a broader term describing a large number of classes/categories of persistent high BP [3–5]. Thus hypertension can be divided into several types based on several criteria which may or may not overlap.

IntechOpen

European Society of Cardiology/European Society of Hypertension (ESC/ESH) criteria for the classification of participants according to office (conventional) BP measurement [4].

Category	SBP (mm Hg)		DBP (mm Hg)
Normal (Normotensive)	120–129	and/or	80–84
High-Normal (Normotensive)	130–139	and/or	85–89
Hypertensive	≥ 140	and/or	≥ 90
Isolated Systolic Hypertensive	≥ 140	and	≤ 90
Isolated Diastolic Hypertensive	≤ 140	and	≥ 90

The America College of cardiology/American Heart Society (ACC/AHA) has more stringent criteria for conventional BP diagnosis of the hypertension categories.

Category	SBP (mm Hg)		DBP (mm Hg)
Normal (Normotensive)	< 120	and	< 80
Elevated (High-Normal)	120–129	and	<80
Grade 1 Hypertension	130–139	and/or	80–90
Grade 2 Hypertension	≥ 140	and/or	≥ 90
Isolated Systolic Hypertensive	≥ 130	and	< 80
Isolated Diastolic Hypertension	< 130	and	≥ 80

The advent of ambulatory BP monitoring (ABPM) has revealed much about other subtypes of hypertension in everyday environments; in fact, some developed countries have called for the application of ABPM as a routine tool in clinical practice [6–9]. The superiority of this technique over office BP measurement has been well documented, particularly with respect to the prediction of cardiovascular events and target organ damage [10, 11]. Another benefit of this method is that it minimises the interference of false BP elevations/reductions that may be influenced by clinical settings or other stimuli, as the case may be with white coat hypertension or masked hypertension [10, 12].

The ABPM technique has been instrumental in the understanding of circadian rhythm of haemodynamics, in particular the phenomena of night-time BP dipping or rising, the early morning BP surge [13] as well as BP variability [8, 12]. In light of all these advantages, it is not surprising that ambulatory techniques are now considered the gold standard in hypertension diagnosis and out of office BP measurement [9, 14]. In fact, the ESH and ESC guidelines recommend that wherever possible this method be used as the basis for hypertension diagnosis [2].

The ESC/ESH and ACC/AHA thresholds for hypertension diagnosis according to ABPM [2, 15].

Category	SBP (mm Hg)		DBP (mm Hg)
Daytime mean	≥ 135	and/or	≥ 85
Night-time mean	≥ 120	and/or	≥ 70
24 hour mean	≥ 130	and/or	≥ 80

Using the above ambulatory blood pressure thresholds, the following subtypes of hypertension have been identified:

Hypertension subtype	Day BP (mm Hg)	Nigh BP (mm Hg)
Isolated Nocturnal Hypertension	< 135/85	≥ 120/70
Isolated Daytime Hypertension	≥ 135/85	< 120/70
Sustained 24-hour Hypertension	≥ 135/85	≥ 120/70

Ambulatory BP has also allowed identification of two abnormal night-time blood pressure patterns. The first one is an attenuated decline in nocturnal BP. Blood pressure varies over 24 hours, it is high during the day and low during the night. Normally, BP decreases by 10% to 20% during the night. Individuals that lack this decline in nocturnal BP are classified as non-dippers. A large body of evidence exists around the strong association between a non-dipping profile and target organ damage at a vascular, cardiac and cerebrovascular level. Another variant BP pattern that is opposite to non-dipping has been identified with ambulatory BP monitoring. Individuals who present with this condition have an abnormally high night-time BP that rises above the daytime BP values. This condition known as reverse dipping has also been associated with cardiovascular target organ damage.

1.1 Isolated systolic hypertension

Isolated Systolic Hypertension is a form of hypertension characterised by elevated SBP ≥ 140 mm Hg and often normal or low DBP < 90 mm Hg [16]. As a result of this, ISH is associated with increased pulse pressure (PP), which is the difference between SBP and DBP [16, 17]. Previous studies of ISH date as far back as 1970 [18], with interest in the subject increasing around the 1980's [19–22]. Most of these earlier studies identified ISH as a disease of the elderly, stemming from the "normal" physiological processes associated with ageing [20, 22, 23]. More recent studies have revealed that ISH does in fact also exist in younger individuals [24–27]. In either age group the condition can have detrimental effects on the cardiovascular system and other vital organs [12, 26, 28].

Systolic BP and PP are both increased in ISH, and are major predictors of heart disease. These haemodynamic parameters are associated with increased risk of myocardial infarction, left ventricular hypertrophy (LVH), renal dysfunction, stroke and cardiovascular mortality to a greater extent than DBP [29–31]. Some data from clinical trials suggest that even small elevations of SBP confer a significant risk of coronary heart disease [32]. The low DBP associated with ISH may lead to impaired tissue perfusion, particularly of the heart itself [29, 31]. In fact, ISH, which was long believed to be a normal and physiologically harmless state associated with the ageing process [30] has been shown to be a stronger predictor of cerebrovascular and cardiovascular events [32] as well as renal disease [29] than elevated DBP. A thorough understanding of the pathophysiology of ISH is necessary in order to manage the condition effectively and possibly reduce its negative effects on target organs.

Systolic BP has been shown to increase with age [33], a phenomenon that has been attributed to "natural" changes occurring in the arterial walls as the body ages. For this reason, most of the physiological mechanisms that are believed to be responsible for ISH are associated with the vascular ageing process [34]. This involves an interplay of several processes typically culminating in increased stiffness of the central arteries [30, 31, 35, 36].

As the vascular system ages - usually from about the age of 50 [17, 30], the arterial walls experience fatigue and the elastin fibres therein begin to fragment. This is associated with increased calcium deposition and subsequent media calcification [17]. In addition to this, more collagen fibres are deposited into this fragile wall. There is an accumulation of Advanced Glycation End products (AGEs), which progressively and irreversibly interlink with collagen and elastin fragments to form a complex matrix [36, 37]. Local inflammation occurs, characterised by the release of pro-inflammatory cytokines and enzymes including some metalloproteases which inhibit the production of Nitric Oxide (NO) an influential vasodilator substance, leading to endothelial dysfunction [35, 36, 38].

The pathophysiology of ISH in young individuals is thought to differ at least to some extent from the mechanisms described for the older population [24, 28]. In some young people, ISH develops following a hyperkinetic pre-hypertensive state which is associated with an increase in sympathetic stimulation. This is associated with adrenergic activation with the release of norepinephrine. In these individuals, an increase in resting heart rate and cardiac output leads to an acceleration of arterial stiffness with an isolated increase of SBP [28]. The findings of McEniery et al. [39] in a study of individuals between 17 and 27 suggest that indeed aortic stiffness is associated with ISH in young people, having similar pathophysiological implications as it does in the elderly. Some researchers have shown that an increase in stroke volume in certain young individuals is the major contributor to an elevated PP leading to premature aortic stiffening [26, 27, 28, 39]. Increased body fat in obese young adults could also be a contributing factor to isolated elevation of SBP as the former has been shown to be a strong predictor of aortic stiffness [24].

Another type of ISH is observed in young active, particularly athletic adults. In this group, the SBP and PP elevations are often isolated to the peripheral arteries (especially in the upper limbs), while central haemodynamics remain normal [28, 40]. This phenomenon has been attributed to the effects of exercise-related bradycardia on stroke volume; which is thought to increase PP by exaggerating the amplification of the pressure wave [28, 40, 41]. This type of ISH is arguably considered spurious and somewhat ‘non-detrimental’ by most researchers [28, 42–44] since most risk is often associated with central rather than peripheral abnormalities [27].

1.2 Ambulatory isolated systolic hypertension

Early studies into ambulatory ISH seemed to suggest that ISH was a form of “white coat” hypertension that was not sustained during day to day activities outside a clinical setting [45, 46]. The work of Staessen et al. [10] compared the predictive ability of ABPM over conventional BP measurement in older ISH patients, and found that ambulatory SBP was a more superior predictor of cardiovascular risk than conventional SBP. Later research using improved technology for ABPM showed that while this may be true to some extent, sustained and masked forms of ISH are also prevalent, particularly in the elderly population [47]. Over time, ABPM became more useful in investigating ISH from several angles. It has been used to investigate postprandial hypotension in elderly ISH patients [48]. Saladini et al. [49] investigated the future risk of sustained hypertension in young, sporty ISH patients diagnosed by ABPM. These studies either used ABPM in people already diagnosed with ISH using conventional BP monitoring or diagnosed ISH with ABPM using only 24-hour BP. None these studies identified the ambulatory ISH subtypes. Therefore, a possibility exists that with ambulatory BP monitoring, different types of ISH can be identified.

With this gap in the current literature, we designed a study using ambulatory BP monitoring, with the aim of identifying different ambulatory ISH subtypes, determining their prevalence and investigating whether these subtypes are associated with preclinical cardiovascular pathology in a population of African ancestry.

2. Methods

2.1 Study group

Participants of African ancestry were recruited from Soweto, a township in the southwest of Johannesburg. The lower age limit for the participants was 18 years and there was no upper age limit. Based on their conventional and ambulatory BP measurements were divided into the following six groups:

i. Normotensives (NT). Those with normal daytime and normal nighttime ambulatory BP (daytime BP < 135/85 mm Hg and nighttime BP < 120/70 mm Hg).

ii. Hypertensives (HT). Those with increased daytime BP and increased nighttime BP (daytime BP ≥ 135/85 mm Hg and night-time BP ≥ 120/70 mm Hg).

iii. Conventional isolated systolic hypertensives (ISHC). Those with increased conventional systolic BP and normal conventional diastolic BP (systolic BP ≥ 140 mm Hg and diastolic BP < 90 mm Hg).

iv. Twenty four-hour ambulatory isolated systolic hypertension (ISH24). Those with increased 24-hour systolic BP and normal 24-hour diastolic BP (24-hour systolic BP ≥ 130 mm Hg and 24-hour diastolic BP < 80 mm Hg).

v. Night-time isolated systolic hypertensives (ISHN). Those with increased night-time systolic BP and normal night-time diastolic BP (night-time systolic BP ≥ 120 and night-time diastolic BP < 70 mm Hg).

vi. Daytime isolated systolic hypertensives (ISHD). Those with increased daytime systolic BP and normal daytime diastolic BP (daytime systolic BP ≥ 135 mm Hg and daytime diastolic BP < 85 mm Hg).

2.2 Blood pressure measurement

Participants were invited to visit the Human Nutrition Clinic at the School of Physiology, Wits Medical School where conventional BP was measured using an automated pressure monitor (Omron, Kyoto, Japan) after they were allowed to rest for 10 minutes. Twenty four-hour ambulatory BP was measured using a 24-hour BP monitor (Spacelab, model 91207). Monitors were set to measure BP every 15 minutes from 06:00–22:00 and every 30 minutes thereafter until 06:00 the next morning. On average, participant bedtime was 19:00 and wake up time was 05:00. Based on this, the 09:00–19:00 and 23:00–05:00 intervals were used to define daytime and night time respectively.

2.3 Anthropometric measurements

Anthropometric measurements were taken while the participants were barefoot and wearing lightweight indoor robes. Weight was measured using a floor scale

(Health o meter® Professional, USA) and was recorded to the nearest 0.1 kg. For this measurement, the participant was asked to stand upright on the middle of the scale with their weight distributed evenly between both feet. Height was measured to the nearest 0.1 m using a wall-mounted stadiometer (Seca®, Germany), with the participant standing upright and the headpiece of the stadiometer was placed horizontally on the vertex (highest point) of the participant's head and the corresponding reading was recorded. Body Mass Index (BMI) was calculated as weight in kilogrammes divided by the square of the height in metres. Participants with a BMI $\geq$ 25 kg/m^2 were considered overweight, and those with a BMI $\geq$ 30 kg/m^2 were considered obese. Waist circumference was measured in at the end of normal expiration using an inextensible measuring tape aligned parallel to the floor at the narrowest point between the costal margin and the upper iliac crest.

2.4 Pulse wave velocity measurement

A high fidelity tonometer interfaced with a SphygmoCor computer software (AtCor Medical Pty. Ltd., West Ryde, New South Wales, Australia - version 9.0) was used to perform pulse wave assessments of pulse wave velocity (PWV), an index of arterial stiffness. Participants were allowed to rest in the supine position for 15 minutes prior to assessment. Using an inextensible measuring tape, distances (in mm) between the relative sampling sites (femoral and carotid) and the suprasternal notch were measured. The difference between the two distances was considered as the pulse wave distance. Applanation tonometry was then used to record sequential wave forms at the participant's dominant carotid and femoral regions. A three lead chest ECG was performed concurrently with the waveform sampling in order to assess the time differences in the generation of the waveforms. The pulse transit time was defined as the average of 10 consecutive beats. The PWV was automatically calculated as the difference between the aforementioned distances (i.e. the pulse wave distance) divided by the pulse transit time.

2.5 Echocardiography

Echocardiography was used to determine the left ventricular mass index for the participants. All echocardiographic measurements were carried out by an experienced technician using an echocardiogram - the Acuson SC2000 Diagnostic Ultrasound System (Siemens Medical Solutions USA, Inc.) linked to a 10-MHz linear array transducer and electrocardiogram. Participants were asked to lie in the left lateral decubitus position. M-mode images were taken at a frame rate of >110 frames per second. M-mode echocardiography of the short axis of the heart was obtained as close to the tip of the mitral valve as possible using the parasternal long axis view (2D). The resulting images were used to measure left ventricular dimensions only when the endocardial surfaces of the septal and posterior walls, as well as both the left and right septal surfaces, could be clearly seen. Wall dimensions, namely the Left Ventricular Internal Diameter at end Diastole (LVIDD), the Posterior Wall Thickness in Diastole (PWTD) and the Interventricular Septal Thickness in Diastole (IVSTD) were obtained from M-mode images. Left ventricular mass values were indexed for body.

3. Statistical analysis

Database management and statistical analyses were performed with SAS software, version 9.4 (The SAS Institute Inc., Cary, North Carolina, USA). Data from individual subjects were averaged and expressed as mean ± SD for continuous variables and categorical variables were expressed as percentages. The differences between the means was calculated using the General Linear Model (GLM) and adjustments were made for the following covariates; age, gender, BMI, alcohol intake and cigarette smoking. A p value <0.05 was considered significant. The Receiver Operator Characteristics (ROC) curve analysis was used to determine how well the different subgroups of ISH would predict an increased PWV and LVMI. The ROC curve analysis is used in clinical prediction to assess how well a test can discriminate between absence or presence of a condition. The analysis yields a curve of sensitivity versus 1-specificity, where the Area Under the Curve (AUC) is a measure of predictive power of the test to a maximum of 1 [50]. The closer the AUC is to 1, the greater the ability of the test in question to discriminate whether the presence of a condition is associated with a change in a given parameter [50].

4. Results

Table 1 shows the demographic, general and clinical characteristics of the population under study. Of the 549 participants, 41 (7.5%) had ISH as measured by conventional means (ISHC). This figure is similar to those obtained for the ambulatory sub-types of ISH, namely 24-hour, Night-time and Daytime ISH which had 39 (7.1%), 42 (7.7%) and 41 (7.5%) participants respectively. Systolic-diastolic hypertension was observed in 161 (29%) of the participants. The mean age of the population was 45.3 ± 18.5 years and the ISHC group was significantly older (65.3 ± 13.5 years) than both normotensives (39.7 ± 17.6 years) and hypertensives (52.1 ± 15.5 years). There were slight reductions in average age within the other ISH subtypes, with ISH24 at 57.8 ± 20.1 years, ISHN at 55.4 ± 24.6 years and ISHD at 53.7 ± 20.9 years. We observed that all the ISH subgroups had greater proportions of female participants than the normotensive or hypertensive groups [51]. Anthropometry revealed significantly higher waist circumference in the ISHC group than in the normotensives, this was also true for all the other ISH subgroups albeit of no known significance. In addition to this, the overall population was overweight with a BMI of 29.1 ± 7.8 kg/m^2. Both ISHC and hypertensives were obese (BMI of 31.4 ± 7.5 kg/m^2 and 30.9 ± 7.5 kg/m^2 respectively), the former group having a significantly higher BMI than the normotensives (BMI = 28.0 ± 7.7 kg/m^2). The average SBPC of the ISHC group (153.1 ± 11.7 mm Hg) was higher than that of the hypertensive group (149.6 ± 20.3 mm Hg), and significantly higher than that of the normotensives (129.7 ± 21.4 mm Hg). Overall, the SBPC values for all ISH sub-types were high. Conventional ISH had an average DBPC of 83.5 ± 4.8 mm Hg, significantly higher than that of normotensives (77.6 ± 7.2 mm Hg) and significantly lower than that of hypertensives (98.6 ± 8.4 mm Hg). Similarly, 24-hour, night-time and daytime ISH all had conventional diastolic blood pressures below those of hypertensives but above those of normotensives. All sub-types of ISH had higher pulse pressure values than both normotensives and hypertensive groups, significantly so for those participants with ISHC (PP = 69.7 ± 12.3 mm Hg).

Tables 2 and **3** show the ROC curve analysis of the relationships between the sub-types of ISH and cardiovascular target organ changes. All subtypes of ISH were significantly associated with increased PWV and LVMI. Conventional ISH strongly predicts arterial stiffness and left ventricular hypertrophy, with area under the curve (AUC) values of 0.88 ± 0.03 (CI: 0.83 to 0.93) and 0.86 ± 0.03 (CI: 0.88 to 0.92), respectively. Daytime ISH was shown to be a strong predictor of both (PWV and LVMI) with all the values exceeding 0.8. all three organ changes under study

	Total sample population	NT	ISHC	ISH24	ISHN	ISHD	HT
Numbers (%)	549	347 (63.2)	41 (7.5)	39 (7.1)	42 (7.7)	41 (7.5)	161 (29.3)
Age (years)	45.3 ± 18.5	39.7 ± 17.6	65.3 ± 13.5	57.8 ± 20.1	55.4 ± 24.6	53.7 ± 20.9	52.1 ± 15.5*#
Female gender (%)	36.6	34.0	51.2	51.3	47.6	56.1	38.5
Waist C (cm)	90.04 ± 16.01	87.02 ± 16.05	98.11 ± 14.27	90.04 ± 60.01	96.86 ± 18.11	95.87 ± 16.23	94.40 ± 14.67*
BMI (kg/m^2)	29.1 ± 7.8	28.0 ± 7.7	31.4 ± 7.5	31.2 ± 8.1	30.9 ± 9.3	31.4 ± 8.9	30.9 ± 7.5*
Smokers (%)	15.1	14.4	19.5	15.4	14.3	21.9	15.5
Alcohol usage (%)	23.3	19.6	24.4	20.5	33	26.8	31.1
SBPC (mm Hg)	129.7 ± 21.4	117.6 ± 11.8	153.1 ± 11.7	151.9 ± 21.7	142.7 ± 23.8	147.7 ± 22.4	149.6 ± 20.3*
DBPC (mm Hg)	84.1 ± 12.0	77.6 ± 7.2	83.5 ± 4.8	88.7 ± 11.9	85.6 ± 10.5	86.7 ± 12.0	98.6 ± 8.4*#
PP (mm Hg)	45.5 ± 14.9	40.1 ± 12.0	69.7 ± 12.3	63.2 ± 16.2	57.1 ± 17.2	61.0 ± 18.0	51.1 ± 17.3*#

BMI, body mass index; NT, Normotensive; ISHC, Conventional Isolated Systolic Hypertension; ISH24, 24 Hour Isolated Systolic Hypertension; ISHN, Night-time Isolated Systolic Hypertension; ISHD, Daytime Isolated Systolic Hypertension; HT, Hypertensive; PP, Pulse Pressure; DBPC, Conventional Diastolic Blood Pressure; SBPC, Conventional systolic blood pressure; Waist C, Waist Circumference.
Data is presented as mean ± SD or percentage.
** depicts significant difference between ISHC and NT,*
 # depicts significant differences between ISHC and HT. $P < 0.05$ for all significant differences.

Table 1.
Demographic and clinical characteristics of participants according to blood pressure status.

ISH subtype	AUC	CI
ISHC	0.88±0.03	0.83 to 0.93
ISH24	0.77±0.04	0.68 to 0.86
ISHN	0.78±0.04	0.70 to 0.85
ISHD	0.83±0.05	0.74 to 60.92

AUC, area under the curve; CI, confidence intervals; ISHC, conventional isolated systolic hypertension; ISH24, 24 hour Isolated systolic hypertension; ISHN, Night-time isolated systolic hypertension; ISHD, Daytime isolated systolic hypertension $P < 0.05$ for all associations. Adjustments were made for age, gender, BMI, the use of antihypertensive medication, smoking and alcohol consumption.

Table 2.
ROC curve analysis of the relationship between ISH and PWV.

ISH subtype	AUC	CI
ISHC	0.86±0.03	0.88 to 0.92
ISH24	0.76±0.03	0.67 to 0.86
ISHN	0.71±0.05	0.62 to 0.80
ISHD	0.80±0.06	0.68 to 0.09

AUC, area under the curve; CI, confidence intervals; ISHC, conventional isolated systolic hypertension; ISH24, 24 hour Isolated systolic hypertension; ISHN, Night-time isolated systolic hypertension; ISHD, Daytime isolated systolic hypertension. $P < 0.05$ for all associations. Adjustments were made for age, gender, BMI, the use of antihypertensive medication, smoking and alcohol consumption.

Table 3.
ROC curve analysis of the relationship between ISH and LVMI.

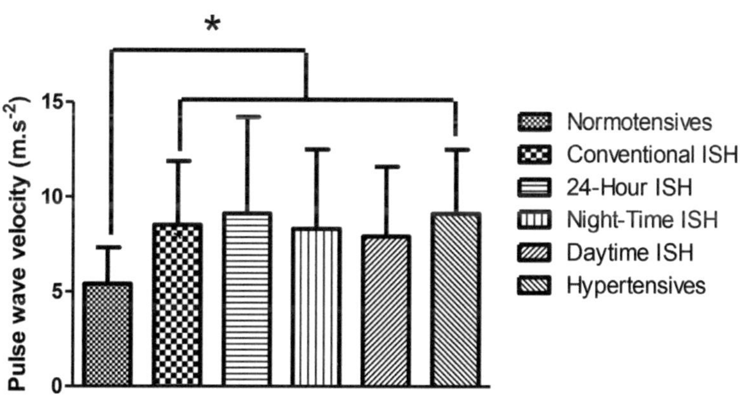

Figure 1.
*Comparison of PWV of ISH subgroups, the hypertensives and the normotensives. This figure shows data of PWV expressed as adjusted means ± SD. The differences between the means was calculated using the general linear model and adjustments were made for the following covariates; age, gender, BMI, alcohol intake and cigarette smoking. There was no significant difference in the PWV of the different ISH subtypes and none of the ISH subtypes was significantly different from the hypertensives. However, the PWV of all the ISH subtypes and hypertensives was significantly higher than that of the normotensives. * = p value <0.05.*

(AUC values all exceeding 0.8). The pattern of association and the significance was maintained even after adjusting for confounding variables.

Figures 1 and **2** shows data of PWV and LVMI respectively expressed as adjusted means ± SD. For both PWV and LVMI, there was no significant difference in the PWV of the different ISH subtypes and none of the ISH subtypes was

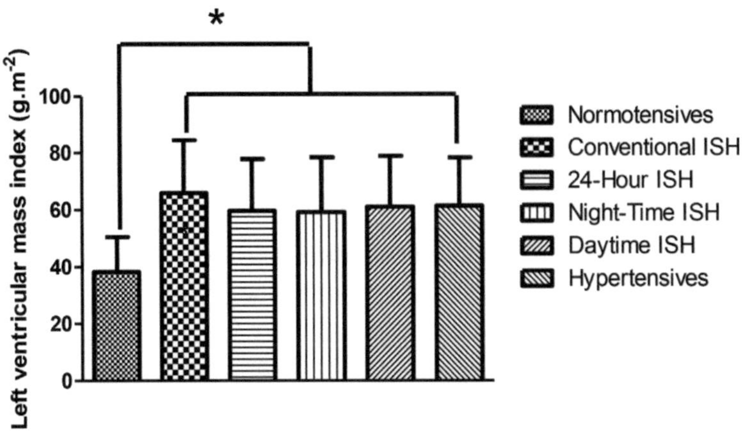

Figure 2.
*Comparison of the LVMI of the ISH subtypes, the normotensives and the hypertensives. This figure shows data of LVMI expressed as adjusted means ± SD. The differences between the means was calculated using the general linear model and adjustments were made for age, gender, BMI, alcohol intake, cigarette smoking and presence of diabetes. There was no significant difference in the LVMI of the different ISH subtypes and none of the ISH subtypes was significantly different from the hypertensives. However, the LVMI of all the ISH subtypes and hypertensives was significantly higher than that of the normotensives. * = p value <0.05.*

significantly different from the hypertensives. However, the PWV and LVMI of all the ISH subtypes were significantly higher than that of the normotensives.

5. Discussion

In the present study, we determined the general characteristics of ISH and went on to divide it into four subtypes namely Conventional ISH, 24-hour ISH, Night-time ISH and Daytime ISH. We proceeded to investigate the associations between each of these subtypes with PWV and LVM. We further investigated the extent to which each of the ISH subtypes predicted the target organ changes mentioned. The results of the present study show that 7.5% of the cohort had ISHC and the same percentage had Daytime ISH. Night-time ISH was found in 7.7% of the population, while 7.1% of the participants had 24-hour ISH. Furthermore, our findings show that all subtypes of ISH are significantly associated with increased PWV and LVMI in measures comparable to general hypertension, The percentage of participants with ISHC in our study is consistent with the work of Gupta *et al.,* [52] who found a similar (7.78%) prevalence of the condition following their study of office workers in a North Indian town. Huang *et al.,* [53] also found a similar prevalence of ISH (7.6%) in a Chinese study. However, all these studies used only conventional BP measurements to determine the prevalence of ISH. Hence our study is the first to identify the three ISH subtypes identified by ambulatory BP monitoring.

5.1 Determinants of ISH

5.1.1 Socio-economic status

Our and other studies indicate that the prevalence of isolated systolic hypertension averages around 8% across populations whether measured by conventional or ambulatory BP techniques. However, Ntuli, et al. [54] investigated a population ethnically similar to our study cohort and their study revealed a much higher prevalence of ISHC (21%). The most likely explanation for this is the socioeconomic difference between their sample population and ours. The study by Ntuli et al. [54] was conducted in rural Limpopo (Dikgale), where unemployment and poverty is high and there is limited access to adequate healthcare [54–56]. Ntuli's study indicates that socio-economic factors could play a role in the prevalence of ISH. Socioeconomic factors have been implicated in contributing to the high prevalence of hypertension in developing countries [57, 58], and it would not be surprising that ISHC would follow the trend.

5.1.2 Age

The mean age of participants in the present study (45.3 years) was similar to that of subjects in the study by Ntuli et al. [54] (44.2 years). Gupta et al. [52] did not report a mean age for their population which was limited to the working age-group under 58 years, while Huang et al. [53] carried out their investigation on participants in the 35–74 age group [52, 53]. The bulk of studies on ISHC have been focused on specific age groups, usually the young (under 35 years of age) or the old (over 50 years old) [27, 49, 59, 60] unlike our population which included all consenting persons over the age of 18. While several studies in recent years have shown that the condition is not at all restricted to the older population [25–27], the relatively high average age associated with ISH (especially the conventional subtype) in our study is consistent with the findings of a number of researchers and with the widely accepted notion that ISH is predominant and naturally occurring in the elderly population [1, 16, 18, 30, 61]. A study by Huang et al. [53] also showed an increase in ISHC with age.

Martins et al. [62] observed an increase in PP and SBP from the age of 45 upward in their analysis of data from the NHANES. Indeed, the most commonly described pathophysiological mechanism for ISH involves changes occurring to the large arteries owing to ageing [13]. With age progression, elastin in the media decreases, leading to a fragmented media [13, 18] which is susceptible to calcium and lipid accumulation. Along with this media calcification occurs the accumulation of smooth muscle cells within the intima, collagen cross linking occurs and all this leads to the thickening and fibrosis of the arterial wall [13, 18, 43]. These changes culminate in arterial stiffness, an increased wall-to-lumen ratio and a reduced cross-sectional area of the lumen of the greater arteries [13, 37, 63]. Due to poor compliance, the large arteries fail to expand and subsequently recoil effectively in systole and diastole of the cardiac cycle, respectively. There is a resultant increase in aortic PP and PWV. Consequently, the reflected wave which would normally return during diastole, returns during late systole and augments systolic pressure; SBP increases while the DBP decreases [43, 63]. In line with this, we observed higher values of average SBPC in the ISH groups than in the normotensive group, and these were comparable to that of hypertensive participants. This was coupled with relatively low DBPC for all ISH sub-types when compared to the hypertensive group. By definition, PP is the difference between SBP and DBP, thus its normal value is approximately 40 mm Hg [64]. Pulse Pressure values exceeding 60 mm Hg are associated with target organ damage which may or may not be asymptomatic [3]. In the present study, PP was markedly increased in participants with ISHC, with an average of 69.7 mm Hg. Wallace et al. [65] also observed similar elevated SBP and PP (67 mm Hg) in their ISHC group. This finding was as expected based on the definition and underlying physiology of the condition [16, 18, 61] since PP is the difference between systolic and diastolic BPs; and an increase in the former and/or decrease in the latter would raise PP.

5.1.3 Obesity

In general, all the ISH groups in this study were obese. Average BMI values ranging from 30.9 to 31.4 were recorded for these groups, all of which exceed the obesity threshold of 30 for BMI [66]. The role of obesity as a risk factor for ISH is well documented [25, 35, 57, 63, 67]. Erhun et al. [68] observed the highest prevalence of ISH among the extremely obese group in their study. The ISH subgroup in the research by Grebla et al. [24] was overweight, and these authors suggested that obesity may be an important determinant of ISH in young adults [25]. A study by Nemes et al. [69] showed that obesity is associated with increased arterial stiffness and that this is true even for young obese adults, whose arterial stiffness they found comparable to that of elderly non-obese individuals. Although all of these studies investigated obesity in ISH by conventional BP measurement, their findings may extend to all the ambulatory subtypes of the condition as well. Our results show that in all participants with any forms of ISH, arterial stiffness as measured by PWV was increased in comparison to normotensives.

Several mechanisms have been described that may explain the role of obesity in ISH. Hyperinsulinaemia and insulin resistance, which are both strongly associated with obesity [70], may mediate aortic stiffness through glycation of vascular wall proteins and subsequent increased cross-linking [69]. Insulin has also been associated with smooth muscle hypertrophy and increased endothelial dysfunction of large arteries likely resulting from oxidant stress, causing increased susceptibility to atherosclerosis [69, 71]. One other significant mechanism that has been implicated in the relationship between obesity and ISH is the activity of leptin [69]. Hyperleptinaemia is associated with endothelial dysfunction in obese individuals [72], which is an underlying cause of arterial stiffness. Schutte et al. [73] reported a strong negative correlation between leptin and arterial compliance coupled with a strong positive relationship between leptin and SBP as well as leptin and PP in obese/overweight hypertensive African women. The high-leptin state of overweight/obese women in our study population, which was predominantly African, has been previously described [74] and may play an important role in ISH.

5.2 Isolated systolic hypertension target and target organ changes

5.2.1 Arterial stiffness

We measured PWV by applanation tonometry, a minimally invasive method which is widely recognised as the 'gold standard' in the determination of arterial stiffness [65, 75]. As far as we know there are no studies which have investigated PWV in ambulatory subtypes of ISH, however, the general association of ISHC with arterial and aortic stiffness has been reported [65, 76, 77]. Antza et al. [77] in their study of arterial stiffness in ISHC observed an increase in arterial stiffness in patients with the condition, and suggested that ISHC may have a role to play in large artery arteriosclerosis.

This observation can be explained in terms of the haemodynamic changes associated with ISH. Since ISH is characterised by elevated systolic and pulse pressures, these parameters exert increased mechanical stress on the arteries over time, leading to elastin fragmentation and subsequent calcification, collagen deposition and smooth muscle cell hypertrophy [34, 37, 76]. In addition to this, endothelial dysfunction associated with the shear stress also triggers the inhibition of NO production and the release of pro-inflammatory cytokines and growth factors such as TGF-β [31, 34, 65]. These augment arterial damage by promoting smooth muscle cell hypertrophy and the increased production of extracellular matrix proteins;

moreover, TGF-β inhibits the activity of those metalloproteases which would otherwise assist by breaking down the collagen build-up, such as MMP-9 [38]. All these factors culminate in arterial stiffening of mainly the central arteries. In essence, ISH speeds up the rate of arterial ageing and increases arterial stiffness, thereby leading to its own exacerbation in a vicious cycle [65]. Several scholars agree that the causal relationship between arterial stiffness and ISH is bidirectional [31, 34, 38].

With this in mind, it is not surprising that we observed significantly elevated PWV in all subtypes of ISH when compared to normotensives. Of interest, is that all ISH groups had an increase in PWV that is comparable to that of the sustained hypertensive group. This suggests that the arterial damage caused by the ISH groups may equal arterial stiffness arising from sustained hypertension in this population. This is contrary to our expectation. We expected the PWV of the ISH24 to be higher than that of the other groups due to the cumulative effects of a high systolic BP that is sustained over a 24-hout period. The explanation for this apparent discrepancy is that 24-hour BP is a combination of both daytime and night-time BP. Since BP decreases at night, that decline in nocturnal BP may have a damping effect on the *overall effect of ISH24 on arterial stiffness.

When we used ROC curve analysis to determine how well the different subgroups of ISH would predict an increased PWV in this population, our results indicate that all ISH subtypes predict PWV. Conventional ISH was the strongest predictor of arterial stiffness with an AUC of 0.88 followed by ISHD at 0.83. In this respect, daytime BP is emerging as the best predictor of ISH in this population as both conventional and daytime ambulatory BP are measured during the day. This is due to the 24-hour pattern of BP in which BP increases during the day and decreases at night. Our results indicate that the increase in daytime systolic BP in people with ISH is exaggerated, resulting in a high PP of 70 mmHg, which is 30 mm Hg the normal value of 40 mm Hg. This is PP value is higher than that of people with sustained hypertension. The same pattern was observed in people with ISHD. As discussed earlier, PP is an independent risk factor for vascular disease. This explains why ISHC and ISHD which have the highest PP, are the strongest predictors of arterial stiffness. Even though ISHN predicts arterial to a lesser extent than ISHC and ISHD, it is still a strong predictor of arterial stiffness with an AUC of 0.78. This highlights the importance of this study which is the first to discover the existence of this clinical entity.

5.2.2 Left ventricular hypertrophy

Left ventricular mass index has been used as an indication of LVH, a major independent predictor of cardiovascular mortality and morbidity [78–80]. We used echocardiography, a well-accepted, efficient and non-invasive tool for the estimation of LVMI [79, 80]. In this study, there were no clear differences in LVMI values obtained for the ambulatory ISH sub-types (ISHD, ISHN and ISH24), suggesting that there are no major differences in the development of LVH among these three subtypes; although the extent of cardiac damage they caused is similar to that associated with hypertension. This implies that even if diastolic BP can be normal, the impact of systolic BP alone is significant has a significant impact on cardiac morphology. The premature return of the reflected wave in ISH is probably the most significant cause of LVM increase [81] in this condition. The augmentation of SBP by the reflected wave results in an increased afterload to the left ventricle. As the left ventricle adapts to the increased workload, concentric hypertrophy of surrounding tissue occurs, resulting in thickening and increase in mass of the left ventricle wall [37]. Poor coronary perfusion owing to low DBP may also exacerbate the effects of increased LVM in ISH as increased oxygen demand of the myocardium becomes difficult to meet [82]. Our results bear some similarity to those obtained by Pearson et al. [83], who reported that ISHC patients exhibited increased LVMI arising from thickened septal and posterior walls of the left ventricle. Lip et al. [84] had related outcomes, they found that LVMI and other echographic parameters were similar between ISHC and full hypertension (SDH) groups. Our study adds significantly to this body of knowledge by showing that ISH has a number of subtypes which are as detrimental to cardiac pathology as both ISHC and sustained hypertension. Some research has shown that increased LVMI even within the "normal" range is clinically relevant i.e. it is associated with significant cardiovascular risk [85]. Since ISH increases the risk of LVH at least twofold, even the preclinical increases in LVM observed in this study may progress to cardiac pathology over time as the elevated SBP persists.

Most ISH studies in the past have been carried out on elderly participants, however, our results show that even after correcting for age the associations and predictions remain unchanged, suggesting that ISH is just as detrimental to the elderly as it is to younger age groups with respect to left ventricle structure and consequently, cardiovascular function. Levy et al. [79] also found that the relationship between increased LVMI and cardiovascular morbidity and mortality was applicable to the middle-aged study group as much as the elderly study group, although their focus was not particularly on ISH. Obesity, which was identified in this ISH population, is thought to increase the risk of LVM and LVH by its tendency to attract other risk factors such as metabolic syndrome and diabetes mellitus [85]. Genetics also plays an important and complex role in the increase of LVM and development of LVH. So, the population under study - being predominantly black, may be at higher risk of LVH. Skelton et al. [86] reported a very high prevalence of increased LVM in an African-American population. This highlights the need for more studies to investigate the impact of ISH subtypes to be investigated.

Similar to PWV, again ISHC and ISHD were the strongest predictors of increased LVMI according to ROC analysis (AUC = 0.86 and 0.80 respectively), followed by ISH24 (AUC = 0.76) and ISHN (AUC = 0.71). This confirms the impact of the increases in daytime systolic BP on cardiovascular organs. There is no comparable research on ISH subtypes predictive power on increased LVMI, however our results provide strong evidence that ISH subtypes, which were not known previous to this study, predict preclinical cardiac pathology similar to hypertension, indicating that these subtypes are clinical entities that require intervention.

6. Conclusion

Our overall findings are that there are three subtypes of ambulatory ISH (24-hour ISH, night-time ISH and daytime ISH) which had not been previously defined. Night-time ISH is the most prevalent form of ISH in this population. Most importantly our results indicate that all these ISH subtypes may be as detrimental to cardiovascular organs as hypertension as they all emerged as good predictors of elevated PWV and LVMI, which are markers of arterial stiffness and left ventricular hypertrophy respectively. This highlights the importance of using both conventional and ambulatory BP techniques for the diagnosis ISH because current strategies that are limited to conventional BP monitoring, are incapable of detecting ambulatory isolated systolic hypertension subtypes. Moreover, since this data shows that night-time ISH is the most prevalent form of ISH, and it predicts both arterial stiffness and left ventricular hypertrophy, diagnosis of nocturnal ISH may be very essential in the management of BP related cardiovascular target organ damage.

Acknowledgements

The authors would like to acknowledge Mokgadi Maseko for her technical support and members of the Soweto community whose voluntary participation made this study possible.

Author details

Muzi Maseko*, Bongubuhle Mlambo, Edgar Phukubje and Thamsanqa Nyundu
University of the Witwatersrand, Johannesburg, South Africa

*Address all correspondence to: muzi.maseko@wits.ac.za

References

[1] Seedat YK, Rayner BL, Veriava, Y. South African Hypertension Practice Guideline 2014. Cardiovascular Journal of Africa. 2014; 25 (6): 288-294.

[2] Williams B, Mancia G, Spiering, W, Rosei, E.A, Azizi M, Burnier M, Clement D.L, Coca A, de Simone G, Dominiczak A. Kahan T. 2018 ESC/ ESH Guidelines for the management of arterial hypertension: The Task Force for the management of arterial hypertension of the European Society of Cardiology and the European Society of Hypertension. Journal of hypertension. 2018;36(10): 1953-2041.

[3] Papademetriou V, Devereux RB, Narayan P, Wachtell K., Bella JN, Gerdts E, Chrysant SG, Dahlöf B.. Similar effects of isolated systolic and combined hypertension on left ventricular geometry and function: the LIFE Study. American journal of hypertension. 200;114(8): 768-774.

[4] Tsimploulis A, Sheriff, HM, Lam PH, Dooley, DJ, Anker, MS, Papademetriou V, Fletcher, RD, Faselis C, Fonarow GC, Deedwania P, White M. Systolic–diastolic hypertension versus isolated systolic hypertension and incident heart failure in older adults: Insights from the Cardiovascular Health Study. International journal of cardiology. 2017; 235: 11-16.

[5] Sulbaran TA, Silva ER, Maestre G. Isolated systolic hypertension: a new challenge in medicine. Journal of human hypertension. 2002; 16(1): 44-47.

[6] Pang TC, Brown MA. Accuracy of ambulatory blood pressure monitors in routine clinical practice. American journal of hypertension. 2006; 19(8): 801-809.

[7] Ommen ES, Schröppel B, Kim JY, Gaspard G, Akalin E, de Boccardo G, Sehgal V, Lipkowitz M, Murphy B. Routine use of ambulatory blood pressure monitoring in potential living kidney donors. Clinical Journal of the American Society of Nephrology. 2007; 2(5): 1030-1036

[8] O' Brien E, Dolan E. Ambulatory blood pressure measurement in the elderly. Hypertension. 2019; 73: 961-964.

[9] Bloch MJ, Basile JN. Ambulatory blood pressure monitoring to diagnose hypertension--an idea whose time has come. Journal of the American Society of Hypertension. 2016; 10(2): 89.

[10] Staessen JA, Thijs L, Fagard R, O'Brien ET, Clement D, De Leeuw PW, Mancia G, Nachev C, Palatini P, Parati G, Tuomilehto J. Predicting cardiovascular risk using conventional vs ambulatory blood pressure in older patients with systolic hypertension. Journal of the American Medical Association. 1999; 282(6): 539-546.

[11] Dolan E, Stanton AV, Thom S, Caulfield M, Atkins N, McInnes G, Collier D, Dicker P, O'Brien E. Ambulatory blood pressure monitoring predicts cardiovascular events in treated hypertensive patients – an Anglo-Scandinavian cardiac outcomes trial substudy. Journal of hypertension. 2009; 27(4): 876-885.

[12] Kocemba J, Kaweka-Jaszcz K, Gryglewska B, Grodzicki T. Isolated systolic hypertension: pathophysiology, consequences and therapeutic benefits. Journal of Human Hypertension. 1998; 12: 621-626.

[13] Snincak M, El-Abdin MZ, Hrabcakova P, Pella J, Kolesar K. Early Morning Surge Blood Pressure and Isolated Systolic Hypertension-A Clinical Importance in Elderly. Journal of Hypertension. 2018; 36: e179.

[14] Hodgkinson J, Mant J, Martin U, Guo B, Hobbs FDR, Deeks JJ, Heneghan C, Roberts N, McManus RJ. Relative effectiveness of clinic and home blood pressure monitoring compared with ambulatory blood pressure monitoring in diagnosis of hypertension: systematic review. British Medical Journal 2011; 342: d3621.

[15] Whelton PK, Carey RM, Aronow WS, Casey DE, Collins KJ, Himmelfarb CD, DePalma SM, Gidding S, Jamerson KA, Jones DW, MacLaughlin E.J. 2017 ACC/AHA/AAPA/ABC/ACPM/AGS/APhA/ASH/ASPC/NMA/PCNA guideline for the prevention, detection, evaluation, and management of high blood pressure in adults: a report of the American College of Cardiology/American Heart Association Task Force on Clinical Practice Guidelines. Journal of the American College of Cardiology. 2018; 71(19): e127-e248.

[16] Hall WD. A rational approach to the treatment of Hypertension in special populations. American Family Physicia. 1999; 60(1): 156-162.

[17] Emeriau JP, Kalula SZ. Management of hypertension in older persons - specific considerations. CME: The SA Journal of CPD. 2013; 31 (10): 358-32.

[18] Colandrea MA, Friedman GD, Nichaman MZ, Lynd CN. Systolic hypertension in the elderly: an epidemiologic assessment. Circulation. 1970; 41(2): 239-245.

[19] Kannel, W.B., Dawber, T.R. and McGee, D.L., 1980. Perspectives on systolic hypertension. The Framingham study. Circulation, 61(6): 1179-1182.

[20] Kannel, W.B., Wolf, P.A., McGee, D.L., Dawber, T.R., McNamara, P. and Castelli, W.P., 1981. Systolic blood pressure, arterial rigidity, and risk of stroke: the Framingham study. Journal of the American Medical Association, 245 (12): 1225-1229.

[21] Curb, J.D., Borhani, N.O., Entwisle, G., Tung, B., Kass, E., Schnaper, H., Williams, W. And Berman, R., 1985. Isolated Systolic Hypertension in 14 Communities. American Journal of Epidemiology, 121(3): 362-370

[22] Saltzberg, S., Stroh, J.A. and Frishman, W.H., 1988. Isolated systolic hypertension in the elderly: pathophysiology and treatment. Medical Clinics of North America, 72(2): 523-547.

[23] Wilking, S.V.B., Belanger, A.L., Kannel, W.B., D'Agostino, R.B. and Steel, K., 1988. Determinants of isolated systolic hypertension. Journal of the American Medical Association, 260(23): 3451-3455.

[24] Grebla, R.C., Rodriguez, C.J., Borrel., L.N. and Pickering, T.G., 2010. Prevalence and Determinants of Isolated Systolic Hypertension among Young Adults: the 1999-2004 U.S. National Health and Nutrition Examination Survey. Journal of Hypertension, 28(1): 15-23.

[25] Jangid, P., Maheshwari, M., Tilwani, K., Nagal, M. and Soni, N.D., 2015. Isolated Systolic Hypertension in Young Healthy Adults – A review. Scholars Academic Journal of Biosciences, 3 (11): 919-921.

[26] Lurbe, E. and Redon, J., 2016. Isolated Systolic Hypertension in Young People is not Spurious and Should Be Treated. Hypertension, 68(2): 276-280.

[27] Eeftinck Schattenkerk, D.W., van Gorp, J., Vogt, L., Peters, R.J. and van den Born, B.J.H., 2018. Isolated systolic hypertension of the young and its association with central blood pressure in a large multi-ethnic population. The HELIUS study. European journal of preventive cardiology, 25(13): 1351-1359.

[28] Palatini, P., Rosei, E.A., Avolio, A., Bilo, G., Casiglia, E., Ghiadoni, L.,

Giannattasio, C., Grassi, G., Jelakovich, B., Julius, S. and Mancia, G., 2018. Isolated systolic hypertension in the young: a position paper endorsed by the European Society of Hypertension. Journal of hypertension, 36(6): 1222-1236.

[29] Chobanian, A.R., 2007. Isolated Systolic Hypertension in the Elderly. New England Journal of Medicine, 357(8): 789-796.

[30] Gavish, B. and Izzo Jr, J.L., 2016. Arterial stiffness: going a step beyond. American Journal of Hypertension, 29(11): 1223-1233.

[31] Cushman, W.C., 1998. The clinical significance of systolic hypertension. American journal of hypertension, 11(S8): 182S–185S.

[32] AlGhatrif, M. and Lakatta, E.G., 2015. The conundrum of arterial stiffness, elevated blood pressure, and aging. Current hypertension reports, 17(2): 12.

[33] Singh R. Isolated Systolic Hypertension. Medicine Update 2012; 22: 111-116.

[34] Park, J.B., Kario, K. and Wang, J., 2015. Systolic Hypertension: An increasing clinical challenge in Asia. Hypertension Research, 38: 227-236.

[35] Bavishi, C., Goel, S. and Messerli, F.H., 2016. Isolated systolic hypertension: an update after SPRINT. The American journal of medicine, 129(12): 1251-1258.

[36] Steppan, J., Barodka, V., Berkowitz, D.E. and Nyhan, D., 2011. Vascular stiffness and increased pulse pressure in the aging cardiovascular system. Cardiology research and practice, 2011.

[37] Ecobici, M. and Stoicescu, C., 2017. Arterial Stiffness and Hypertension–Which Comes First? Maedica, 12(3): 184.

[38] Schiffrin, E.L., 2004. Vascular stiffening and arterial compliance: implications for systolic blood pressure. American journal of hypertension, 17(S3): 39S–48S.

[39] McEniery, C.M., Yasmin, Wallace, S., Maki-Petaja, K., McDonnell, B., Sharman, J.E., Retallick, C., Franklin, S.S., Brown, M.J., Lloyd, R.C. and Cockcroft, J.R., 2005. Increased stroke volume and aortic stiffness contribute to isolated systolic hypertension in young adults. Hypertension, 46(1): 221-226.

[40] Mahmud, A. and Feely, J., 2003. Spurious systolic hypertension of youth: fit young men with elastic arteries. American journal of hypertension, 16(3): 229-232.

[41] Bursztyn, M., 2018. Isolated systolic hypertension in young adults: a heterogeneous finding. Journal of hypertension, 36(9): 1791-1792.

[42] O'Rourke, M.F., Vlachopoulos, C. and Graham, R.M., 2000. Spurious systolic hypertension in youth. Vascular medicine, 5(3): 141-145.

[43] Hulsen, H.T., Nijdam, M.E., Bos, W.J., Uiterwaal, C.S., Oren, A., Grobbee, D.E. and Bots, M., 2006. Spurious systolic hypertension in young adults; prevalence of high brachial systolic blood pressure and low central pressure and its determinants. Journal of hypertension, 24(6): 1027-1032.

[44] Krzesinski, J.M. and Saint-Remy, A., 2006. Spurious systolic hypertension in youth: what does it really mean in clinical practice? Journal of hypertension, 24(6): 999-1001.

[45] Silagy, C.A., McNeil, J.J. and McGrath, B.P., 1990. Isolated systolic hypertension: does it really exist on ambulatory blood pressure monitoring? Clinical and Experimental Pharmacology and Physiology, 17(3): 203-206.

[46] Sega, R., Cesana, G., Milesi, C., Grassi, G., Zanchetti, A. and Mancia, G., 1997. Ambulatory and home blood pressure normality in the elderly: data from the PAMELA population. Hypertension, 30(1): 1-6.

[47] Franklin, S.S., 2012. Elderly Hypertensives: How Are They Different? Journal of Clinical Hypertension, 14(11): 779-786.

[48] Grodzicki, T., Rajzer, M., Fagard, R., O'Brien, E.T., Thijs, L., Clement, D., Davidson, C., Palatini, P., Parati, G., Kocemba, J. and Staessen, J.A., 1998. Ambulatory blood pressure monitoring and postprandial hypotension in elderly patients with isolated systolic hypertension. Journal of human hypertension, 12(3): 161-165.

[49] Saladini, F., Fania, C., Mos, L., Garavelli, G., Mazzer, A. and Palatini, P., 2018. Risk of Developing Sustained Hypertension in Isolated Systolic Hypertension of the Young Identified with Ambulatory Blood Pressure Monitoring. Journal of Hypertension, 36: e7.

[50] Chung, C.M., Cheng, H.W., Chang, J.J., Lin, Y.S., Hsiao, J.F., Chang, S.T. and Hsu, J.T., 2014. Relationship between resistant hypertension and arterial stiffness assessed by brachial-ankle pulse wave velocity in the older patient. Clinical interventions in aging, 9: 1495.

[51] Maseko J., Woodiwiss A., Majane O., Libhaber C., Brooksbank R., Norton G. Journal of Hypertension 2013. 31 (7): 1379-1386.

[52] Gupta, A.K., Negi, P.C., Gupta, B.P., Bhardwaj, A. and Sharma, B., 2006. Isolated Systolic Hypertension among Office Workers in North Indian Town. Indian Journal of Community Medicine, 31(2): 109-110.

[53] Huang, J., Wildman, R.P., Gu, D., Muntner, P., Su, S. and He, J., 2004. Prevalence of isolated systolic and isolated diastolic hypertension subtypes in China. American Journal of Hypertension, 17 (10): 955-962.

[54] Ntuli, S.T., Maimela, E., Alberts, M., Choma, S. and Dikotope, S., 2015. Prevalence and Associated Risk Factors of Hypertension amongst adults in a rural community of Limpopo Province, South Africa. African Journal of Primary Healthcare and Family Medicine, 7(1): 1-5.

[55] Alberts, M., Urdal, P., Steyn, K., Stensvold, I., Tverdal, A., Nel, J.H. and Steyn, N.P., 2005. Prevalence of cardiovascular diseases and associated risk factors in a rural black population of South Africa. European Journal of Cardiovascular Prevention & Rehabilitation, 12(4): 347-354.

[56] Kanjala, C., Alberts, M., Byass, P. and Burger, S., 2010. Spatial and temporal clustering of mortality in Digkale HDSS in rural northern South Africa. Global Health Action, 3(1), 5236.

[57] Seedat, Y.K., 1999. Hypertension in black South Africans. Journal of Human Hypertension, 13: 97-103.

[58] Gómez-Olivé, F.X., Alix, S.A., Made, F., Kyobutungik, C., Nonterah, E., Micklesfield, L., Alberts, M., Boua, R., Hazelhurst, S., Debpuur, C, Mashinya, F., Dikotope, S., Sorgho, H., Cook, I., Muthuri, S., Soo, C., Mukomana, F., Agongo, G., Wandabwa, C., Afolabi, S., Oduro, A., Tinto, H., Wagner, R.G., Haregu, T., Wade, A., Kahn, K., Norris, S.A., Crowther, N.J., Tollman, S., Sankoh, O. and Ramsay, M., as members of AWI-Gen and the H3Africa Consortium, 2017. Regional and sex differences in the Prevalence and Awareness of Hypertension: An H3Africa AWI-Gen Study Across 6 Sites in Sub-Saharan Africa. Global Heart, 12 (2): 81-90.

[59] Ming, J., Sheng, L.L., Zhang, L.G., De Ren, Q., Xueyan, C., Fen,

Z.J., Ru, F.S. and Ling, W.S., 1993. Abnormal renal function in isolated systolic hypertension correlation with ambulatory blood pressure. International journal of cardiology, 41(1): 69-75.

[60] Chaudhry, S.I., Krumholz, H.M. and Foody, J.M., 2004. Systolic hypertension in older persons. Journal of the American Medical Association, 292(9): 1074-1080.

[61] Stokes, G.S., 2006. Treatment of Isolated Systolic Hypertension. Current Hypertension Reports, 8: 377-383.

[62] Martins, D., Nelson, K., Pan, D., Tareen, N. and Norris, K., 2001. The effect of gender on age-related blood pressure changes and the prevalence of isolated systolic hypertension among older adults: data from NHANES III. The Journal of Gender-specific medicine, 4 (3): 10-3, 20.

[63] Tan, J.L. and Thakur, K., 2019. Systolic Hypertension. In StatPearls [Internet]. StatPearls Publishing.

[64] Homan, T.D. and Cichowski, E., 2019. Physiology, pulse pressure. In StatPearls [Internet]. StatPearls Publishing.

[65] Wallace, S.M., Yasmin, McEniery, C.M., Mäki-Petäjä, K.M., Booth, A.D., Cockcroft, J.R. and Wilkinson, I.B., 2007. Isolated systolic hypertension is characterized by increased aortic stiffness and endothelial dysfunction. Hypertension, 50(1): 228-233.

[66] Janssen, I., Katzmarzyk, P.T. and Ross, R., 2004. Waist circumference and not body mass index explains obesity-related health risk. The American journal of clinical nutrition, 79(3): 379-384.

[67] He, F.J., Markandu, N.D., MacGregor, G.A., 2005. Modest Salt Reduction Lowers Blood Pressure in Isolated Systolic Hypertension and Combined Hypertension. Hypertension, 46 (1): 66-70.

[68] Erhun, W.O., Olayiwola, G., Agbani, E.O. and Omotoso, N.S., 2005. Prevalence of hypertension in a university community in South West Nigeria. African Journal of Biomedical Research, 8:15-19

[69] Nemes, A., Gavallér, H., Csajbók, É., Forster, T. and Csanády, M., 2008. Obesity is associated with aortic enlargement and increased stiffness: an echocardiographic study. The international journal of cardiovascular imaging, 24(2): 165-171.

[70] Brunzell, J.D. and Hokanson, J.E., 1999. Dyslipidemia of central obesity and insulin resistance. Diabetes care, 22: C10.

[71] Arcaro, G., Cretti, A., Balzano, S., Lechi, A., Muggeo, M., Bonora, E. and Bonadonna, R.C., 2002. Insulin causes endothelial dysfunction in humans: sites and mechanisms. Circulation, 105(5): 576-582.

[72] Leung, Y. and Kwan, C., 2008. Dual vascular effects of leptin via endothelium: hypothesis and perspective. Chinese Journal of Physiology, 51(1): 1-6.

[73] Schutte, R., Huisman, H.W., Schutte, A.E. and Malan, N.T., 2005. Leptin is independently associated with systolic blood pressure, pulse pressure and arterial compliance in hypertensive African women with increased adiposity: the POWIRS study. Journal of human hypertension, 19(7): 535.

[74] Maseko, M., Mashao, M., Bawa-Allah, A., Phukubje, E., Mlambo, B. and Nyundu, T., 2018. Obesity masks the relationship between dietary salt intake and blood pressure in people of African ancestry: the impact of obesity on the relationship between sodium and blood

pressure. Cardiovascular journal of Africa, 29(3): 172-176.

[75] Stoner, L., Young, J.M. and Fryer, S., 2012. Assessment of Arterial Stiffness and Endothelial Function Using Pulse Wave Analysis. International Journal of Vascular Medicine, 2012.

[76] O'Rourke, M.F. and Nichols, W.W., 2005. Aortic Diameter, Aortic Stiffness, and Wave Reflection Increase with Age and Isolated Systolic Hypertension. Hypertension, 45(4): 652-658.

[77] Antza, C., Papakatsika, S., Dimopoulos, C., Mikoudi, K., Stabouli, S. and Kotsis, V., 2015. 7C. 01: Arterial Stiffness in Isolated Office Systolic Hypertension. Journal of hypertension, 33: e96.

[78] Savage, D.D., Garrison, R.J., Kannel, W.B., Levy, D., Anderson, S.J., Stokes, J.3., Feinleib, M. and Castelli, W.P., 1987. The spectrum of left ventricular hypertrophy in a general population sample: The Framingham Study. Circulation, 75(1): 26-33.

[79] Levy, D., Garrison, R.J., Savage, D.D., Kannel, W.B. and Castelli, W.P., 1990. Prognostic implications of echocardiographically determined left ventricular mass in the Framingham Heart Study. New England Journal of Medicine, 322(22): 1561-1566.

[80] Ofili E.O., Cohen, J.D., Vrain, J.A.S., Pearson, A., Martin, T.J., Uy, N.D., Castello, R. and Labovitz, A.J., 1998. Effect of treatment of isolated systolic hypertension on left ventricular mass. Journal of the American Medical Association, 279(10): 778-780.

[81] Karpetas A, Sarafidis PA, Georgianos PI, Protogerou, A, Vakianis P, Koutroumpas G, Raptis V, Stamatiadis DN, Syrganis C, LiakopoulosV, EfstratiadisG. Ambulatory recording of wave reflections and arterial stiffness during intra-and interdialytic periods in patients treated with dialysis. Clinical Journal of the American Society of Nephrology. 2015; 10(4): 630-638.

[82] Nichols WW, Edwards DG. Arterial elastance and wave reflection augmentation of systolic blood pressure: deleterious effects and implications for therapy. Journal of cardiovascular pharmacology and therapeutics. 2001; 6(1): 5-21.

[83] Pearson AC, Gudipati C, Nagelhout D, Sear J, CohenJD, LabovitzAJ. Echocardiographic evaluation of cardiac structure and function in elderly subjects with isolated systolic hypertension. Journal of the American College of Cardiology. 1991; 17(2): 422-430.

[84] Lip GY, Blann AD. and Beevers DG. Prothrombotic factors, endothelial function and left ventricular hypertrophy in isolated systolic hypertension compared with systolic-diastolic hypertension. Journal of hypertension. 1999; 17(8): 1203-1207.

[85] Foppa M, Duncan BB, Rohde LE. Echocardiography-based left ventricular mass estimation. How should we define hypertrophy? Cardiovascular ultrasound. 2005; 3(1): 17.

[86] Skelton TN, Andrew ME, Arnett DK, Burchfiel CM, Garrison RJ, Samdarshi TE, Taylor HA, Hutchinson RG. Echocardiographic left ventricular mass in African-Americans: The Jackson cohort of the Atherosclerosis Risk in Communities Study. Echocardiography. 2003; 20(2): 111-120.

Chapter 6

Inter Arm Blood Pressure and Cardiovascular Risk in Young Adults at Ellisras

Betty Sebati, Kotsedi Monyeki, Hlengani Siweya and Susan Monyeki

Abstract

Cardiovascular disease is a notable cause of death globally. When undetected, varying measurements of BP between arms can lead to inaccuracies in the interpretation and management of blood pressure consequently putting individuals in an avoidable risk through sub-optimal blood pressure control. The aim of the study was to determine the difference in blood pressure between the arms and its association to cardiovascular risk in young adults at Ellisras. A total of 624 young adults aged 18 to 29 years old participated in the study. Blood pressure measurements and blood analysis were done according to standard procedures. Multivariate logistic regression was used to determine the association between interarm blood pressure and cardiovascular risk factors. There was significant ($p \leq 0.05$) mean difference of diastolic blood pressure of the <10 mmHg and ≥ 10 mmHg groups. There was a positive significant association between systolic inter arm blood pressure difference and hypertension (B = 5.331; 95%CI = 12.260–23.183; P = 0.026) while no significant association was found between diastolic blood pressure and interarm diastolic differences in diastolic blood pressure (B = 1.081; 95%CI = 1.032–1.131; P = 0.920). The current study showed positive associations between inter arm differences and a few cardiovascular risk factors including BMI and gender. Detection of an inter-arm BP difference should motivate the need for a thorough cardiovascular/health assessment.

Keywords: inter arm blood pressure, young adults, cardiovascular risk, cross-sectional study, association

1. Introduction

Cardiovascular disease (CVD) is a notable cause of death globally [1]. One main contributing factor to cardiovascular disease development is arteriosclerosis and it is the key cause of morbidity and mortality [2]. Blood pressure (BP) measurement is the most commonly utilized method of assessing arteriosclerosis activity [3]. Systolic blood pressure (SBP) difference between arms (inter-arm difference/IAD) is one risk marker that is easy to measure since it does not require extra equipment and seems acceptable to patients. Circumstances in which differences in BP were found in clinical settings were infrequent [4, 5].

When undetected, varying measurements of BP between arms can lead to inaccuracies in the interpretation and management of blood pressure consequently putting individuals in an avoidable risk through sub-optimal blood pressure control [6]. Furthermore it has been reported that systolic BP difference of 10 mmHg or greater between both arms was related with cardiovascular risk/complications [7, 8]. Moreover an inter arm difference is mostly encountered with differences in systolic of 10 mmHg or greater prevalent in 11% of hypertensive patients, 7% diabetic patients as well as 4% of the general population [5].

Past studies have discovered a rise in the incidence of big inter arm difference in hypertensive [9] and diabetic patients [10]. The association between inter arm difference and atherosclerosis-related diseases, such as coronary artery disease [11], and other peripheral artery disease were also reported [12, 13]. Nevertheless, the majority of these studies took place in populations that were Westernized/urbanized with little sample sizes and comprising of certain disease groups. The prevalence of selected cardiovascular risk factors has been reported in young adults at Ellisras including BP/hypertension [14], but the inter arm BP difference was not investigated. Furthermore as far as we are aware, such a study was not reported among black South Africans in Limpopo Province. Therefore the study aimed to determine the blood pressure difference between arms and its association to cardiovascular risk in young adults at Ellisras.

2. Methods and materials

2.1 Sample

The study constituted of 624 young adults (306 males; 318 females) aged 18 to 29 years old from the Ellisras Longitudinal Study (ELS) in Lephalale, Limpopo province in South Africa. The details of ELS are explained elsewhere [15]. The study was approved by the Ethics Committee at the University of Limpopo prior to the study commencing. Consent forms were also signed by the participants.

Participants with factors that could influence the reliability of the study including pregnancy and chronic diseases or hospitalization were excluded.

2.2 Blood pressure measurements

Prior to being measured the participants rested for approximately 5 minutes. Afterwards, three blood pressure (BP) readings of systolic blood pressure (SBP) And diastolic blood pressure (DBP) were measured five minutes apart in both the left and right arms using an electronic Micronta monitoring kit, [16, 17]. Average BP was calculated for both arms. Then the difference between the average SBP and DBP in the left and right arms was calculated.

2.3 Cardiovascular risk factor measurements

All participants underwent height and weight measurements according to the standard procedures [18]. The weight and height were then used to determine the body mass index (BMI) [18].

There was fasting of between 8–10 hours before the collection of blood samples. All blood sample collections were carried out in schools by qualified nurses from the

Witpoort Hospital at Ellisras in the morning. The samples were collected, stored, transported, and analyzed according to standard procedures [14].

Blood glucose (fasting) was drained into fluoride tubes and measured using an Accu-chek [19]. The total cholesterol (TC) and high-density lipoprotein cholesterol (HDL-C) levels were both measured using standard procedure that utilizes spectrophotometry. The Friedewald equation was then used to determine low density lipoprotein cholesterol (LDL-C) (LDL-C = TC - HDL-C - TG/2.2) [20]. Triglycerides (TG) measurement was done through standard enzyme-based colorimetric technique. These measurements were all accomplished using an AU480 Chemistry System from Beckman Coulter (Brea, Calif).

All apparatuses underwent calibration based on standard procedures. These blood analysis was carried out by workers in the Department of Pathology and Medical Science Unit at University of Limpopo.

The cut-off points were as follows: hypertension was defined as systolic and diastolic blood pressure ≥ 140/90 mmHg. Diabetes was defined as elevated FBG ≥7.8 mmol/L while obesity was defined as BMI (kg/m2) ≥25 kg/m^2 [21].

2.4 Statistical analysis

Inter arm systolic blood pressure difference (IASBPD) and inter arm diastolic blood pressure difference (IADBPD) were described as the absolute value of the left arm SBP/DBP minus the right arm SBP/DBP respectively. Both the IASBPD and IADBPD were grouped into two categories based on a cut-off point: <10 mmHg which is normal and ≥ 10 mmHg which is the category increasing cardiovascular risk [22]. Continuous variables were articulated as mean ± standard deviation while categorical variables were articulated as frequencies and percentages. Moreover comparisons of the variables were performed between the two cut-off groups using independent *t* test for continuous variables, and chi-square test for categorical variables. A multivariate logistic regression model was used to analyze the association between IASBPD and IADBPD, height, weight, BMI, SBP, DBP, fasting glucose, TC, TG, HDL-C, LDL-C, diabetes and hypertension. All analyses were performed using SPSS software version 14.0 and P-value of ≤0.05 was considered statistically significant.

3. Results

Table 1 represents the Descriptive statistics of the general characteristics. There was significant (p ≤ 0.05) mean difference of diastolic blood pressure of the <10 mmHg and ≥ 10 mmHg groups. The prevalence of obesity, diabetes and hypertension was insignificantly (p > 0.05) higher in the <10 mmHg group (1.8–30.9%) than the ≥10 mmHg (0–16.7%).

Table 2 shows the association between risk factors and inter arm differences in systolic blood pressure among Ellisras young adults. There was a positive significant association between IASBPD and hypertension (B = 5.331; 95%CI = 12.260–23.183; P = 0.026). There was also a positive significant association found between gender and IASBPD (B = 1.998; 95%CI = 0.022–3.903; P = 0.043).

Table 3 shows the association between risk factors and interarm differences in diastolic blood pressure among Ellisras young adults. There was a positive significant association found between SBP and IADBPD (B = 1.003; 95%CI = 0.967–1.041; P = 0.001) while there was no significant association found between DBP and IADBPD (B = 1.081; 95%CI = 1.032–1.131; P = 0.920).

Variables	<10 mmHg	≥10 mmHg	P-value
Height (cm)	168.26 ± 13.15	169.52 ± 10.19	0.743
Weight (Kg)	66.99 ± 14.22	67.74 ± 22.54	0.859
BMI (Kg/m^2)	23.51 ± 5.47	23.58 ± 7.39	0.964
SBP (mmHg)	119.99 ± 12.88	117.92 ± 20.38	0.585
DBP (mmHg)	70.03 ± 9.62	81.50 ± 15.41	0.000
Fasting glucose (mmol/L)	5.54 ± 1.27	5.38 ± 0.87	0.677
TC (mmol/L)	4.14 ± 1.03	4.39 ± 1.05	0.406
TG (mmol/L)	1.01 ± 0.59	1.05 ± 0.48	0.827
HDL-C(mmol/L)	1.15 ± 0.34	1.18 ± 0.33	0.724
LDL- C (mmol/L)	2.80 ± 0.87	3.00 ± 0.84	0.429
Gender	m = 301(49.2%) f = 311(50.8%)	m = 5 (41.7%) f = 7(58.3%)	0.606
Obesity	189(30.9%)	2(16.7%)	0.716
Diabetes	10(1.66%)	0(0%)	0.655
Hypertension	11(1.8%)	1(8.3%)	0.103

P ≤ 0.05.

Table 1.
Descriptive statistics showing general characteristics.

Variables	B	95%CI		P-value
		Lower	upper	
Age (years)	0.929	0.825	1.046	0.222
Gender	1.998	0.022	3.903	0.043
Height (cm)	1.002	0.981	1.024	0.853
Weight (kg)	1.038	0.986	1.092	0.159
BMI (Kg/m^2)	0.882	0.764	1.018	0.087
SBP (mmHg)	1.000	0.974	1.026	0.983
DBP (mmHg)	1.012	0.980	1.045	0.464
Fasting glucose(mmol/L)	1.093	0.822	1.454	0.540
TC(mmol/L)	0.000	0.000	—	1.000
TG (mmol/L)	23.905	0.000	—	1.000
HDL-C (mmol/L)	1174525.430	0.000	—	1.000
LDL-C (mmol/L)	7854389.463	0.000	—	1.000
Diabetes	0.000	0.000	—	0.999
Hypertension	5.331	12.260	23.183	0.026

P ≤ 0.05.

Table 2.
The association between risk factors and inter arm differences in SBP.

Variables	B	95%CI		P-value
		Lower	upper	0.105
Age (years)	0.858	0.713	1.032	0.203
Gender	1.970	0.963	5.596	0.596
Height (cm)	1.023	0.940	1.113	0.851
Weight (kg)	1.013	0.889	1.153	0.654
BMI (Kg/m^2)	0.920	0.640	1.323	0.853
SBP (mmHg)	1.003	0.967	1.041	0.001
DBP (mmHg)	1.081	1.032	1.131	0.920
Fasting gucose(mmol/L)	1.024	0.624	1.632	1.000
TC(mmol/L)	187307.604	0.000	—	1.000
TG (mmol/L)	0.072	0.000	—	1.000
HDL-C (mmol/L)	0.000	0.000	—	1.000
LDL-C (mmol/L)	0.000	0.000	—	1.000
Diabetes	0.000	0.000	—	0.999
Hypertension	0.261	0.022	3.132	0.290

$P \leq 0.05$.

Table 3.
The association between risk factors and inter arm differences in diastolic blood pressure among Ellisras young adults.

4. Discussion

In the current study, 12 participants (5 males and 7 females; 1.92% of the sample size) showed an inter arm difference ≥ 10 mmHg. A previous study has suggested that interarm BP difference was more usual among young healthy study participants, with an interarm blood pressure difference > 10 mm Hg reported in 111 (12.6%) and 77 (8.8%) participants for SBP and DBP respectively [23]. The current study did not find similar results due to a low prevalence found. Another study conducted among hypertensive patients reported a prevalence of 7.7% (285 patients with a systolic interarm difference of ≥10 mm Hg), while 1.5% (57 patients) had a ≥ 10 mmHg diastolic interarm blood pressure difference. Furthermore, a study by Kim et al. [22] reported a 0.6% (21 patients) prevalence for both systolic and diastolic interarm difference ≥ 10 mmHg.

The different findings found between the current and other related studies could be because of the varying age groups, diseases profile of the participants (some being healthy and others suffering from hypertension and other chronic diseases) or even the different methods used to measure the interarm BP difference. The difference in systolic blood pressure between arms is considered a risk marker and advantageous due to that it is easy to measure clinically without additional equipment and is more acceptable to patients. Furthermore, studies have associated a systolic inter arm difference ≥ 15 mmHg [24], and ≥ 10 mmHg with cardiovascular risk and mortality [7]. The inability to detect the interarm BP difference may result in insufficient treatment of people suffering from hypertension and interrupt hypertension diagnosis. Hence, it is vital to measure blood pressure in both arms.

A previous study has reported that blood pressure measured in only one arm would lead to approximately 30% misdiagnosis of hypertensive patients being wrongfully classified as normotensive [25].

In multivariate logistic regression of the current study, a positive significant association was found between systolic interarm blood pressure and hypertension as well as gender. In addition there was also a positive significant association found between SBP and diastolic interarm blood pressure difference in the current study. A previous study by Kimura et al. [26], reported a positive association between systolic interarm systolic blood pressure > 10 mm Hg and SBP and BMI. This was different from the findings of the current study since we found a non-significant association between BMI and both IASBPD and IADBPD. Furthermore, another study by Grossman et al. [27], reported that interarm BP difference was not associated with age, BMI, and heart rate, but was in association with SBP in both young and healthy patients [27]. The latter findings are similar to the current study since we found an association between SBP and IADBPD. Moreover, A study by Grossman et al. [27] which is supported by another study by Ma et al. [28], reported that high inter arm systolic blood pressure difference seems to be more common in older than in younger people.

The study had several limitations. The study had limited variables to broadly represent the large spectrum of cardiovascular risk/health. The effect of controlling interarm blood pressure difference on cardiovascular risk could not be evaluated at this stage. The study did not have a large range in terms of the age hence the effect of age on the inter arm blood pressure difference could not be adequately determined. The cardiovascular health status of the participants was determined on a cross sectional basis hence some factors that can temporarily affect measurements may have affected the readings. The nature of the study cannot fully establish a cause and effect relationship, hence possible bias cannot be ruled out.

5. Conclusions

The current study found a low prevalence of interarm BP difference and showed positive associations between inter arm differences and a few cardiovascular risk factors including hypertension and gender. More similar studies should include a variety of risk factors and diseases as well as a broader age group. Carrying out such an investigation on a longitudinal basis is also necessary for exclusion of factors that can temporarily affect the findings. Detection of an interarm BP difference that is $\geq$10 mmHg should motivate the need for a thorough cardiovascular/health assessment to prevent late diagnosis and other related complications.

Acknowledgements

The Ellisras Longitudinal Study (ELS) administrators, Mr. Makata, Mrs. Makgae, as well as Mr. T Tselapedi are greatly acknowledged. The ELS participants and community coordinators are gratefully recognized for their assistance.

Abbreviation

ELS	Ellisras Longitudinal Study

Author details

Betty Sebati[1], Kotsedi Monyeki[1*], Hlengani Siweya[2] and Susan Monyeki[1]

1 Department of Physiology and Environmental Health, University of Limpopo, Sovenga, South Africa

2 Executive Dean Faculty of Science and Agriculture, University of Limpopo, Sovenga, South Africa

*Address all correspondence to: kotsedi.monyeki@ul.ac.za

References

[1] Clark CE, Boddy K, Warren FC, Taylor RS, Aboyans V, Cloutier L, McManus RJ, Shore AC, Campbell JL. Associations between interarm differences in blood pressure and cardiovascular disease outcomes: protocol for an individual patient data meta analysis and development of a prognostic algorithm. BMJ Open. 2017; 7:e016844. doi:10.1136/bmjopen-2017-016844.

[2] Kusunose K, Sato M, Yamada H, Saijo Y, Bando M, Hirata Y, Nishio S, Hayashi S, Sata M. Prognostic implications of non-invasive vascular function tests in high-risk atherosclerosis patients. Circ J. 2016; 80:1034-40.

[3] Shimamoto K, Ando K, Fujita T, Hasebe N, Higaki J, Horiuchi M, Imai Y, Imaizumi T, Ishimitsu T, Ito M, Ito S, Itoh H, Iwao H, Kai H, Kario K, Kashihara N, Kawano Y, Kim-Mitsuyama S, Kimura G, Kohara K, Komuro I, Kumagai H, Matsuura H, Miura K, Morishita R , Naruse M, Node K, Ohya Y, Rakugi H, Saito I ,Saitoh S, Shimada K, Shimosawa K, Suzuki H,Tamura K ,Tanahashi N, Tsuchihashi T, Uchiyama M , Ueda S, Umemura S. The Japanese Society of Hypertension Guidelines for the Management of Hypertension (JSH 2014). Hypertens Res. 2014; 37:253-390.

[4] Tanaka Y, Fukui M, Tanaka M, Fukuda Y, Mitsuhashi K, Okada H, Yamazaki M, Hasegawa G, Yoshioka K, Nakamura N. The inter-arm difference in systolic blood pressure is a novel risk marker for subclinical atherosclerosis in patients with type 2 diabetes. Hypertens Res. 2014; 37:548-52.

[5] Clark CE, Taylor RS, Shore AC, Campbell JL. Prevalence of systolic inter-arm differences in blood pressure for different primary care populations: system- atic review and meta-analysis. Br J Gen Pract. 2016; 66:e838-47.

[6] McDonagh, S, Clark, CE. Inter-arm differences in blood pressure: a brief summary. Diabetes and Primary Care. 26 September 2019.

[7] Cao KW, Xu JS, Qing SG, Hu WT, Li P, Cheng XS, Su H. Association of an inter-arm systolic blood pressure difference with all-cause and cardiovascular mortality: an updated meta-analysis of cohort studies. Int J Cardiol. 2015; 189: 211-9.

[8] Zhou M, Gao Z, Chen F, Xu HJ, Dong X, Ma L. The inter-arm systolic blood pressure difference and risk of cardiovascular mortality: a meta-analysis of cohort studies. Clin Exp Hypertens. 2016; 38:317-24.

[9] Fonseca-Reyes S, Forsyth-MacQuarrie AM, Garcia de Alba-Garcia JE. Simultaneous blood pressure measurement in both arms in hypertensive and nonhypertensive adult patients. Blood Press Monit. 2012; 17:149-54.

[10] Clark CE, Steele AM, Taylor RS, Shore AC, Ukoumunne OC, Campbell J. Interarm blood pressure difference in people with diabetes: measurement and vascular and mortality implications: a cohort study. Diabetes Care. 2014; 37:1613-20.

[11] Igarashi Y, Chikamori T, Tomiyama H, Usui Y, Hida S, Tanaka H, Nagao T, Yamashina A. Clinical significance of interarm pressure difference and ankle-brachial pressure index in patients with suspected coronary artery disease. J Cardiol. 2007; 50:281-9.

[12] Clark CE. Difference in blood pressure between arms might reflect peripheral vascular disease. BMJ. 2001; 323:399-1399.

[13] Clark CE, Campbell JL, Powell RJ. The interarm blood pressure difference

as predictor of cardiovascular events in patients with hypertension in primary care: cohort study. J Hum Hypertens. 2007; 21:633-8.

[14] Sebati B, Monyeki K ,Kemper HCG, Sekgala MD, Mphekgwana P. 2019. Anthropometric indices for predicting cardiovascular risk factors: Ellisras longitudinal study. AM J HUM BIOL. 2019; e23293.

[15] Monyeki KD, Van Lenthe FJ, Steyn NP. Obesity: does it occur in African children in a rural community in South Africa?. Int j epidemiol. 1999; 28: 287-292.

[16] National High Blood Pressure Education Program (NHBPEP). Update on the 1987 task force report on high blood pressure in children and adolescents: a working group report from the National High Blood Pressure Education Program. Paediatrics. 1996; 98: 649-658.

[17] National High Blood Pressure Education Program NHBPEP. National High Blood Pressure Education Program Working Group on High Blood Pressure in Children and Adolescents. The fourth report on the diagnosis, evaluation, and treatment of high blood pressure in children and adolescents. Pediatrics. 2004; 114: 555-576.

[18] Norton K, Olds, T. (Eds.). Anthropometrica: a textbook of body measurement for sports and health courses. UNSW press: 1996.

[19] Barrett SC, Huffman FG, Johnson, P. Validation of finger-prick testing of fasting blood glucose, total cholesterol, and HbA1c in adolescents. Point of Care. 2011; 10: 51-58.

[20] Friedewald WT, Levy RI, Fredrickson DS. Estimation of the concentration of low-density lipoprotein cholesterol in plasma, without use of the preparative ultracentrifuge. Clinical chemistry. 1972; 18: 499-502.

[21] Ho SY, Lam TH, Janus ED. Waist to stature ratio is more strongly associated with cardiovascular risk factors than other simple anthropometric indices. Ann epidemiol. 2003; 13(10): 683-691.

[22] Kim SA, Kim JY, Park JB. Significant interarm blood pressure difference predicts cardiovascular risk in hypertensive patients. Medicine. 2016: 95(24).

[23] Grossman A, Prokupetz A, Gordon B, Morag-Koren N, Grossman E. Inter-arm blood pressure differences in young, healthy patients. *J Clin Hypertens (Greenwich)*. 2013;15:575-578.

[24] Clark CE, Taylor RS, Shore AC, Ukoumunne OC, Campbell JL. Association of a difference in systolic blood pressure between arms with vascular disease and mortality: a systemic review and meta-analysis. The Lancet. 2012; 379 (9819):905-914.

[25] Poon LC, Kametas N, Strobl I, Pachoumi C, Nicolaides KH. Inter-arm blood pressure differences in pregnant women. *BJOG*. 2008; 115:1122-1130.

[26] Kimura A, Hashimoto J, Watabe D, Takahashi H, Ohkubo T, Kikuya M, Imai Y. Patient characteristics and factors associated with inter-arm difference of blood pressure measurements in a general population in Ohasama, Japan. *J Hypertens*. 2004; 22:2277-2283.

[27] Grossman A, Weiss A, Beloosesky Y, Morag-Koren N, Green H, Grossman E. Inter-arm blood pressure difference in hospitalized elderly patients-is it consistent? *J Clin Hypertens (Greenwich)*. 2014; 16:518-523.

[28] Ma W, Zhang B, Yang Y, Qi L , Meng L, Zhang Y, Huo Y. Correlating the relationship between interarm systolic blood pressure and cardiovascular disease risk factors. *J Clin Hypertens*. 2017;19:466-471. https://doi.org/10.1111/jch.12987

Chapter 7

Association of Anthropometric Parameters with Blood Pressure and Blood Glucose among Ellisras Children

Moloko Matshipi, Hlengani James Siweya and Phuti Joanna Makgae

Abstract

Obesity as directly measured by anthropometric parameters has been demonstrated to be associated with hypertension and type 2 diabetes mellitus, which are common risk factors for CVD. The study aimed at assessing the relationship between blood pressure, blood glucose and anthropometric parameters in Ellisras children. A total of 492 children aged 6 to 11 years, participated in the study. Neck circumference, waist circumference, body mass index, waist-to-height ratio, fasting blood glucose, systolic and diastolic blood pressure were measured using standard procedures. Linear regression showed significant association ($P < 0.05$) of anthropometric parameters (except waist-to-height ratio) with blood pressure. Fasting blood glucose was significantly associated with neck circumference when adjusted for age and gender. Positive correlation was found for systolic blood pressure with neck and waist circumference and body mass index in both genders and for diastolic blood pressure, the correlation was only found in boys. Fasting blood glucose was negatively correlated with neck circumference. Waist circumference ($P = 0.025$, $\beta = 1.208$, 95% CI = 1.017–1.285) was better than BMI ($P = 0.046$, $\beta = 1.340$, 95% CI = 1.005–1.788) in predicting elevated systolic blood pressure. These findings suggest that it is crucial to manage anthropometric parameters in the Ellisras community in order to decelerate the increase of hypertension and diabetes mellitus.

Keywords: body mass index, neck circumference, waist circumference, waist to height ratio, fasting blood glucose and blood pressure

1. Introduction

Obesity is a key global public health alarm with about 500 million people worldwide affected [1, 2]. In epidemiological studies, anthropometric parameters, body mass index (BMI), waist circumference (WC), neck circumference (NC) and waist-height ratio (WHtR) are often used as measures of obesity [2–5]. Obesity as directly measured by anthropometric technique has been demonstrated to be associated with hypertension and type 2 diabetes mellitus, common risk factors for CVD [6, 7].

IntechOpen

The diagnosis of diabetes is often based on a fasting plasma glucose, random plasma glucose, a 2-hour plasma glucose value in a 75 g oral glucose tolerance test or a glycated hemoglobin (A1C) measurement, but generally on fasting plasma glucose, partly because of its better sensitivity to diagnose diabetes [5, 8]. Hypertension uses information about systolic blood pressure (SBP) and/or diastolic blood pressure (DBP) to derive an estimate for diagnosis [9].

In view of the burden of obesity, hypertension and diabetes and their impact on children and the scarcity of information on the relationship of blood glucose, blood pressure with anthropometric parameters in rural South African communities, more especially in Ellisras, the present study aimed to determine the relationship of blood pressure and blood glucose with anthropometric parameters among Ellisras rural children aged 6 to 11 years and to determine which of the anthropometric parameters is associated with greater odds of high blood pressure and high blood glucose levels in this population.

2. Methodology

2.1 Geographical area

Ellisras, also known as Lephalale, is a relatively deep rural area located within the North- western area of Limpopo province, South Africa. The population consist of approximately 50000 people residing in 42 settlements and are adjacent to the Botswana border. Majority of residence in this population work at Iscor coal mine and Matimba electricity power station, whereas the remaining work class is involved in subsistence farming, while the minority is in civil services and education [10].

2.2 Sampling and study design

Research design and sampling method for the Ellisras Longitudinal study (ELS) have been reported elsewhere [10].

In this study, a total of 492 children (n = 296 boys; n = 196 girls) aged 6 to11 who are part of the ELS, participated in this study. Ethical approval prior to this study was obtained from Ethics Committee of the University of Limpopo. Guardians were provided with, and signed, written informed assent.

2.3 Anthropometry

Anthropometric measurements were done according to the International Society for the Advancement of Kin-anthropometry (ISAK). Weight was measured on an electronic scale to the nearest 0.1 kg, and a Martin anthropometry was used to measure height to the nearest 0.1 cm. Flexible steel tape was used to measure NC and WC. Waist circumference was measured midway between the lower costal margin and iliac crest immediately after exhalation. Neck circumference was measured directly below the thyroid cartilage perpendicular to the long axis of the neck. All measurements were taken with the participants standing in an anatomical position.

Children with BMI $<$85th, $\geq$85th and $\geq$ 95th percentile were considered normal, overweight and obese, respectively [7]. Children with WC $\geq$90th percentile were considered to have abdominal obesity, and those with NC 90th $\geq$ were considered to have obesity [3, 11]. BMI was calculated as weight in kilograms (kg) divided by the square of height in metres (m), whereas waist to height ratio was calculated as waist circumference divided by height.

2.4 Blood pressure

To measure blood glucose, the participants were first made comfortable, by sitting on the chair for at least five minutes before measurements. From each subject at least three reading blood pressure (systolic and diastolic) measurements were taken, at an interval of five minutes apart. Blood pressures readings were taken using electronic Micronta monitoring kit. The device has a bladder which contains an electronic infrasonic transducer that monitors the blood pressure and pulse rate, thus displaying these on the screen. Hypertension was defined by systolic and diastolic blood pressure ≥ 95th percentile of age and sex adjusted reference level [6].

2.5 Blood glucose

To measure blood glucose level all subjects were asked to do an 10 hours overnight fasting prior to the test, in the morning their capillary blood sample were obtained by a finger prick and blood was caught up in little cuvettes, which were prepared with below mentioned reagents (glucose oxidase and reagents to measure the generation of hydrogen peroxide such as non-toxic phenol red and horseradish peroxidase was bonded to filter paper). After mixing with the reagents, fasting blood glucose was measured using Hemocue® [8]. Type 2 diabetes mellitus was defined by fasting blood glucose ≥7.1 mmol/L of sex and age adjusted reference level.

2.6 Statistical analysis

All the statistical analyses were performed using the Statistical Package for the Social Sciences (SPSS) version 25. Data comparison was done using student t-test for 2 groups. Descriptive statistics were performed for age, anthropometric parameters, fasting blood glucose and blood pressure (systolic and diastolic). The Linear regression model was used to assess the association between blood pressure (systolic and diastolic), blood glucose and anthropometric parameters after adjusting for potential confounders. The logistic regression was used to determine the risk of developing hypertension and type 2 diabetes mellitus using anthropometric parameters. Statistical significance was set at a probability level of 0.05 (**Figures 1** and **2**).

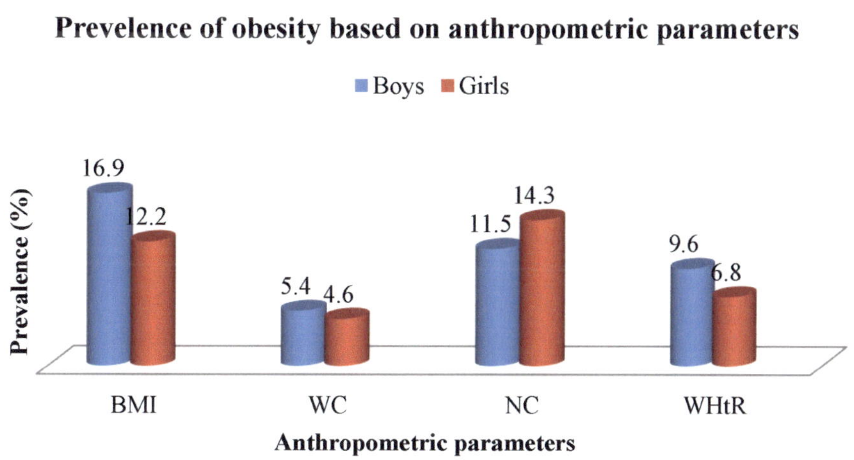

Figure 1.
Gender specific prevalence of obesity based on WC, BMI, WHtR and NC among Ellisras children aged 6 to 11 years. The prevalence of obesity was higher in boys measured by BMI (16.9%), WC (5.4%) and WHtR (9.6%), as compared to girls BMI (12.2%), WC (4.6%) and WHtR (6.2%) and that measured by NC was higher in girls (14.3%) than in boys (11.5%).

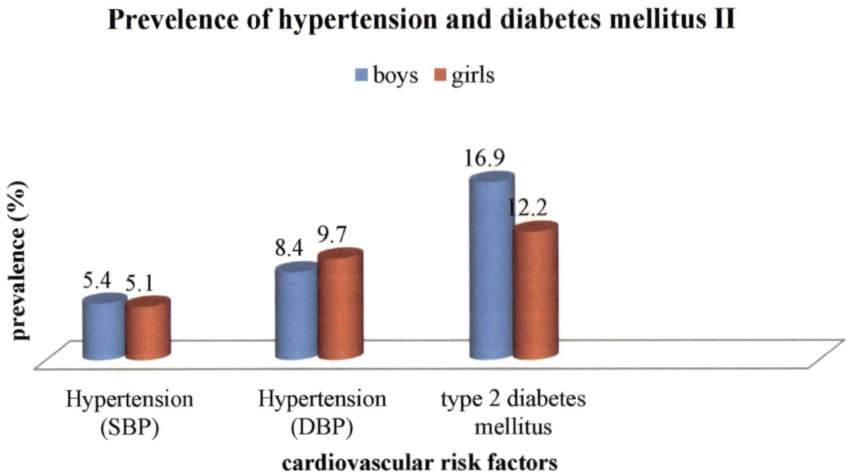

Figure 2.
Gender-specific prevalence of hypertension and type 2 diabetes mellitus among Ellisras children age 6 to 11 years. The prevalence of hypertension defined by SBP was higher in boys (5.4%) than in girls (5.1%), hypertension defined by DBP was higher in girls (9.7%) than in boys (8.4%) and that of type 2 diabetes mellitus was higher in boys (16.9%) as compared to girls (12.2%).

3. Results

Table 1 showed descriptive statistics of anthropometric parameters, blood pressure and fasting blood glucose stratified by gender. The study population comprised predominately boys (60%) with boy to girl ratio of 1.51:1. Boys showed higher mean values of age NC, WC, BMI and WHtR than girls. In contrast, girls had higher mean SBP, DBP and FBG values.

Table 2 showed positive correlation for systolic blood pressure with NC (0.261** and 0.252**), WC (0.276** and 0.208**) and NC (0.264** and 0.233**) in boys and girls respectively. Positive correlation was found for diastolic blood pressure with NC (0.176**), WC (0.272**) and BMI (0.212**) in boys. Negative correlation was found for fasting blood glucose with NC (−0.147*) and positive correlation for fasting blood glucose with BMI (0.176*)

Variables	Boys	Girls
Age (years)	9.637 (1.351)	9.341 (1.086)
SBP (mmHg)	96.621 (11.569)	97.740 (10.540)
DBP(mmHg)	65.426 (8.930)	66.300 (9.216)
FBG (mmol/L)	4.542 (1.900)	4.707 (1.160)
BMI (kg/m^2)	14.411 (1.203)	14.182 (1.368)
NC (cm)	25.850 (1.350)	25.287 (1.275)
WHtR	0.411 (0.022)	0.407 (0.023)
WC (cm)	54.720 (3.153)	53.853 (3.354)

M = Mean; SD = standard deviation; NC = Neck Circumference (cm); WC = waist circumference (cm); BMI = body mass index (kg/m^2); WHtR = waist to height ration; SBP = systolic blood pressure (mmHg); DBP = diastolic blood pressure (mmHg); FBG = fasting blood glucose (mmol/L).

Table 1.
Descriptive statistics of anthropometric parameters, systolic and diastolic blood pressure and blood glucose of Ellisras children age 6 to 11 years.

	SBP		DBP		FBG	
	Boys	**Girls**	**Boys**	**Girls**	**Boys**	**Girls**
FBG	−0.029	0.075	0.044	0.131		
NC	0.261**	0.252**	0.176**	0.102	−0.147*	−0.027
WC	0.276**	0.208**	0.272**	0.065	−0.065	0.111
BMI	0.264**	0.233**	0.212**	0.096	−0.004	0.176*
WHtR	−0.046	0.058	0.064	0.025	0.031	0.035

***$p < 0.001$; *$p < 0.05$ statistical significant; NC = Neck Circumference (cm); WC = waist circumference (cm); BMI = body mass index (kg/m^2); WHtR = waist to height ration.*

Table 2.
Pearson correlation coefficient (r) of blood pressure (systolic and diastolic) and blood glucose with anthropometric parameters.

	Unadjusted			Adjusted for age and sex		
Para meters	**β**	**P-value**	**95%CI**	B	**P-value**	**95%CI**
Systolic blood pressure						
BMI	0.244	<0.001	1.390–2.901	0.161	<0.001	0.942–2.529
WC	0.240	<0.001	0.528–1.120	0.186	<0.001	0.296–2.072
WHtR	−0.009	0.838	−49.434–40.129	0.069	0.135	−10.957–80.784
NC	0.242	<0.001	1.294–2.724	0.197	<0.001	0.780–2.485
Diastolic blood pressure						
BMI	0.156	<0.001	0.487–1.731	0.072	0.004	0.319–1.640
WC	0.177	<0.001	0.249–0.734	0.171	<0.001	0.190–0.758
WHtR	0.043	0.337	−18.486–53.846	0.091	0.053	−0.463–75.012
NC	0.134	0.003	0.307–1.488	0.120	0.026	0.098–1.515
Fasting blood glucose						
BMI	0.046	0.312	−0.056–0.173	0.083	0.081	−0.014–0.229
WC	−0.018	0.692	−0.054–0.036	0.034	0.516	−0.035–0.070
WHtR	0.027	0.551	−4.582–8.586	0.011	0.824	−6.137–7.704
NC	−0.120	0.008	−0.254–−0.039	−0.104	0.054	−0.257–0.002

P value < 0.05 = statistical significant; CI = confidence interval; β = beta; NC = Neck Circumference (cm); WC = waist circumference (cm); BMI = body mass index (kg/m^2); WHtR = waist to height ration.

Table 3.
Linear regression analysis for the association of anthropometric parameters with, blood glucose and blood pressures.

Table 3 shows the linear regression for the association of anthropometric parameters (NC, BMI, WC and WHtR) with DBP, SBP and FBG. There was a significant association of SBP with BMI (β = 0.244, 95%CI = 1.390–2.901), WC (β = 0.240, 95%CI = 0.528–1.120) and NC (β = 0.242, 95%CI = 1.294–2.724).

Table 4 showed binary logistic regression analysis for determining the odds of high blood pressure and high blood glucose using anthropometric parameters. After multivariate adjustment by age and gender, BMI (P = 0.046, β = 1.340, 95% CI = 1.005–1.788) showed to have significantly greatest odds for high SBP followed by WC (P = 0.025, β = 1.143, 95% CI = 1.017–1.285).

	Unadjusted		Adjusted for age and gender
		Systolic blood pressure	
Parameters	**OR(95% CI)**	**P value**	**OR (95% CI)**
BMI	1.340 (1.005–1.788)	0.046	1.258(0.925–1.709)
NC	1.208 (0.903–1.617)	0.203	1.080(0.763–1.530)
WC	1.143 (1.017–1.285)	0.025	1.115(0.975–1.276)
WHtR	1.510 (1.106–1.666)	0.579	1.413(0.752–1.777)
Diastolic blood pressure			
BMI	1.150 (0.909–1.456)	0.244	1.210(0.941–1.558)
NC	1.076 (0.856–1.354)	0.529	1.189(0.901–1.571)
WC	1.069 (0.973–1.174)	0.164	1.120(1.004–1.249)
WHtR	1.042 (0.144–1.317)	0.092	0.172(0.093–3.181)
Fasting blood glucose			
BMI	0.987 (0.827–1.177)	0.884	1.009(0.838–1.215)
NC	0.831 (0.701–0.986)	0.034	0.813(0.663–0.998)
WC	0.975 (0.910–1.045)	0.479	0.983(0.907–1.066)
WHtR	0.137(0.124–1.432)	0.083	0.978(0.809–1.183)

P value < 0.05 = statistical significant; CI = confidence interval; OR = odds ratio; NC = Neck Circumference (cm); WC = waist circumference (cm); BMI = body mass index (kg/m^2); WHtR = waist to height ration.

Table 4.
Binary logistic regression analysis of anthropometric parameters with systolic and diastolic blood pressure.

4. Discussion

The main purpose of the study was to determine the relationship of blood pressure, blood glucose with anthropometric parameters among Ellisras children aged 6 to 11 years old and several major findings emerged.

The present study showed that NC is significantly associated with blood glucose, which corroborates the previous findings that increased NC is an emerging risk factor for high blood glucose [12]. However, it is difficult to explain in the present study why only NC was associated with fasting blood glucose, although BMI, WC and WHtR are also anthropometric parameters. One possible explanation for these findings may be that different anthropometric parameters have varied impact on blood glucose. The mechanism linking anthropometric parameters with blood glucose levels is not clear but main schools of thought on the matter suggest different mechanisms. Firstly, in obesity (i.e WHR >0.90 or BMI >30 kg/m2), abundance of circulating fatty acids and liver-derived triglyceride (VLDL) provide an excellent fuel for muscle, decreasing their requirement for glucose [13]. People with obesity tend to be sedentary, and thus muscle consumes less glucose [14]. In obesity, increased delivery of fatty acids to the liver (as in visceral obesity) enhances gluconeogenesis and thus leading to production of glucose [15]. In obesity the increased fatty acid cause insulin resistance directly by activating enzymes that decrease the response to insulin, thereby aggravates the pre-existing insulin resistance which results in elevated blood glucose level and eventually type 2 diabetes mellitus [16].

The study also demonstrated that NC, WC and BMI are significantly associated with blood pressure, which confirms the observations of the previous findings around the relationship between mean anthropometric parameters and blood pressure values [4, 7, 17]. However, the precise mechanism by which anthropometric parameters act to increase blood pressure is not fully understood. One possible mechanism is linked to the prognostic importance of visceral adipose tissue assessments by WC rather than general obesity assessments by BMI [18, 19]. Visceral adipose tissue produces angiotensinogen, interleukin-6 and leptin [20]. An imbalance in production of these adipokines, particularly angiotensinogen leads to the activation of the rennin-angiotensin system, causing vasoconstriction and reabsorption of sodium [20]. The constriction of blood vessels increases blood pressure and eventually the development of high blood pressure.

This study has several limitations. Firstly this is a cross sectional study and does not allow establishment of cause-effect relationship, secondly the study model does not provide information regarding the ability of anthropometric parameter to future health outcome, and lastly the study was conducted in rural areas in Ellisras so the findings might not be generalizable to the overall Ellisras population.

5. Conclusion

The study shows that both blood glucose and blood pressure are associated with some anthropometric parameters. These findings suggest that it is crucial to manage and control traditional risk factors in rural South African communities in Ellisras in order to decelerate the increase in obesity, hypertension and type 2 diabetes mellitus and to reduce the burden of cardiovascular disease. The present study highlights the need of incorporating body mass index (BMI), waist circumference (WC), neck circumference (NC) and waist-height ratio (WHtR) while evaluating the association of easily accessed anthropometric parameters with CVD risk factors.

Acknowledgements

The ELS administrators T.T. Makata, L. Majadibodu, and U.T. Motlogelwa are greatly acknowledged for coding the ELS data.

Conflict of interest

The authors declare no conflict of interest.

Author details

Moloko Matshipi[1*], Hlengani James Siweya[2] and Phuti Joanna Makgae[1*]

1 Department of Physiology and Environmental Health, University of Limpopo, Polokwane, South Africa

2 Faculty of Science and Agriculture, University of Limpopo, Polokwane, South Africa

*Address all correspondence to: moloko.matshipi@ul.ac.za; phutimakgae@gmail.com

DOI: http://dx.doi.org/10.5772/intechopen.95938

References

[1] Finucane MM, Stevens GA, Cowan MJ, Danaei G, Lin JK, Paciorek CJ. National, regional, and global trends in body-mass index since 1980: systematic analysis of health examination surveys and epidemiological studies with 960 country-years and 9• 1 million participants. The Lancet, 12: 57-67.

[2] Zhu Y, Shao Z, Jing J, Ma J, Chen Y, Li X, Yang W, Guo L, Jin Y. Body mass index is better than other anthropometric indices for identifying dyslipidaemia in Chinese children with obesity. 2016.

[3] Ribas SA and Santana da Silva LC. Anthropometric indices; predictors of dyslipidaemia in children and adolescents from north of Brazil. Nutricion Hospitalaria 2012; 27: 1228-1235.

[4] Priyanka NP, ArunKavana GV, Nayanatara A, Anupama N and Ramesh B. Association of anthropometric indices of obesity with dyslipidemia: A study from South India. European Journal of Biotechnology and Bioscience 2014; 2: 59-62.

[5] Rao J, Bhat AN, and Bhati AS. Relationship of anthropometric variables with fasting blood sugar in moderate and sedentary workers. International Journal of Basic and Applied Physiology 2017; 6: 112-118.

[6] Ramoshaba NE, Monyeki KD, Zatu MC, Hay L and Mabata LR. The Relationship between Blood Pressure and Anthropometric Indicators in Rural South African Children: Ellisras Longitudinal Study. Journal of Obesity and Weight Loss Therapy 2015; 12: 135-142.

[7] Kondolot M, Horoz D, Poyrazoğlu S, Borlu A, Öztürk A, Kurtoğlu S and Mazıcıoğlu MM. Neck Circumference to Assess Obesity in Preschool Children. Journal of Clinical Research in Paediatric Endocrinology 2017; 9: 17-23.

[8] Matshipi M, Monyeki KD and Kemper H. The Relationship between Physical Activity and Plasma Glucose Level amongst Ellisras Rural Young Adult Males and Females: Ellisras Longitudinal Study. International Journal of Environmental Research and Public Health 2017; 14:

[9] Cassani RSL, Fernando N, Pazin-Filho A and Schmid A. Relationship between blood pressure and anthropometry in a cohort of Brazilian men: A Cross-Sectional Study. American Journal of Hypertension 2009; 22: 980-984.

[10] Monyeki KD, Kemper HGC and Makgae PJ. The association of fat patterning with blood pressure in rural South African children: the Ellisras Longitudinal Growth and Health Study. International Journal of Epidemiology 2005; 35: 114-120.

[11] Kurtoglu S, Hatipoglu N, Mazicioglu MM and Kondolot M. Neck circumference as a novel parameter to determine metabolic risk factors in obese children. European Journal of Clinical Investment 2012; 42: 623-630.

[12] Ben-Noun L and Laor A. Relationship between changes in neck circumference and cardiovascular risk factors. Clinical Cardiology 2006; 11: 14-20.

[13] Mittendorfer B, Yoshino M, Patterson BW, and Klein S. VLDL Triglyceride Kinetics in Lean, Overweight, and Obese Men and Women. J Clin Endocrinol Metab 2016; 101:4151-4160.

[14] Strasser B. Physical activity in obesity and metabolic syndrome. Ann N Y Acad Sci 2013; 1281: 141-159.

[15] Ghosh A. Comparison of anthropometric, metabolic and dietary fatty acids profiles in lean and obese dyslipidaemic Asian Indian male subjects. Eur J Clin Nutr 2007; 61: 2-9.

[16] Marshall WJ and Bangert SJ. ISBN 9780723434603. "Obesity. Clinical Chemistry", 6th ed. Ch.14.London: Mosby Elsevier, 2008: 271.

[17] Deshmukh PR, Gupta SS, Dongre AR, Bharambe MS, Maliye C, Kaur S and Gar BS. Relationship of anthropometric indicators with blood pressure levels in rural Wardha. Indian Journal of Medical Research 2006; 123: 657-664.

[18] Thompson M, Dana T, Bougatsos C, Blazina I and Norris SL. Screening for hypertension in children and adolescents to prevent cardiovascular disease. Paediatrics 2013; 131: 490-525.

[19] Gupta N, Goel K, Shah P, Misra A. Childhood obesity in developing countries: epidemiology, determinants, and prevention. Endocr Rev. 2012; 33: 48-70.

[20] Weisberg SP, McCann D, Desai M, Rosenbaum M, Leibel RL, Ferrante AW., Jr. Obesity is associated with macrophage accumulation in adipose tissue. The Journal of Clinical Investigation 2003; 11:1796-1808.

Chapter 8

Factors Associated with Overweight and Obesity among Women Aged 15-49 Years in Zimbabwe: Evidence from the 2005/6, 2010/11 and 2015 Zimbabwe Demographic and Health Survey

Kudzaishe Mangombe, Naomi Wekwete, Amos Milanzi, Ronald Musizvingoza and Charles Lwanga

Abstract

Overweight and obesity have increasingly become a health concern globally and, in particular, developing countries such as Zimbabwe. Obesity is associated with an increased risk of non-communicable diseases such as diabetes and cardiovascular diseases. Previous studies in the country have controlled for other factors, but none have examined the relationship between household assets ownership and body mass index. This study examines the association between demographic, socioeconomic factors and household assets ownership and obesity among Zimbabwean women of reproductive age over the 10-year period from 2005 to 2015 based on three Demographic and Health Surveys. The analytical sample consisted of non-pregnant women aged 15–49 years who were *dejure* household residents. Logistic regression models were used to examine the association between background variables and Body Mass Index. Women in urban areas, with higher education, working and from richer households are more likely to be at risk of overweight and obesity. However, possession of household assets such as television, radio and telephone were not associated with overweight/obesity, except for the television in 2010/11. Thus, there is need for constant awareness programmes on healthy eating food, and physical activity especially among older women and those working.

Keywords: obesity, overweight, household assets, trends, Zimbabwe

1. Introduction

Obesity has become a public health problem that has shifted from being a problem in rich countries to one that is found across all income levels. Worldwide obesity has nearly tripled and it is estimated that 4.7 million people died prematurely in 2017 due to obesity-related causes [1]. The number of premature deaths due to obesity-related causes is projected to increase to 5.5 million in 2025 [2]. Sub-Saharan Africa has the lowest prevalence of obesity in comparison to other regions of the world [3]. However, the prevalence of obesity and overweight is projected to increase in the next two decades [4] and Southern Africa is disproportional affected [5]. In response to this, World Health Organisation (WHO) came out with "Global action plan on physical activity 2018–2030: more active people for a healthier world" which is aimed at providing effective and feasible policy actions to increase physical activity globally [6]. In Zimbabwe, the prevalence of overweight and obesity increased substantially over the decade from 25% in 2005 to 36.6% in 2015 [7]. Obesity is likely to lead to death, high blood pressure/hypertension, high cholesterol coronary, diabetes, cardiovascular diseases (CVDs), hypertension, coronary heart disease, and stroke [6].

Evidence from several research studies indicated that socio-economic background factors increased the likelihood for individuals to end up being obesity. The emerging prevalence of overweight and obesity in Africa has been largely attributed to the rising level of urbanisation in the region and its attendant global nutrition transition [8]. Urbanisation in Africa is increasing rapidly and African countries are projected to have 50% urbanisation by 2020 [9]. These risk factors of obesity are similar to those found in several studies across the world as accounting for the increasing overweight and obesity epidemic in developing countries and the stall in the phenomenon in developed countries [10, 11]. Literature is showing differences in overweight and obesity to the disadvantage of those in urban settings [5]. These rural–urban disparities could be explained by the differences in lifestyle such as time spent watching television, mechanisation of occupation and dietary pattern in Africa [5, 12, 13]. Studies elsewhere have confirmed that women who were informally employed and listened to the radio were less likely to be overweight or obese compared to those who were unemployed and did not listen to the radio, respectively [14].

Research had shown socioeconomic differences in overweight and obesity by the level of education and wealth to the detriment of those with lower socio-economic status in most countries across Africa similar to those found in other previous studies [15]. Studies have argued that cultural norms that favour fatter body size contribute significantly to the socio-economic status differences in overweight and obesity in developing countries, particularly in Africa [16]. Women of higher socioeconomic status have the resources and knowledge of the importance of physical activity and healthy diet but they also face several socio-cultural barriers that may prevent them from putting those into use [17]. With specific reference to those with no education, research had shown that the odds of being overweight/obese significantly increased with the level of education [18].

Studies have revealed a significant association between overweight/obesity and age [14, 19, 20]. Studies have shown the likelihood of obesity and overweight to be high among older women and the possible reason for this finding maybe that old age is likely to be characterised by high physical inactivity as well as the consumption of more energy-dense foods, which may result in overweight and obesity [14]. Another possible explanation for this could be that, as people grow, the composition of their body changes, which results in an increase in fat mass and a decline in fat-free mass [19, 20]. Overweight and obesity vary greatly between men and women, with women across the globe disproportionately affected [21]. Generally, women with higher parities have been found to have higher retention of gestational weight gain and consequently the onset of overweight and obesity [16, 22]. The real impact of parity and associated reproductive factors could, however, be modest and intertwined in a complex pattern with socio-cultural, demographic and socio-economic factors, as well as other risk factors [22].

Researches have shown an association between religious affiliation and obesity and overweight. This finding can be explained in the context of a study by Kahan (2015) in 38 countries that found high rates of physical inactivity among Muslim women, as well as Benjamin and Donnelly (2013) who conducted a study on barriers and facilitators influencing the physical activity of Arabic adults [23, 24]. Married women are more susceptible to being overweight or obese, thus marital status is a strong predictor of obesity [25]. Hormonal contraception use has been found to increase the risk of obesity and injected depot medroxyprogesterone acetate also increased weight [26, 27].

The rapidly changing role of women in African societies, with their increasing involvement in the labour force, especially in urban areas contribute to the dramatic changes in dietary patterns and food supply occurring in these settings [28]. In addition, in these settings, a direct relationship between socioeconomic status and obesity has been observed, since higher socioeconomic groups are more likely to buy extra food and achieve their desire to look healthy and strong [29]. Therefore, this paper aim to investigate the problem of obesity and included household assets as part of the background variables.

2. Methods

2.1 Source of data

This paper utilises pooled data from 3 consecutive Zimbabwe Demographic and Health Surveys (ZDHS) from the following years; 2005/6, 2010/11 and 2015. The ZDHS is a nationally representative sample survey of women aged 15–49 years, which is conducted every five years. Permission to use the data sets was sought from Measure DHS. The data collected covers: individual and household level socio-demographic; health and sexual activity; maternal and child health; mortality; fertility; family planning; and nutrition.

2.2 Study participants and sample size

The sample sizes of the interviewed women aged 15–49 were selected based on a master sampling plan, which was provided by the Central Statistics Office (1988–2005) and Zimbabwe National Statistics Agency (ZIMSTAT) (2010–2015). A two-stage cluster sampling process was used. Firstly, enumeration areas were selected from a list of clusters obtained from the master sampling plan provided by ZIMSTAT, followed by a selection of households from each cluster. All women aged 15–49 years were selected from each selected household and interviewed. Informed consent was obtained from the respondents before being interviewed. The analysis was limited to currently non-pregnant women aged 15–49 years who were *dejure* household members: survey year 2005/6, n = 7,798; 2010/11, n = 7,612; and 2015, n = 8,552). All data sets from the three surveys were weighted.

3. Variables

3.1 Dependent variable

Overweight and obesity was the outcome variable and the measurement of obesity is based on the Quetelet Index, also known as body mass index (BMI). BMI is weight divided by height squared (kg/m^2). The biomarkers took the weight and height measurements during the face-to-face interviews. The study adopted the widely accepted definition of overweight and obesity as a BMI of ≥25.0 kg/m^2 and 30 kg/m^2, respectively. Overweight and obesity were combined as one category to ensure enough cases for the analysis. We use a binary variable to classify respondents whose BMI was ≥25.0 kg/m^2 as overweight and obesity and coded "1" while those below 25.0 kg/m^2 were classified otherwise and coded "0".

3.2 Independent variables

The independent variables used in this study were categorised into two groups: demographic factors and socioeconomic status (SES). The demographic factors were: age (15–19, 20–24, 25–29, 30–34, 35–39, 40–49); parity (<2, 2–3, 4–5, 6+); marital status (never in a union, currently in a union, and formerly in a union); religion (Roman Catholic, Protestant, Pentecostal and others). SES was measured using six indicators: wealth (poorest, poorer, middle, richer and richest); the level of education (no education and primary were collapsed for easy analysis), secondary, higher education); employment status (unemployed and employed); place of residence (rural or urban); region or province all (ten Zimbabwean provinces were included); and household assets (radio, television and telephone).

3.3 Data analysis

We used frequency distributions to describe and summarise the characteristics of the respondents across all three survey years under study. In addition, the bivariate relationship between the background characteristics and the dependent variable were examined using the Chi-square test of independence. In the last part, three binary logistic regression models were fitted to examine the associations between the independent variables and the outcome variable.

4. Findings

About a quarter (25.2%) of the women were either overweight or obese in 2015, 31.3% in 2010 and 34.9% in 2015 (**Table 1**). The majority of women sampled were from rural areas, 59.8% in 2005, 61.7% in 2010 and 61.9% in 2015. More than two-thirds of women came from households that had wealth between middle and richest, 66.4% in 2005, 65.8% in 2010 and 65.8% in 2015. At least sixty percent of women had at least secondary education, 63.3% in 2005, 59.6% in 2010 and 72.8%. Most respondents were aged between 15 and 34 years, 74.5% in 2005, 72.1% in 2010 and 51% in 2015. The majority of women had parity <2, 46.9% in 2005, 44.1% in 2010, 41.2 in 2015. The most common religion was Apostolic sect, 29.2% in 2005, 37.4% in 2010 and 41.4% in 2020. More than half of women were currently in a union, 54.6% in 2005, 59.5% in 2010 and 59.5% in 2015. In terms of employment, most women were not working, 62.4% in 2005, 62.2% in 2010 and 57.9% in 2015. The highest proportions of women were from Harare province, 17% in 2005, 18.4% in 2010 and 17.8% in 2015. The least proportion of women was from Matebeleland South province, 5.0% in 2005, 5.2% in 2010 and 4.2% in 2015. Close to half of the women reported that their household owned a radio (55.2% in 2005, 41.3% in 2010 and 55.6% in 2015). Around 40% of women reported that their household owned a television set (39.2% in 2005, 43.2% in 2010 and 44.3% in 2015). Ownership of a telephone was low, 11.4% in 2005, 4.9% in 2010 and 3.9% in 2015.

Variables	2005/06(%)	2010/11(%)	2015(%)
Place of Residence			
Urban	3,136 (40.2)	2911(38.3)	3,260(38.1)
Rural	4661(59.8)	4,700(61.7)	5,292 (61.9)
Household wealth			
Poorest	1,340 (17.2)	1288(16.9)	1,468 (17.2)
Poorer	1,271 (16.3)	1,320(17.4)	1,452(17.0)
Middle	1,345 (17.2)	1382(18.2)	1,536(18.0)
Richer	1765 (22.6)	1,697 (22.3)	1,945(22.7)
Richest	2077(26.6)	1922(25.3)	2,151(25.1)
Level of Education			
No Education/Primary	2869(36.8)	2310 (30.4)	2,328(27.2)
Secondary	4690(60.2)	4933 (54.8)	5,603(65.5)
Higher	238(3.1)	368(4.8)	620(7.3)
Age			
15–19	1880 (24.1)	1638(21.5)	1,912 (2.3)
20–24	1605 (20.6)	1452 (19.1)	1,381 (16.5)
25–29	1249(16.0)	1,317(17.3)	1,381 (16.5)
30–34	1,073 (13.8)	1084(14.2)	1,345(15.7)
35–39	769(9.9)	874(11.5)	1095(12.8)
40-44	652(8.4)	673(8.9)	907(10.6
45-49	570(7.3)	574(7.5)	528(6.2)
Parity			
<2	3654 (46.9)	3353(44.1)	3,524 (41.2)
2–3	2288(29.3)	2550(33.5)	2,977 (34.8)
4–5	1118(14.4)	1158(15.2)	1,508 (17.6)
6+	738(9.5)	551 (7.2)	543 (6.4)
Religion			
Roman Catholic	793 (10.2)	653(8.6)	575 (6.7)
Protestant	2042 (26.2)	1290 (17.0)	1,390 (16.3)
Pentecostal	1384 (17.8)	1643 (21.6)	2,138 (25.0)
Apostolic sect	2278 (29.2)	2,844(37.4)	3,542 (41.4)
Others	1300(16.7)	1181 (15.2)	906 (10.6)
Marital Status			
Never in Union	2253 (28.9)	1964(25.8)	2,278(26.6)
Currently in Union	4260 (54.6)	4523(59.5)	5,089(59.5)
Formerly in Union	1285 (16.5)	1121 (14.7)	1,186(13.9)
Employment status			
Working	2942 (37.8)	2875 (37.8)	3,598(42.1)
Not Working	4841(62.4)	4737(62.2)	4,954(57.9)

Variables	2005/06(%)	2010/11(%)	2015(%)
Province of Residence			
Manicaland	912(11.7)	1007(13.2)	1,069(12.5)
Mashonaland central	707(9.1)	731(9.6)	738 (8.6)
Mashonaland east	624(8.0)	699(9.2)	839 (8.7)
Mashonaland west	721(9.3)	878 (11.5)	997 (11.7)
Matabeleland north	474 (6.1)	377 (5.0)	405 (4.7)
Matabeleland south	393(5.0)	398(5.2)	357 (4.2)
Midlands	1,031(13.2)	937(12.3)	1,073 (12.6)
Masvingo	970(12.4)	741 (9.7)	1,036(12.1)
Harare	1322 (17.0)	1340(18.4)	1,525 (17.8)
Bulawayo	643(8.2)	443 (5.8)	513(6.00)
household has: radio			
No	3494 (44.8)	4,464 (58.7)	4,773 (55.8)
Yes	4300 (55.2)	3,148(41.3)	3,7789(44.1)
household has: television			
No	4740 (60.8)	4,319 (56.7)	4,767(55.7)
Yes	3052 (39.2)	3,293 (43.2)	3,785(44.3)
household has: telephone			
No	6906 (88.6)	7,240 (95.1)	8,218 (96.1)
Yes	887 (11.4)	372(4.9)	334(3.9)
Total, n	**7798(100)**	**7,612 (100)**	**8,552(100)**

Table 1.
Percentage distribution of the characteristics of women in Zimbabwe, 2005–2015.

The results show that there has been an increasing trend in the percentage of women in Zimbabwe who were either overweight or obese from 2005/06 (25.2%) to 2015 (34.9%) (See **Table 2**).

The results of the bivariate analysis reveal a significant association between background variables and overweight/obesity (**Table 2**). Women from urban areas were more likely to be overweight or obese (35.8 in 2005, 40.3% in 2010 and 46.7% in 2015) compared to those from rural areas (18% in 2005/06, 25.4% in 2010/11 and 27.7% in 2015) ($p = 0.000$). Similarly, urban provinces such as Harare and Bulawayo were more likely to have women who were obese and overweight compared to women in rural provinces ($p = 0.000$). Women from richest households were at higher risk of overweight/obesity over the period, 39.1% in 2005, 42.5% in 2010 and 50% in 2015 compared to women from the poorest households (13.6, 17.4 and 18.7%, respectively) ($p = 0.000$). Similarly, the level of education was associated with the prevalence of overweight/obesity ($p = 0.000$). Women with higher education were more likely to be obese/overweight (57.4% in 2005, 48% in 2010 and 57% in 2015) compared to women with primary or no education (22.6%, 29.5% and 28.2%, respectively) ($p = 0.000$). Obesity/overweight increased with parity, for 2005/06 and 2010/11, the highest prevalence of overweight/obesity was among women with 4–5 children while for 2015, the highest prevalence was among women

Variables	2005/06(%)		2010/11(%)		2015(%)	
Prevalence of Obesity						
Obese/Overweight	1963(25.2)		2,383(31.3)		2,984(34.9)	
Normal	5,835(74.8)		5,229(68.7)		5,568(65.1)	
Place of Residence						
Urban	1121 (35.8)	0.00	1189 (40.3)	0.00	1521 (46.7)	0.00
Rural	842 (18.0)		1194 (25.4)		1527 (27.7)	
Household wealth						
Poorest	182(13.6)	0.00	224(17.4)	0.00	279 (18.7)	0.00
Poorer	194 (15.3)		314(23.8)		355(24.5)	
Middle	251(18.7)		394(28.5)		472 (30.7)	
Richer	524(29.7)		635 (37.4)		802 (41.2)	
Richest	812 (39.1)		817(42.5)		1076 (50.0)	
Level of Education						
No Education/Primary	647 (22.6)	0.00	681 (29.5)	0.00	656(28.2)	0.00
Secondary	1179 (25.1)		1525 (30.9)		1972 (35.2)	
Higher	137 (57.4)		177(48.1)		356(57.4)	
Age						
15–19	214 (11.4)	0.00	200 (12.2)	0.00	251 (13.1)	0.00
20–24	293 (18.3)		305 (21.0)		331(24.0)	
25–29	322 (25.8)		432 (32.8)		481(34.8)	
30–34	334 (31.2)		430 (39.7)		621(46.2)	
35–39	302(39.3)		389 (43.8)		529(48.2)	
40-44	270(41.4)		336 (49.9)		491(54.1)	
45-49	229 (40.1)		297 (51.7)		281(53.2)	
Parity						
<2	635 (17.4)	0.00	705 (21.0)	0.00	806(22.9)	0.00
2–3	688(30.1)		930 (36.5)		1272 (42.7)	
4–5	389(34.7)		511 (44.2)		659(43.7)	
6+	251(34.1)		237 (43.0)		248 (45.7)	
Religion						
Roman Catholic	254 (32.0)	0.00	258 (39.4)	0.00	226(39.4)	0.00
Protestant	643 (31.5)		496(38.5)		556(40.7)	
Pentecostal	388 (28.0)		565(34.4)		849 (39.7)	
Apostolic sect	431(18.9)		741(26.1)		1037 (29.3)	
Others	248(19.1)		324(27.4)		307(33.8)	
Marital Status						
Never in Union	342(15.2)	0.00	328 (16.7)	0.00	420(18.4)	0.00
Currently in Union	1248 (29.3)		1648(36.4)		2075 (40.8)	
Formerly in Union	374 (29.1)		407(36.3)		489(41.3)	

Variables	2005/06(%)		2010/11(%)		2015(%)	
Employment status						
Working	932(31.7)	0.00	1270 (26.8)	0.00	1608 (44.7)	0.00
Not Working	1031 (21.3)		1313 (38.7)		1377 (27.8)	
Province of Residence						
Manicaland	258(28.3)	0.00	231(31.9)	0.00	330 (30.9)	0.00
Mashonaland central	89(12.6)		165 (22.6)		216(29.2)	
Mashonaland east	135(21.6)		200(28.7)		278(33.1)	
Mashonaland west	164 (22.7)		253 (28.8)		310(31.6)	
Matabeleland north	78 (16.6)		88 (23.3)		116 (28.6)	
Matabeleland south	98 (25.0)		102(25.6)		100(27.9)	
Midlands	227 (22.0)		278(29.7)		342(31.9)	
Masvingo	192(19.8)		214 (28.9)		320 (31.0)	
Harare	491 (37.1)		601 (43.0)		736 (48.2)	
Bulawayo	231 (35.9)		160 (36.2)		237 (46.2)	
Household has: radio						
No	631 (18.0)	0.00	1285 (28.8)	0.00	1614 (33.8)	0.05
Yes	1332 (31.0)		1098 (34.9)		1370 (36.3)	
Household has: television						
No	878 (18.5)	0.00	1064 (24.6)	0.00	1310 (27.5)	0.00
Yes	1085(35.5)		1320 (40.1)		1675 (44.2)	
Household has: telephone						
No	1589 (23.0)	0.00	2218 (30.6)	0.00	2831 (34.5)	0.00
Yes	374 (42.0)		165 (44.3)		154 (46.0)	
Overall	**1963(25.2)**		**2,383(31.3)**		**2985 (34.9)**	

Table 2.
Prevalence of overweight and obesity by background variables.

with 6+ children (p = 0.000). Women currently in a union or formerly in the union were more likely to be overweight or obese compared to women who have never been in union (p = 0.000). For 2005/06 and 2015, women who were working were at higher risk of overweight/obesity (31.7% in 2005 and 44.7% in 2015) compared to women not working (21.3% and 27.8%, respectively) p = 0.000). For 2010/11, women who were not working were more likely to be overweight or obese (38.7%) than those not working (26.8%) (p = 0.000) in 2010.

Household asset ownership was associated with the prevalence of overweight/obesity. Women from households with radios were more likely to be overweight/obese (31% in 2005/06, 34.9% in 2010/11) compared to women from households without a radio had prevalence of (18.0% in 2005, and 28.8% in 2010) (p = 0.00). Women from households with television were more likely to be overweight or obese (35.5% in 2005, 40.1% in 2010 and 44.2% in 2015) compared to women from households without a television (18.5%, 26.6% and 27.5%, respectively) (p = 0.000). Women from households which owned a telephone had the highest prevalence of overweight/obesity, 42.0% in 2005, 44.3% in 2010 and 46.0% in 2015

Variables	2005 aOR(95% CI)	2010 aOR(95% CI)	2015 aOR(95% CI)
Place of Residence			
Urban (ref)			
Rural	0.95 (0.72-1.22)	0.80(0.64-0.99)**	1.11 (0 .87-1.42)
Household wealth			
Poorest(ref)			
Poorer	1.18 (0.93- 1.49)	1.58(1.28- 1.95)***	1.46(1.17-1.81)***
Middle	1.44(1.12-1.84)**	1.95 (1.56-2.47)***	1.95(1.58-2.41)***
Richer	2.35(1.70-3.20)***	2.38 (1.82-3.10)***	3.06 (2.32-4.05)***
Richest	3.06 (2.06-4.56)***	3.92(2.11-4.04)***	4.56 (3.20-6.51)***
Level of Education			
No Education/Primary(ref)			
Secondary	1.05(0.89-1.25)	1.08 (0.92-1.27)	1.17 (1.01-1.35)**
Higher	1.89(1.37-2.60)***	1.19(0.89-1.60)	1.32 (1.01- 1.72)**
Age			
15–19(ref)			
20–24	1.37 (1.06-1.75)**	1.44 (1.12-1.84)**	1.42(1.12- 1.80)**
25–29	1.96(1.48- 2.59)***	2.41 (1.87-3.12)***	2.25(1.69-3.00)***
30–34	2.44 (1.82-3.28)***	2.99 (2.29- 3.92)***	3.38(2.53-4.50)***
35–39	3.24(2.41-4.36)***	3.58 (2.65- 4.84)***	3.70(2.71-5.05)***
40-44	3.69(2.73- 5.00)***	4.43 (3.21-6.11)***	4.75 (3.50-6.46)***
45-49	4.16 (3.94-6.88)***	5.04(3.61-7.03)***	4.74(3.31-6.78)***
Parity			
<2 (ref)			
2–3	1.25 (1.04-1.51)**	1.18 (0.97-1.44)	1.19(0.99- 1.43)*
4–5	1.49(1.15- 1.92)**	1.60 (1.26- 2.07)***	1.22(0.96- 1.56)*
6+	1.50(1.11-2.03)**	1.56(1.16-2.09)**	1.58 (1.17- 2.15)**
Religion			
Roman Catholic(ref)			
Protestant	1.00 (0.82-1.22)	0.97 (0.76-1.24)	1.07 (0.82-1.37)
Pentecostal	0.85 (0.69-1.06)	0.85(0.67-1.08)	1.00 (0.79-1.27)
Apostolic sect	0.75 (0.61-0.92)**	0.68 (0.54-0.86)***	0.87 (0.67-1.14)
Others	0.67(0.54-0.85)**	0.71(0.55-0.931)**	1.02(0.78-1.33)
Marital Status			
Never in Union(ref)			
Currently in Union	1.44 (1.14-1.83)**	1.68 (1.32-2.14)***	1.65(1.36-2.01)***
Formerly in Union	1.13(0.86-1.49)***	1.35(1.02-1.79)**	1.39(1.10- 1.75)**
Employment status			
Not Working(ref)			
Working	1.23 (1.06- 1.44)**	1.04(0.91-1.19)	1.15 (1.00-1.31)**

Variables	2005 aOR(95% CI)	2010 aOR(95% CI)	2015 aOR(95% CI)
Province of Residence			
Manicaland(ref)			
Mashonaland Central	0.44 (0.27-0.70)**	0.64(0.50-0.85)***	1.03(0.79-1.34)
Mashonaland East	0.66(0.50-0.87)**	0.84 (0.60-1.18)	0.97(0.75-1.24)
Mashonaland West	0.66 (0.51- 0.86)**	0.83 (0.68-1.01)	0.85(0.66-1.10)
Matabeleland North	0.69 (0.52-0.93)**	0.85 (0.63-1.12)	1.10 (0.82- 1.44)
Matabeleland South	1.00 (0.75-1.31)	0.94 (0.74-1.20)	0.90 (0.68-1.19)
Midlands	0.64 (0.51-0.81)***	0.92 (0.72-1.18)	0.96 (0.72-1.28)
Masvingo	0.89(0.67- 1.20)	1.05(0.84-1.31)	1.00 (0.78-1.30)
Harare	0.97(0.74-1.26)	1.02 (0.80-1.31)	1.16 (0.89-1.52)
Bulawayo	0.85(0.66-1.10)	0.78 (0.59-1.05)	1.12 (0.85- 1.42)
household has: radio			
No			
Yes	1.09(0.92-1.30)	1.02(0.89-1.15)	1.00 (0.88-1.14)
household has: television			
No			
Yes	1.08(0.90-1.29)	1.25 (1.05-1.47)**	1.07(0.89-1.29)
household has: telephone			
No			
Yes	1.38(1.12-1.69)	1.20 (0.92-1.58)	0.91 (0.65-1.29)

Notes: aOR, adjusted odds ratio.
$^{*}p < 0.1$.
$^{**}p < 0.05$
$^{***}p < 0.001$

Table 3.
Odds ratio estimates for overweight /obesity women aged 15-49 years from 2005-2015 in Zimbabwe.

compared to women with households without a telephone (23%, 30.6% and 34.5%, respectively) ($p = 0.000$).

Table 3 shows the results of the multiple regression, indicating variables that are statistically significant after controlling for other factors. Women from rural areas were less likely to be overweight/obese compared to those from urban areas only in 2010 (aOR = 0.80, $p < 0.05$). Household wealth was associated with being overweight/obese, with women from richest households were three times (aOR = 3.06), four times (aOR = 3.92) and five times (aOR = 4.56) more likely to be overweight/obese compared to those from poorest households in 2005, 2010 and 2015, respectively ($p < 0.001$). In 2005/06, women with higher education had a significantly higher likelihood of being overweight/obese compared to those with no/primary education (1.89 times higher, $p < 0.001$), while in 2015, women with secondary and higher education were 1.17 and 1.32 more likely to be overweight/obese, respectively than those with primary or no education ($p < 0.05$). Older women aged 45–49 years had increased odds of overweight/obesity compared to the young women aged 15–19 years, four times (aOR = 3.06) in 2005, five times (aOR = 5.04) in 2010 and five times (aOR = 4.74) in 2015 ($p < 0.001$). Parity also increased the likelihood of overweight/obesity, women with parity of 6+ had more than 50%

higher chances of being overweight/obese compared to those with parity of <2 in three periods, 2005, 2010 and 2015 ($p < 0.05$). Women currently in union were more likely to be overweight/obese compared to those never in union, 44% higher chances in 2005 ($p < 0.05$), 68% higher chance in 2010 ($p < 0.001$) and 65% higher chance in 2015 ($p < 0.001$) (**Table 3**).

Working increased odds of overweight/obesity compared to those not working, aOR = 1.23 in 2005, and aOR = 1.15 in 2015 ($p < 0.05$). Household ownership of radio and telephone did not show a statistically significant association with women's chances of being overweight or obese. Household ownership of television showed a significant increased likelihood of overweight/obesity in 2010 only (aOR = 1.25) ($p < 0.05$) with no significant likelihood in 2005 and 2015.

5. Discussion

The aim of the study was to examine factors associated with overweight and obesity among women aged 15–49 years in Zimbabwe. Our study found that rural women were less likely to be overweight and obese than urban women. Similar findings were also reported by Neupane, Prakash and Doku 2015 who found obesity to be more prevalent in urban setups [5]. Neupane et al. [5] attributed this disparity to differences in lifestyle, dietary pattern and type of occupation. Women in rural areas tend to be involved in activities that call for their energy use such as farming, collecting firewood and fetching water and thus use up lots of calories. The study findings also reveal that women from richer households had higher odds of overweight and obesity than women from the poorest households. Similar findings were reported by Neupane et al. [5]. We found higher education and working status to be constantly associated with overweight/obesity in 2005 and 2015 and not in 2010/11. Studies elsewhere concur with current findings [18]. This could be related to the fact that these highly educated women are more likely to be working and more likely to come from richer households, and thus use energy saving devices at home to execute their daily domestic chores or can afford to employ domestic workers. In addition, some women tend to afford eating western food outlets at work which are perceived to be 'junk' and fatty food. However, the period 2010/11 has no statistically significant relationships as the period comes immediately after the economic challenges that occurred in 2008, spilling the effects into this period, such that education and working were overridden by other factors, thus diluting the relationship of these factors with overweight/obesity. Ownership of household assets was not associated with overweight or obesity except for television in 2010/11. This is contrary to other studies which found asset ownership such as radio and telephone to be associated with obesity. It is not surprising that a sedentary lifestyle has been observed to closely relate to time spent watching television as a leisure activity [13, 18]. Subsequently, reduced energy expenditure because of this leisure activity is closely associated with overweight and obesity.

Age was a constant predictor of overweight and obesity in all three surveys. With increasing age, women tend to be at higher odds ratios of becoming overweight and obese. Elsewhere in similar settings, the prevalence of overweight and obesity was also reported to be higher among older women [14, 19, 20]. Other studies associate obesity in old age to be characterised by high physical inactivity as well as the consumption of more energy-dense foods, which may result in overweight and obesity [14]. The current study found parity to be significantly associated with overweight/obesity. Similarly, several studies found multiparous women had the highest odds of being obese [7, 14] as well associated with the onset of higher retention of gestational weight gain [16, 22]. Marital status also emerged as a key factor in influencing overweight/obesity as women who were in a union or had been in a union had higher odds of overweight and obesity. Similar studies have found married women are more susceptible to being overweight or obese [25]. This could be due to childbearing as married women tend to have children, as the tradition implies marriage with childbearing and thus as parity increases in marriage, so the risk of overweight/obesity.

6. Limitations

The study used cross-sectional data and reported factors associated with which might not imply a causative relationship. Consequently, results are restricted to how individuals were responding at one moment in time rather than over a period of time. Second, sampling procedures rely on archival data that may contain counting, collection, and recording errors. As a result, selection and recall biases may perhaps have been introduced during data collection. Third, the explanatory variables included in the study were limited to the ones collected as part of the demographic and health survey. The Zimbabwe Demographic Health Surveys lack key variables which can be sued as proxy to lifestyle behaviours such as diet preferences and physical exercises. The majority of the variables in our study were either biological (age, sex, parity) or socioeconomic (education, marital status, wealth, employment status and education). It is difficult to interpret our results in the absence of key factors such as type of food consumed and level of exercise.

7. Conclusion

The study has shown that demographic and socio-economic variables are more likely to be associated with overweight and obesity. Women in urban areas, with higher education, working and from richer households are more likely to be at risk of overweight and obese. Also, older women and those currently in a union or had been in union are more likely to be overweight/obese. However, possession of household assets such as television, radio and telephone were not associated with overweight/obesity, except for the television in 2010/11. This calls for interventions that address the socio-economic factors. Thus, there is need for constant awareness programmes on healthy eating food, and physical activity especially among older women and those working.

Author details

Kudzaishe Mangombe[1]*, Naomi Wekwete[1], Amos Milanzi[1], Ronald Musizvingoza[2] and Charles Lwanga[3]

1 Center for Population Studies, University of Zimbabwe, Zimbabwe

2 Independent Researcher

3 School of Statistics and Planning, Makerere University, Uganda

*Address all correspondence to: kudzimangobee@gmail.com

References

[1] Roser, M. and Ritchie, H. Obesity-Our World in Data. Published online at OurWorldInData.org (2017).

[2] Lin, X. et al. Global burden of noncommunicable disease attributable to high body mass index in 195 countries and territories, 1990–2017. Endocrine (2020). doi:10.1007/s12020-020-02352-y

[3] Dake, F. A. A. & Fuseini, K. Recreation, transportation or labour saving? Examining the association between household asset ownership and body mass index among Ghanaian women. BMC Obes. (2015). doi:10.1186/s40608-015-0075-z

[4] Ellulu, M., Abed, Y., Rahmat, A., Ranneh, Y. & Ali, F. Epidemiology of obesity in developing countries: challenges and prevention. Glob. Epidemic Obes. (2014). doi:10.7243/2052-5966-2-2

[5] Neupane, S., Prakash, K. C. &Doku, D. T. Overweight and obesity among women: Analysis of demographic and health survey data from 32 Sub-Saharan African Countries. BMC Public Health (2016). doi:10.1186/s12889-016-2698-5

[6] Word Health Organization. Global Action Plan on Physical Activity 2018–2030. Journal of Policy Modeling (2018).

[7] Mukora-Mutseyekwa, F., Zeeb, H., Nengomasha, L. &Adjei, N. K. Trends in prevalence and related risk factors of overweight and obesity among women of reproductive age in Zimbabwe, 2005–2015. Int. J. Environ. Res. Public Health (2019). doi:10.3390/ijerph16152758

[8] Popkin, B. M., Lu, B. &Zhai, F. Understanding the nutrition transition: measuring rapid dietary changes in transitional countries. Public Health Nutr. (2002). doi:10.1079/phn2002370

[9] Kennedy, G., Nantel, G. & Shetty, P. Globalization of food systems in developing countries: impact on food security and nutrition. in FAO food and nutrition paper (2004).

[10] Astrup, A. & Brand-Miller, J. Diet composition and obesity. The Lancet (2012). doi:10.1016/S0140-6736(12)60456-5

[11] Archer, E., Hand, G. A. & Blair, S. N. Validity of U.S. Nutritional Surveillance: National Health and Nutrition Examination Survey Caloric Energy Intake Data, 1971–2010. PLoS One (2013). doi:10.1371/journal.pone.0076632

[12] Mangemba, N. T. & San Sebastian, M. Societal risk factors for overweight and obesity in women in Zimbabwe: A cross-sectional study. BMC Public Health (2020). doi:10.1186/s12889-020-8215-x

[13] Seidu, A.-A., Ahinkorah, B. O., Agbaglo, E. &Nyaaba, A. A. Overweight and obesity among women of reproductive age in Mali: what are the determinants? Int. Health (2020). doi: 10.1093/inthealth/ihaa094

[14] Ahmed, K. Y. et al. Trends and determinants of underweight and overweight/obesity among urban Ethiopian women from 2000 to 2016. BMC Public Health 20, 1276 (2020).

[15] Cohen, E., Boetsch, G., Palstra, F. P. &Pasquet, P. Social valorisation of stoutness as a determinant of obesity in the context of nutritional transition in Cameroon: The Bamiléké case. Soc. Sci. Med. (2013). doi:10.1016/j.socscimed.2013.07.004

[16] Gupta, N., Goel, K., Shah, P. & Misra, A. Childhood obesity in developing countries: Epidemiology, determinants, and prevention.

Endocrine Reviews (2012). doi:10.1210/er.2010-0028

[17] Robinson, W. R., Cheng, M. M., Hoggatt, K. J., Stürmer, T. &Siega-Riz, A. M. Childbearing is not associated with young women's long-term obesity risk. Obesity (2014). doi:10.1002/oby.20593

[18] Tuoyire, D. A. Television exposure and overweight/obesity among women in Ghana. BMC Obes. 5, 8 (2018).

[19] Gallagher, D. et al. Appendicular skeletal muscle mass: Effects of age, gender, and ethnicity. J. Appl. Physiol. (1997). doi:10.1152/jappl.1997.83.1.229

[20] Villareal, D. T., Apovian, C. M., Kushner, R. F. & Klein, S. Obesity in older adults: Technical review and position statement of the American Society for Nutrition and NAASO, the Obesity Society. Obes. Res. (2005). doi:10.1038/oby.2005.228

[21] Flegal, K. M., Carroll, D., Kit, B. K. & Ogden, C. L. Prevalence of obesity and trends in the distribution of body mass index among US adults, 1999–2010. JAMA - J. Am. Med. Assoc. (2012). doi:10.1001/jama.2012.39

[22] Koch, E. et al. Impact of parity on anthropometric measures of obesity controlling by multiple confounders: A cross-sectional study in Chilean women. J. Epidemiol. Community Health (2008). doi:10.1136/jech.2007.062240

[23] Kahan, D. Prevalence and correlates of adult overweight in the Muslim world: analysis of 46 countries. Clin. Obes. (2015). doi:10.1111/cob.12089

[24] Benjamin, K. & Donnelly, T. Barriers and facilitators influencing the physical activity of Arabic adults: A literature review. Avicenna (2013). doi:10.5339/avi.2013.8

[25] Sikorski, C. et al. Obesity and associated lifestyle in a large sample of multi-morbid German primary care attendees. PLoS One (2014). doi:10.1371/journal.pone.0102587

[26] Sugiharti, S., Hadi, H. & Julia, M. Hormonal contraception as a risk factor for obesity. Med. J. Indones. (2005). doi:10.13181/mji.v14i3.191

[27] Adebowale, S. A., Fagbamigbe, F. A. &Bamgboye, E. A. Contraceptive use: implication for completed fertility, parity progression and maternal nutritional status in Nigeria. Afr. J. Reprod. Health (2011).

[28] Collinson, M. A. Striving against adversity: the dynamics of migration, health and poverty in rural South Africa. Glob. Health Action (2010). doi:10.3402/gha.v3i0.5080

[29] Mokhtar, N. et al. Diet culture and obesity in northern Africa. in Journal of Nutrition (2001). doi:10.1093/jn/131.3.887s

Chapter 9

Smoking and Non-Communicable Diseases in Sub-Saharan Africa: The Nigeria Scenario

Abayomi Ayodapo and Babalola Ibisola

Abstract

Smoking remains a strong factor in the emergence of Non-Communicable Diseases (NCDs) and it contributes to the development of cardiovascular diseases, cancers, diabetes mellitus and chronic respiratory disease which are the four leading NCDs worldwide. Non-Communicable Diseases has been implicated in about two thirds of the global premature deaths. However despite the strong evidence of link of smoking to NCDs, the prevalence of smoking is still high among the youths and adults, with an attendant adverse health effects. Nigeria, though a signatory to WHO Framework Convention on Tobacco Control (WHO FCTC) of 2005, and its recent domestication in National Tobacco Act of 2015, effective operationalization and implementation is still a mirage.

Keywords: Prevalence, Smoking, non-communicable diseases, Nigeria, Africa

1. Introduction

Non-communicable diseases (NCDs) as at 2015 already account for more than 80 percent of premature deaths in developing countries and the reported single largest preventable risk factor for NCDs is tobacco smoking [1]. The transition of tobacco hubs from the West to the African continent is of paramount importance, and Nigeria lies at the forefront of the shift from a tobacco-producing to a tobacco-consuming nation [2]. Smoking is the inhalation of the smoke of burning tobacco encased in cigarettes, pipes, and cigars. Most smokers begin smoking during their adolescent years, and they grow into the habit making nicotine addiction difficult to curb [3]. As these adolescents become adults, they serve as role models to youths, reinforcing a vicious cycle [3]. The health consequences of tobacco smoking depend on the duration and quantity of the smoking behaviour. Starting to smoke early in life increases the risk of NCDs and adolescent smokers are at greatest risk of future morbidity and mortality [4].

This chapter will highlight the prevalence and determinants of smoking in Nigeria, its measured effects on the health and well-being of the citizens, its economic burden, governmental and institutional efforts towards the control of tobacco smoking and the success, if any, of these measures.

Historical Background: Cigarette smoking is a mode of consumption of tobacco, *an agricultural* product derived from the leaves of plant *nicotiana*^{sp}. Tobacco was first grown as a cash crop in America in 1962 by settlers in James town

Virginia USA. Tobacco consumption gradually gained wide publicity through 1880s, through chewing, smoking pipes and hand rolled cigar or cigarettes. However, the invention of the first cigarette–making machine by James Bonsack capable of milling 120,000 sticks of cigarette per day revolutionised the trade, spread and consumption of this product worldwide [5].

There was an astronomic growth in the industry across the globe and consumption was freely rising until 1964 when it witnessed its first set back. The Surgeon General of the USA, Luther L. Terry (MD) issued the first warning dangers on cigarette smoking on January 11th 1964, relating the tar and nicotine content as causes of cancer. His Advisory Committee made their observations and conclusions based on the findings of more than 7,000 articles relating to smoking and disease available at that time in the biomedical literature [6]. They concluded that cigarette smoking was responsible for lung and laryngeal cancers in men, probable cause of lung cancer in women and the most important cause of chronic bronchitis.

The guided restrictions placed on the use of tobacco in Nigeria and other parts of the world were the results of the early steps taken by Luther L. Terry who insisted on warning labels on every cigarette pack [7] which forced tobacco industries to modifying their products by introducing filters and reducing the nicotine contents in their products. The warning labels transformed over years [7] and most developed countries made a stricter conditionality that forced many cigarette companies outside the shores of the US to the developing countries especially in Asia, Africa and South America where they found safe haven to establish their industries.

Generally, the 19th Century was associated with improvement in health research which further revealed other adverse effects of smoking. Subsequently, its ban or reduction in use gained a global attention. Despite the known adverse consequences of tobacco consumption, it is only in the Kingdom of Bhutan (South Asian country) that the sales of tobacco are illegal [8].

Historically, the agenda for a national policy on tobacco control in Nigeria dates back to the pre independence era, it however was not until a decade after the 2005 signing of the World Health Organisation Framework Convention for Tobacco Control (WHO FCTC) [9, 10]. Economic challenge such as lack of fund and loss of employment by the citizens were some of the reasons cited for the delay in implementing the tobacco compliant policy. This is in difference to the observation by Egbe et al. in their 2017 report that focused on and implicated the tobacco industry as the major influence against the implementation of the WHO FCTC since 2005 when Nigeria ratified the FCTC, until 2015 when the National Tobacco Control Act (NTCA) was signed into law [9, 11].

2. Prevalence of smoking in Nigeria

Globally, it is estimated that the number of smokers will increase from the present prevalence of 1.3 billion to 1.6 billion people in 2025. Its associated mortality is estimated to increase to 8.3 million persons in 2030 from 4.8 million persons in 2006 [12]. In 1990, Obot reported a prevalence of 26.8% of current smokers and 4.7% of past smokers among Nigerian adults [13]. According to the 2012 GATS conducted in Nigeria, the overall prevalence of adults who currently smoked was 3.7% [(3.1 million people): 7.2% - males; 0.3% - females)] [14]. The average age at initiation of daily smoking, according to the report showed that majority began after 16 years old [14]. More recent studies among medical, pharmacy and nursing students in Southwest Nigeria had life time prevalence of 17.9% and 5.04% for lifetime and current smokers [15]. The undergraduate university students study in Ilorin, North-central

Nigeria recorded a similar result, 17.1 and 5.7 prevalence for lifetime and current smokers respectively [16]. The male to female prevalence ratio among current smokers were 3.8:1, male 7.7% and female 2.0%. The mean age at initiation of smoking for males (15.5 ± 2.9, range 10–22 years) was not significantly different from that of females (15.6 ± 3.3, range 10–19 years). A common factor in all the Nigerian studies is male predominance among all categories of smokers [9, 13, 15, 16]. The gender difference may be attributed to societal perception as most African communities see smoking as a sign of masculinity or even specific to manhood and vigour, while social values discourages smoking among women. This is also true in some other African studies such as Ghana [17] and Sudan [18]. Few Nigerian studies and findings from systematic review studies conducted across Sub-Saharan African countries shows no consistent disparity in smoking prevalence between rural and urban populations [19, 20]. Hence, tobacco control policies should be strengthened across all Nigerian societies regardless of geography or existing health or socioeconomic inequalities.

3. Determinants of cigarette smoking

A substantial body of literature has emerged over the last few decades which examined the determinants of smoking behaviour in an economic framework of demand incorporating cigarette prices. Most studies in Nigeria were focused mainly on the determinants without much emphasis on the effect of cigarette pricing. Some of the determinants highlighted include the age of onset, peer group, parental influences, media influence etc. The Nigeria climate and weather favours the cultivation of tobacco in large commercial scale, especially in the South-western part of the country. This agricultural setting may influence tobacco smoking, but little is known about the influence of tobacco leave plantation (agricultural setting) on the incidence and prevalence of tobacco among children and adults in Nigeria.

3.1 Age

One important determinant of cigarette smoking with perhaps the highest immediate and long term consequences is the age. Early age at debut implies that the smoker will not only have longer time over which his/her tolerance levels can increase but also that the period of exposure to cigarette smoking with subsequent complications will be high. On the average, at the turn of thirty years of age, the rate of decline in the functional capacities of human organ-system is at about 0.1% annually. This modest decline is lost and the downward trend as high as 1% annual decline is seen in those with one form of existing morbidities or harmful lifestyle practices such as cigarette smoking.

Age of smoking debut is around 15 years in Nigeria and by age 17, a persistent smoking pattern is already established and a significant 15% smoking prevalence among the adolescents [21, 22]. The male to female prevalence ratio among current smokers were 3.8:1, male 7.7% and female 2.0%. The mean age at initiation of smoking for males (15.5 ± 2.9, range 10–22 years) was not significantly different from that of females (15.6 ± 3.3, range 10–19 years) [16]. The driving force for the onset age of smoking among Nigerian children depends on the population being under study, whether out-of-school youths or in-school youths. For the out-of-school youths, psychosocial factors such as belonging to a polygamous home, low level of fathers' education, feeling loneliness in the face of weak family bonds and harsh survival realities plays an initial dominant factor, coupled with peer pressure with the attendant high prevalence of smoking among the group [20, 23]. Since these psychosocial problems are usually due to physical, emotional and sexual abuse and neglect, they usually resort to tobacco smoking or other forms of substance abuse as a coping mechanism to ameliorate their condition. And among the in-school youths, the onset age of smoking is influenced by peer pressure and media influences. Additional risk factors in both groups are family conditions, such as low parental education, polygamy, not living with parents, having a parent who smokes and having divorced or separated parents [20]. Older studies in Nigeria and other developing countries in Africa were in agreement with the findings regarding early initiation of the youths into the act of cigarette smoking. Early commencement of smoking in high schools within Nigeria was reported in several works in this field [24–26]. The path to addiction commonly commences from this stage (the initiation phase) and by the age of 21 (in the university), the cigarette uptake process is mostly completed [27]. This trend of early initiation into cigarette smoking has been related to the highly addictive nature of cigarette and tobacco related substances.

Studies suggest that age at smoking initiation is related to subsequent aspects of smoking behaviour, such as cigarette consumption, nicotine dependence and smoking cessation [28]. Breslau predicted that the probability of smoking cessation among adults is inversely related to age at initiation [29].

Reports have shown that initiation into smoking and other dangerous life styles majorly occurs at the adolescent age [24–26, 30]. The disease burden emanating from chronic cigarette smoking is quite enormous. A recent report placed the current cost of medical treatment and low productivity emanating from cigarette smoking in Nigeria at five hundred and ninety-one million dollars ($591 M) per annum [31]. This is capable of significantly eroding the gains and advantages of a young population in growing economy like ours. Therefore the policy formulators must painstakingly exercise every right to inform and protect this group of individuals at all times.

3.2 Parental factors

Environmental factors also known as behavioural factors that are important in smoking prevalence can be found in the familiar (shared) or individual-specific (unshared) environment. The familiar environment is more likely to influence a smoker if anyone in his immediate environment is smoking such the parent(s). Parental influence could be direct (when the parent is a smoker) or indirectly (when parents are uninvolved in the affairs of their children).

A study in Port Harcourt Nigeria attributed 6.3% of the adolescent smokers, in their recent survey, to parental influence [32]. This factor ranked fourth behind Experimental exposition, Peer Influence and Advertisement. They reiterated the role of parents in moulding the characters of their children/wards against cigarette smoking, a factor though not as strong as peer influences and experimental expositions [32]. There is also some contribution by religiosity and the culture of the region which can influence the family/societal values and traditions and in the long run an individual's smoking habit.

A study among secondary school students in the Southwest Nigeria established a very strong relationship between the students smoking behaviour and those of their parents among other factors [24]. The study posited that parental influence ($p = 0.002856$) played significant role in the adoption of smoking behaviour by youths. They further advised that enlightenment and rehabilitation programmes targeted against cigarette smoking should also involve parent smokers to ensure effective outcome [24].

3.3 Peer influence

The peer influence has been observed to have a higher influence on smoking initiation and persistence [33, 34]. Powell et al., used the peer effect model in their study on tobacco control policies and youth smoking behaviour; to establish that peer effects play a significant role in youth smoking decisions [35].

3.4 Media influences

The numbers of hours people watch television have also been shown to influence the smoking habits and initiation [26]. Television programs depicting tobacco usage may encourage smoking among adolescents, however the converse was observed in an Iraq study [36]. Although bans have prevented direct tobacco advertising on television, studies have indicated the widespread portrayal of smoking on television on prime-time programming, movies, music videos, and sporting events. Rarely is smoking portrayed as a negative influence or unattractive, thus making television an indirect means of smoking advertising [33].

3.5 Legislation

The presence of legislation against smoking also determines smoking habits. This will limit the availability and youth access to cigarettes, elevate the age of onset of smoking, ensure a smoke-free indoor air and thus reduce the adverse effects of tobacco on the smoker and passive smokers. Chaloupka studied the effects of limits on youth access on smoking rates controlling for their enforcement and compliance [38]. He found that most state and local tobacco control policies did not have statistically significant effects on youth smoking except when strong restrictions exist. However, the combined effect of all non-tax policies on smoking participation was significant [37, 38]. Studies have concluded that strong smoking restrictions significantly reduced both smoking prevalence and average daily cigarette consumption among young adults [39, 40]. In fact a strict enforcement against cigarette smoking for 20 years in Brazil resulted in a 50% cut in prevalence of smoking among the young adults [40]. This is probably why in developed countries, where there is strong political will against the act of smoking, a decreasing prevalence of smoking is being documented [35].

3.6 Health status

Furthermore, individual-specific environmental factors include factors like mood and general state of health play significant role. Depressed individuals tend to smoke more and a history of major depressive disorder is associated with a lower chance to quit smoking [41]. Personal feeling of insecurity, insomnia, loneliness and feeling of grandeur all increase affiliation to cigarette smoking. On the other hand, sudden diagnosis of an ailment can encourage a current smoker to quit.

Some people may associate a particular status with smoking. They feel that smoking brings respect and is an acknowledgment of superiority. Finally, defiance to authority can be a factor that influences smoking. Some children tend to show disagreement/rebellion against parents, teachers or designated authorities through smoking [36]. These factors cannot be quantified and may confound with one another.

4. Adverse effects of smoking

Cigarette smoke is a complex mixture of chemicals. It is believed that the reason why people smoke is due to the active ingredient in the tobacco, nicotine which acts as a stimulant and a relaxant through its effects on the central nervous system, adrenals and the sympathetic nervous system [42, 43]. When a cigarette is smoked, nicotine-rich blood passes from the lungs to the brain within seven seconds and immediately stimulates the release of many chemical messengers including acetylcholine, norepinephrine, epinephrine, vasopressin, arginine, dopamine, autocrine agents, and beta-endorphin [42, 43]. This release of neurotransmitters and hormones is responsible for most of the effects of nicotine. Nicotine appears to enhance concentration and memory due to the increase of acetylcholine. It also appears to enhance alertness due to the increases of acetylcholine and norepinephrine. Arousal is increased by the resultant elevated level of norepinephrine. Pain is reduced by the increases of acetylcholine and beta-endorphin. Anxiety is reduced by the increased beta-endorphin. Nicotine also extends the duration of positive effects of dopamine and increases sensitivity in brain reward systems [44, 45]. This is one of the key reasons why cigarette is very addictive.

Some smoke components, such as carbon monoxide (CO), hydrogen cyanide (HCN), and nitrogen oxides, are gases. Others, such as formaldehyde, acrolein, benzene, and certain N-nitrosamines, are volatile chemicals contained in the liquid-vapour portion of the smoke aerosol. Still others, such as nicotine, phenol, polyaromatic hydrocarbons (PAHs), and certain tobacco-specific nitrosamines (TSNAs) are contained in the submicron-sized solid particles that are suspended in cigarette smoke. In view of this chemical complexity, cigarette smoke has been shown to have multiple and highly diverse effects on human health. These adverse effects have been documented in literature to involve every organ in the human body culminating in various cancers, chronic obstructive pulmonary airway disease to various cardiovascular diseases. It has also been linked with auditory problems [46] while in India and China it has been associated with increased prevalence in pulmonary tuberculosis [47].

The use of tobacco has been reported to be associated with increased chronic lung diseases, asthma, angina depression, arthritis, diabetes, hypertension and cerebrospinal accidents [45–51]. The adverse economic effect of tobacco smoking is huge [5, 52, 53]. In the United States, an estimated $96 billion per annum were being incurred from tobacco use and related medical expenses due to loss of productivity and over $2 billion would be saved annually from healthcare insurance if all smokers in the US were to quit smoking [54].

5. Control of tobacco use through legislation

The Youths are the most effective groups targeted by public/health policy makers and economists for smoking prevention programmes, since almost all first use of cigarettes occur at this age and the development of addictive habits also begins at this age. Health policy designed to discourage the use of Tobacco products especially in this age group was signed and approved by many countries including Nigeria, under the aegis of the WHO Framework Convention on Tobacco Control (WHO FCTC) of 2005. The WHO Framework Convention on Tobacco Control (FCTC), was adopted by the 56th World Health Assembly on May 21, 2003, and implemented on February 27, 2005. In this treaty, WHO recommends a four-pronged strategy for the control of smoking. The first prong advocates a ban on all forms of advertising and an increase in public health information with special attention to youths. By

2008, WHO revealed a six evidenced-based policy package known as "MPOWER" through which the FCTC could be implemented. This acronym stands for (i) Monitor tobacco use and prevention policy, (ii) Protect people from tobacco smoke, (iii) Offer help to quit tobacco use, (iv) Warn people about the dangers of tobacco, (v) Enforce bans on tobacco advertising, promotion and sponsorship, and (vi) Raise taxes on tobacco.

The MPOWER also seeks to enhance price and excise tax policy, smoke-free indoor air laws, laws restricting access of minors to tobacco (including retail tobacco licencing), advertising and promotion restrictions on tobacco products, requirements for warning labels on tobacco products, and requirements for product ingredient disclosure [55]. It provides a practical measure for countries wishing to reduce demand for tobacco in line with WHO FCTC [55]. According to the 2013, WHO Report on the Global Tobacco Epidemic, a third of the world's population is covered by at least one measure of the MPOWER at the highest level. Turkey is the only country at present protecting its entire population with all MPOWER measures at the highest level [56].

Global Adults Tobacco Survey (GATS) report, a component of the Global Tobacco Surveillance System (GTSS), an initiative of the WHO is used by countries to collect data on adult tobacco use and MPOWER measures [14]. In Nigeria, the 2012 survey report which targeted adults aged 15 and older, showed a generally below average indices to the MPOWER measures [14]. This was compounded by the prolonged delay in signing the tobacco smoking bill into law and currently the procrastination in the operationalization and enforcement of the law.

One of the factors that influence consumers in a market economy is price, and the law of demand that defines the typical relationship between price and quantity demanded states that 'consumers will demand more of a particular product at a lower price, and less at a higher price' [37]. This may not entirely apply to cigarette smoking due the associated addiction. The price elasticity of demand measures the responsiveness or sensitivity of the quantity demanded of a particular product to changes in its price [37]. In relation to smoking, there is need to understand how price adjustment will affect the demand for cigarettes. Hence, this will help define the influence of price adjustment as control measure for control of cigarette smoking among the youths.

With effective control measures in place, the rate of tobacco consumption has been stabilised in developed nations between 1970 and 2000. Unfortunately, there has been tremendous increase in consumption rate in the developing countries. Leder and Esson had projected that within the next 25 years the rate of smoking would have increased by 60% and 100% respectively in countries of Medium and Low level human developments respectively [55]. Fifty percent of the mortality from cigarette smoking was projected to involve the productive age groups (35–69 years) which is a great set back to the socioeconomic development of these countries. Nigeria being a part of the WHO FCTC and in the bid to curb this trend, it is necessary to find out the impact of this anti-smoking policy on smoking behaviour of young people.

It will be sufficed to say that; passive smoking is also a challenge in Nigeria as overall prevalence in the home was 24.1%, while it stands at 43.0% in non-home areas including public places [57]. The health impact of this is also enormous which include but not limited to lung cancers, stroke, triggering of asthmatic conditions, TB infections and progression to TB diseases, stroke, chronic obstructive pulmonary diseases, cardiovascular diseases [58]. In 2008, Federal Capital Territory (FCT), Abuja passed most comprehensive public ban on smoking, followed by Lagos State [57]. This ban outlawed smoking in all communal areas including restaurants, bars and workplaces. The National Tobacco Act later provide new opportunities for broad scale reduction in passive smoking exposure in public places at the national level.

In Nigeria, the first law on tobacco regulation was in the Section 6 of the Nigeria (Constitution) Order-in Council of 1954 but it was essentially designed to make provisions for licencing and payment of duties of Tobacco importation. Presently, the only law in-place which also legislates on the consumption and advertisement of tobacco is the "Tobacco Smoking (Control) Decree No. 20 of 1990". It prohibits smoking in public places including schools, public transportation, stadium, theatres, medical establishment etc. It also stipulates restrictions on tobacco advertisements and provides penalties for smokers, sellers and advertisers that do not conform to the provisions [20]. Unfortunately a smoking age limit and the restriction of cigarette sales to or by minor are not provided for in this law. The presence of the so called warnings like: "The Federal Ministry of health warns that Tobacco smoking is dangerous to health" or "Smokers are liable to die young"; appear insufficient since the minors do not understand the implications. The enforcement of the existing law is another questionable issue. The agitations on the existing inefficient anti-smoking laws in Nigeria culminated in the recent commencement of legislative process for the review of the present Tobacco Smoking (Control) Decree No. 20 of 1990. This bill sort for an act to repeal the Tobacco smoking Control Act 1990, CAP. T6 Laws of the Federation and to enact the National Tobacco Control bill 2012 to provide for the regulation and control of production, manufacturing, sale, advertising, promotion and sponsorship of tobacco products in Nigeria and other related matters. The public hearing was held at the National Assembly Complex on 15th October 2014. It was finally passed into law by the legislatures and received the presidential assent on May 27th 2015. The Nigeria National Tobacco Control Act of 2015, was passed to domesticate the WHO FCTC; however, implementation has been poor as most public places are yet to be smoke free, and no funds have been dedicated for tobacco law enforcement. Currently the bureaucratic processes involving the operationalization of the Act is ongoing. The operationalization of this Act needed to be given a deserved attention as report shows half of adolescent smokers become regular smoking adults, and a further half of this population is expected to die of tobacco-associated illnesses, further highlighting the great burden smoking in young poses and the need to end this habit [20]. Hopefully, when the law becomes effectively operationalised and implementation enforced, it will help in reducing the tides of smoking with its attendant health risk.

The health hazards of smoking and the impact on quality of life should be part of focus on tobacco control initiatives for youths. Former smokers should be involved in active antismoking campaigns and the factors that made them quit should be taken into consideration when designing anti-smoking measures.

6. Conclusion

Tobacco smoking poses a huge burden to Nigerian youths (the most populous country in Africa) and the high prevalence and various determinants were reported. Following the 2003 World Health Organisation (WHO) Framework Convention on Tobacco Control (FCTC), Nigeria ratified the convention agreement in 2005, and in 2015 signed into law the National Tobacco Control (NTC) Act that regulates all aspects of tobacco control including advertising, packaging, and smoke-free areas. A thriving tobacco market raises serious public health concerns, particularly for a country with a relatively weak health system.

Careful implementation of smoke-free legislation (targeted at reversing tobacco epidemic) beyond the national level to state and local levels may complement successful measures like taxes, health education and media campaigns. Besides, Nigeria needs to develop comprehensive surveillance systems to monitor the production, sales, and consumption of cigarettes to effectively achieve control targets. It is imperative that all stakeholders engage in concerted efforts in tobacco control strategies.

Author details

Abayomi Ayodapo* and Babalola Ibisola
Department of Family Medicine, University College Hospital, Ibadan, Nigeria

*Address all correspondence to: aayodapo@gmail.com

References

[1] World Health Organization. Global action plan for the prevention and control of noncommunicable diseases, 2013±2020. Geneva, Switzerland: World Health Organization; 2013.

[2] MeÂndez D, Alshanqeety O, Warner KE. The potential impact of smoking control policies on future global smoking trends. Tobacco Control. 2013; 22:46±51. https://doi.org/10.1136/tobaccocontrol-2011-050147 PMID: 22535364

[3] Eriksen M, Mackay J, Schluger N, Islami F, Drope J. The tobacco atlas, 5thed. Atlanta, Georgia: American Cancer Society; 2015.

[4] World Health Organization. Youth and health risks. WHA64.28. 2011. http://www.who.int/hac/events/wha_a64_r28_en_youth_and_health_risks.pdf

[5] Jacobs M. From the First to the Last Ash. The Histroy, Economics and Hazards of Tobacco. Vol. 1. 1995. 1-112 p.

[6] Centers for Disease Control and Prevention. History of the Surgeon General. 2012.

[7] Golden RN, Fiore MC. The 50th anniversary of the Surgeon General's Report on smoking and health. Wis Med J. 2014;113(2):81-82.

[8] The International Tobacco Control Policy Evaluation Project ITC Bhutan Project Report May 2011 (MoH, RGoB, ITC Bhutan Project Report). available from:https://itcproject.org/files/Report_Publications/National_Report/itcbhutanreportapr27v20web.pdf

[9] Oladepo O, Oluwasanu M, Abiona O. Analysis of tobacco control policies in Nigeria: historical development and application of multi-sectoral action. BMC Public Health. 2018;18(Suppl 1): 77-88.

[10] WHO. WHO framework convention on tobacco control. Geneva:World Health Organization; 2003.

[11] Egbe CO, Bialous SA, Glantz SA. Original investigation Avoiding " A Massive Spin-Off Effect in West Africa and Beyond ": The Tobacco Industry Stymies Tobacco Control in Nigeria. Nicotine Tob Res. 2017;19(7): 877-887.

[12] Lim HK, Ghazali SM, Kee CC, Lim KK, Chan YY, Teh HC, et al. Epidemiology of smoking among Malaysian adult males: Prevalence and associated factors. BMC Public Health. 2013;13(1):2-11.

[13] Obot IS. The use of tobacco products among Nigerian adults: a general population survey. Drug Alcohol Depend. 1990;26:203-208.

[14] Health, O F, Ministry of health, WHO, CDC N. Global Adults tobacco survey: Country report 2012. Abuja; 2012.

[15] Awopeju O, Erhabor G, Awosusi B, Awopeju O, Adewole O, Irabor I. Smoking prevalence and attitudes regarding its control among health professional students in South-Western Nigeria. Ann Med Health Sci Res. 2013;3(3):355.

[16] Fawibe AE, Shittu AO. Prevalence and characteristics of cigarette smokers among undergraduates of the University of Ilorin, Nigeria. Niger J Clin Pract. 2011;14(2):201-205.

[17] Mamudu HM, Veeranki SP, John RM. Tobacco use among school - going adolescents (11-17 years) in Ghana. Nicotine Tob Res. 2013;15(8):1355-1364.

[18] Atari DO. Gender differences in the prevalence and determinants of tobacco use among school-aged adolescents (11 - 17 years) in sudan and south sudan. Pan Afr Med J. 2014;18:1-10.

[19] Braithewaite R, Addo J, Smeeth L,Lock K. A systematic review of tobacco smoking prevalence and description of tobaccocontrol strategies in Sub-Saharan African countries; 2007-2014.PLoSONE.2015; 10(7):e0132401

[20] Oyewole BK, Animasahun VJ, Chapman HJ. Tobacco use in Nigerian youth: a systematic review. PLos ONE 2018;13(5):e0196362. doi:10.1371/journal.pone.0196362

[21] Abikoye GE, Kashimawo AJ, Eze CU. Tobacco smoking and awareness of smoking-cessation products in a university community. J Public Heal Epidemiol. 2013;5(8):351-356.

[22] Ebirim CIC, Amadi AN, Abanobi OC, Iloh GUP. The Prevalence of Cigarette Smoking and Knowledge of Its Health Implications among Adolescents in Owerri, South-Eastern. Health (Irvine Calif). 2014;(6):1532-8.

[23] Adeloye D, Anta A, Fawibe A, Gadanya M, Ezeigwe N, Mpazanje RG. Current prevalence pattern of tobacco smoking in Nigeria: a systematic review and meta-analysis BMC Public Health (2019) 19:1719 https://doi.org/10.1186/s12889-019-8010-8

[24] Osungbade KO, Oshiname FO. Determinants of cigarette smoking among senior secondary school students in a rural community of southwest Nigeria. Niger J Med. 2008;17(1):40-44.

[25] Omokhodion FO, Faseru BO. Perception of cigarette smoking and advertisement among senior secondary school students in Ibadan, Southwestern Nigeria. Vol. 26, West African Journal of Medicine. 2007. p. 206-9.

[26] Odeyemi KA, Osibogun A, Akinsete AO, Sadiq L. The Prevalence and Predictors of Cigarette Smoking among Secondary School Students in Nigeria. Niger Postgrad Med J. 2009;16(1):40-45.

[27] Ross H, Chaloupka FJ, Wakefield M. Youth Smoking Uptake Progress: Price and Public Policy Effects. East Econ J. 2003;32(2):355-367.

[28] Morley KI, Lynskey MT, Madden PAF, Treloar SA, Heath AC, Martin NG. Exploring the inter-relationship of smoking age-at-onset, cigarette consumption and smoking persistence: Genes or environment? Psychol Med. 2007;37(9):1357-1367.

[29] Breslau N, Fenn N, Peterson EL. Early smoking initiation and nicotine dependence in a cohort of young adults. Drug Alcohol Depend. 1993;33(2):129-137.

[30] Owoeye A. "Nigeria Tobacco Control Bill, The World is Watching" 2010. A comment on Nigerian Business day Newspaper

[31] Owoeye OB, Olaniyan O. Economic cost of Tobacco-Related Diseases in Nigeria. a study of three Hospitals in Ibadan, Southwest Nigeria. 2015. MPRA Paper No.88054 pgs 1-30. https://mpra.ub.uni-muenchen.de/88054/MPRA Paper No. 88054

[32] Okagua J, Opara P, Alex-Hart BA. Prevalence and determinants of cigarette smoking among adolescents in secondary schools in Port Harcourt, Southern Nigeria. Int J Adolesc Med Health. 2016;28(1):19-24.

[33] Gidwani PP, Sobol A, Dejong W, Perrin JM, Gortmaker SL. Television viewing and initiation of smoking among youth. Pediatrics. 2002;110(3):505-508.

[34] Gecková AM, Stewart R, Van Dijk JP, Orosová O, Groothoff JW,

Post D. Influence of socio-economic status, parents and peers on smoking behaviour of adolescents. Eur Addict Res. 2005;11(4):204-209.

[35] Powell LM. Peer Effects, Tobacco Control Policies, and Youth Smoking Behavior Research Paper Series, No. 24. Tob Control. 2003;(24).

[36] Siziya S, Muula AS, Rudatsikira E. Correlates of current cigarette smoking among in-school adolescents in the Kurdistan region of Iraq. Confl Health. 2007;1(1):13.

[37] Chaloupka FJ, Grossman M. Price, Tobacco Control Policies and Youth Smoking. J Health Econ. 1996;16(3):359-373.

[38] Chaloupka FJ. Youth Smoking Uptake Progress: East Econ J. 2006;32(2):355-367.

[39] Levy DT, Cho S Il, Kim YM, Park S, Suh MK, Kam S. SimSmoke model evaluation of the effect of tobacco control policies in Korea: The unknown success story. Am J Public Health. 2010;100(7):1267-1273.

[40] Levy D, de Almeida LM, Szklo A. The Brazil SimSmoke Policy Simulation Model: The Effect of Strong Tobacco Control Policies on Smoking Prevalence and Smoking-Attributable Deaths in a Middle Income Nation. PLoS Med. 2012; 9(11).

[41] Aubin HJ, Tilikete S, Barrucand D. Depression and Smoking. Encephale.1996; 22(1);17-22. PMID: 8681871

[42] Middlekauff HR, Park J, Moheimani RS. Adverse effects of cigarette and non-cigarette smoke exposure on the autonomic nervous system: mechanism and implications for cardiovascular risk. Journal of American College of Cardiology 2014; 64(16):1740-1750.

[43] Pierce JP, Evans N, Farkas A J, Cavin SW, Berry C, Kramer M, et al. Tobacco Use in California: An Evaluation of the Tobacco Control Program, 1989-1993. 1994 *La Jolla, California*; University of Calif. San Diego; 164-167.

[44] D'Souza MS, Markou A. Neuronal mechanism underlying development of nicotine dependence: implications for novel smoking-cessation treatments. Addiction Science Practice 2011; 6(11):4-6.

[45] Kenny P, Markou A.2006. Nicotine self-administration acutely activates brain reward systems and induces a long-lasting increase in reward sensitivity. Neuropsychopharmacology 2006; 31:1203-1211.

[46] Kumar A, Gulati R, Singhal S, Hasan A, Khan A. The effect of smoking on the hearing status-A hospital based study. Journal of clinical and diagnostic research 2013;7(2): 210-214. doi:10.7860/jcdr/2013/4968.2730

[47] Gajalakshmi V, Peto R, Kanaka TS, Jha P. Smoking and mortality from tuberculosis and other diseases in India:retrospective study of 43000 adult male deaths and 35000 controls. The Lancet 2003;362;9383:507-515. DOI: https://doi.org/10.1016/S0140-6736(03)14109-8

[48] Yawson AE, Baddoo A, Hagan-seneadza NA, Calys-tagoe B, Hewlett S, Dako-gyeke P, et al. Tobacco use in older adults in Ghana: sociodemographic characteristics, health risks and subjective wellbeing. BMC Public Health. 2013;13:1-8.

[49] Ibekwe R. Modifiable risk factors of hypertension and socio-demographic profile in Oghara, Delta State; prevalence and correlates. Ann Med Health Sci Res. 2015;5(1):71.

[50] Ige OK, Owoaje ET, Adebiyi OA. Non communicable disease and risky

behaviour in an urban university community Nigeria. Afr Health Sci. 2013;13(1):62-67.

[51] Oladimeji AM onisol., Fawole O, Nguku P, Nsubuga P. Prevalence and factors associated with hypertension and obesity among civil servants in Kaduna, Kaduna State, June 2012. Pan Afr Med J. 2014;18(June 2012):13.

[52] Onyekwena C, Chukwuemelie Akanonu P, Ishaku J. The economics of tobacco control in Nigeria: modelling the fiscal and health effects of a tobacco excise tax change in Nigeria. Tob Induc Dis. 2018;16(1).

[53] Owoeye OB, Olaniyan O. Economic cost of tobacco-related diseases in Nigeria: a study of three hospitals in Ibadan, Southwest Nigeria. 2018;(88054).

[54] Medicine NL of. Tobacco use and dependence Guideline Panel. Treating Tobacco use and dependence: 2008 Update. Rockville (MD); 2008.

[55] WHO. WHO Framework Convention on Tobacco Control. 2004.

[56] WHO. WHO report on the global tobaccco epidemic 2013: Enforcing bans on tobacco advertising, promotion and sponsorship. 2013.

[57] Omaduvie U, Adisa A. Exposure to Secondhand Smoke in the Home and Public areas among Adolescents in Abuja, Nigeria: Tobacco control implications. Tob. Prev. Cessation 2015; 1(8):1-6. http://dx.doi.org/10.18332/tpc/61178

[58] Iloh GU, Amadi AN, Iro OK. Epidemiology of exposure to secondhand smoke from cigarettes among innocent neversmoked adult Nigerians in a resource-poor environment of a primary care clinic in Southeastern Nigeria. Arch Med Health Sci 2017; 5:59-64.

Section 3

Lifestyle and Cardiovascular Diseases

Chapter 10

Lifestyle and Epidemiology: Poverty and Cardiovascular Diseases a Double Burden in African Populations

Franck Ngowa Nzali, Mazou Ngou Temgoua, Joel Noutakdie Tochie and Simeon Pierre Ckoukem

Abstract

Cardiovascular diseases (CVDs), ranked top non-communicable diseases (NCDs), are the second leading cause of mortality in Africa, especially in sub-Saharan Africa (SSA) where they account for 73·4% global deaths and 80% of all premature deaths yearly. The ill-health due to CVDs in SSA is equivalent to the combined burden due to communicable, maternal, neonatal and nutritional diseases. Un-addressed, it is extrapolated that the Sustainable Development Goal 3.4 which targets NCDs will not be achieved. The preponderance of CVDs in SSA is due to determinants such as the epidemiological transition of diseases, aging, stress, illiteracy, poor health systems and poverty. This is quite worrisome for SSA dubbed "one of the most poverty stricken region on the globe". As such, poverty in Africa may adversely affect CVDs, but this has been less examined. This chapter explores the impact of poverty on CVDs and healthcare systems related to CVDs in Africa.

Keywords: epidemiology, poverty, cardiovascular, disease, Africa

1. Introduction

Cardiovascular diseases (CVDs) such as heart failure, cerebrovascular diseases, and ischemic heart diseases are major plaques in Africa. The burden of CVDs is high in Africa and particularly in sub-Saharan Africa (SSA) where the magnitude of CVDs is equivalent to the combined magnitude due to communicable, maternal, neonatal and nutritional diseases. In Africa the burden of CVDs, is partly flued by poverty which is often overlooked. This chapter discusses the impact of poverty on CVDs and healthcare systems related to CVDs in Africa.

2. Epidemiological transition and cardiovascular diseases in Africa

Epidemiological transition can be defined as the transition, under the influence of socio-economic development and aging, from predominantly infectious diseases to mainly chronic non-communicable diseases [1]. This concept was first introduced in the 1971's by Omrad and Olshansky, and Ault later on refined its meaning [2]. The transition process according to Omrad was in three ages or phases [2]: The age of pestilence and famine, the age of receding pandemics, and the age of degenerative and man-made diseases.

The age of pestilence and famine is characterized by a period of high infant and child mortality with a low mean life expectancy of less than 30 years. This stemmed from the high rate of malnutrition and infectious diseases or communicable disease like tuberculosis, pneumonia, and diarrheal diseases in Africa; with less than 10% of the mortality rate due to cardiovascular diseases [2, 3]. The age of receding pandemics is characterized by an improvement in public health policies and nutrition patterns leading to a decrease in the rate of infant and child deaths from to malnutrition and infectious diseases. This decrease in mortality was accompanied by a rise in the life expectancy from 30 to 50 years or more [2, 3]. The age of degenerative and man-made diseases is marked by an excessive intake of fat and calories with a decrease in physical activity leading to the emergence of non-communicable diseases (NCDs) such as ischemic heart diseases and heart failure. An increase in life expectancy as a result of a reduction in the mortality rate of infectious or communicable diseases tremendously marked the age of degenerative and man-made diseases. On the other hand, there is a higher death rate shift in NCD, more specifically cardiovascular diseases (CVDs). The death rate due to CVDs varies between 35 and 65% of the overall mortality rate [2, 3]. The challenges entail strengthening the prevention and improvement of the management of CVD.

Low- to middle-income countries (LMICs) in Sub-Saharan Africa (SSA) are of the epidemiological transition process [4]. A 20-year assessment of the disease burden in SSA between 1990 to 2010 shows a decline in premature mortality and disability attributable to neonatal, nutritional and maternal communicable diseases, including lower respiratory infections and diarrhoeal diseases [4]. It is worth mentioning that there were communicable diseases that occur permanently with the same high mortality rate over these 20 years-periods [4]. With only 12% of the world's population in Africa, Africa bears a considerable proportion of the global burden of tuberculosis, HIV/AIDS and malaria with rates of 31%, 62% and 70% respectively [5]. Besides communicable diseases, the disease burden due to NCDs is not trivial. Between 1990 to 2010, the disease burden from several NCDs increased, particularly stroke, depression, diabetes, and ischemic heart disease [4]. An assessment made in SSA from 1990 to 2017 shows a 67% growth in the total number of disability-adjusted lives (DALYS) due to NCDs (90.6 million in 1990 and 151.3 million in 2017) [6]. The increment in NCDs in SSA was mainly flued by CVDs, ranked as the second leading cause of the NCD burden in 2017, resulting in 22.9 (21.5–24.3) million DALYs (15.1% of the total NCD burden), after the group of disorders categorized as other NCDs (28.8 million [25.1–33.0] DALYs, 19.1%) [6]. This data show the progressive and increasing installation of NCDs in Africa and their impact on morbidity and mortality.

3. Poverty in Africa

Poverty is a multidimensional concept. According to the United Nations Development Programme (UNDP), poverty is not only the lack of income necessary to meet food and non-food needs (clothing, energy, housing) but also a lack of basic human capabilities (illiteracy, malnutrition, reduced life expectancy, poor maternal health, illness) [7]. Therefore poverty should not be considered only under the spectrum of financial income; as a result, the concept of poverty is difficult to quantify. But for a global assessment of poverty, a monetary scale has been developed as a common denominator between the different regions of the world in order to be able to assess poverty. According to the World Bank, the poverty line is considered to be 1.90 dollars per day per inhabitant since 2011 [8]. In 2015, the rate of the world's population living in poverty was 10%, representing 736 million people, more than half of whom live in SSA, on less than US$1 a day [8, 9]. The advent of industrialization in China and India tremendously decreased the poverty rate unlike in SSA where progress in poverty has been limited. Of these 736 million poverty stricken population living on earth in 2015, 80% resided in SSA [10]. According to the World Bank's estimates, the global poverty rate slightly dipped to 8.6% in 2018. No isolated figure was reported for SSA. But since 2018, the World Bank has repeatedly reported that SSA will consistently record a poverty rate of at least two figures till the year 2030 unless very drastic interventions are put into place to address the problem of poverty in SSA [10].

In several SSA countries, the direct care costs, are high in relation to household income, a major factor in poverty. The cost of HIV/AIDS treatment for an adult, combined with the loss of income due to absence from work, can push an entire household below the poverty line. Therefore, just as good health can stimulate economic growth, poor health can lead to poverty from which it is very difficult to escape. The vicious cycle of poverty and poor health is observed in many African countries. About 76% of people in SSA have an income of less than US$2 per day and 46.5% have an income of less than US$1.08 per day [9]. While poverty has been declining in other parts of the world such as East and South Asia over the two decades the trend is clearly reversed in SSA. Between 1981 and 2001, the domestic product of SSA countries fell by 13% and the number of people in this region living on less than US$1 per day doubled from 164 million to 314 million. While Africans accounted for only 16% of the world's poor population in the year 1985, the proportion rose to 31% by 1998, and this trend is expected to continue [9].

4. Cost of management of cardiovascular disease in Africa

In Africa, the cost of management is variable. With regard to hypertension, the overall average daily cost of drug treatment for uncomplicated hypertension is estimated at 368 ± 234.6 FCFA, i.e. 0.68 ± 0.44 dollars, representing more than a third of the daily income (1.90 dollars) [11]. In view of the cost of treatment, the absence of symptoms associated with hypertension is often the cause of non-adherence to treatment. Also, some patients who often reach the stages of complications of CVDs often experience the cost of treatment increased by the additional cost of treating the associated complications [12].

In Africa, 60–70% of health expenditure is paid by households directly to health facilities, compared to a global average of 46%. This may be due to the preponderance of the informal sector (farmers, craftsmen,...) which groups together more than 70% of the African population who are not covered by health insurance. Contrary to those in the informal sector, some African governments are setting up compulsory health insurance systems for the formal sector, civil servants or employees of private companies, financed through employee and employer contributions [13].

5. Poverty, malnutrition and cardiovascular disease: a vicious cycle

Poverty is one of the socio-economic factors at the root of malnutrition in Africa. The prevalence of malnutrition in SSA rose from 181 million in 2010 to 222 million in 2016 [14]. Poverty and malnutrition are part of a vicious circle. Poverty leads to malnutrition, especially maternal malnutrition, which causes low birth weight, stunted infants and adolescents. These individuals will be disadvantaged later in life because they may show a reduction in physical and mental development leading to low skills and reduced human capital. Competence is one of the faculties developed through adequate nutrition of children and adolescents. Wachs has defined competence as the ability to adapt and interact with one's environment [15]. Human capital refers to well-nourished, healthy, educated, skilled and alert individuals - an improved human condition - resulting in a workforce that could be the most productive asset of any country. However, the absence of this productivity, particularly economic productivity, perpetuates poverty [16]. Alongside poverty, we also have a trend towards the Westernization of the African lifestyle, which is not the least compounding factor for the emergence of CVDs in Africa.

The African population is experiencing an increasing rate of urbanization, with a shift in migration from rural to urban areas, with changes in lifestyle habits in particular, as the traditional diet rich in fruits and vegetables is gradually being replaced by a diet rich in calories densed foods from snacks, sweetened beverages, animal fats and low in complex carbohydrates. This change in diet is accompanied by weight gain (overweight and obesity) and a decrease in physical activity due to the abolishment of traditional agriculture for sedentary work [9]. This change in lifestyle is contributing to an increase in the prevalence of cardiovascular risk factors in Africa, with a tendency to equalize the prevalence in high-income countries. The prevalences of some cardiovascular risk factors in SSA are given below in comparison with high-income countries (HICs): Smoking rates are 10% in SSA versus 30% in HIC; hypertension prevalence in individuals ≥18 years old is 30% in SSA (40% in urban and 20% in rural populations) versus 20% in HIC; diabetes mellitus prevalence in persons aged above 17 years is 7.1% in adult males and females in SSA compared with up to 8% in males and up to 6% in women in HIC. Also, dyslipidemia prevalence in adults is 25% in SSA versus 40–60% in HICs; physical inactivity prevalence is 22% in SSA versus 29–40% in HIC; and obesity whose prevalence rates are variable in SSA and higher among women (2–40%) compared with men (1–15%) versus 18–35% in women and 12–30% among men in HIC [17]. Poverty has several consequences, including the development of communicable and non-communicable diseases.

In the 1980s, a real revolution in the understanding of chronic diseases in adults was initiated with the pioneering work of an English epidemiologist named David Barker. During an observational study, he found that regions of UK that had a high rate of cardiovascular mortality, also had a high infant mortality rate [18]. Then a meticulous study of patients with NCDs [18], allowed him to put forward a hypothesis on the "origin of the development of health and disease" or early origin of adult diseases based on the premise that environmental factors during foetal life have a considerable impact on the susceptibility to various pathologies later in life of these exposed persons [18]. More precisely; malnutrition occuring in utero permanently changes the body's structure and function in ways that "programme" the appearance of disease in childhood, adolescenthood or adulthood [18].

At present it has been recognized that malnutrition during pregnancy is the cause of an alteration in the fetus in the short term of the programmed metabolism of carbohydrates and lipids and of the functions of the genes. In the long term, these changes will lead to reduced cognitive development, decreased educational performance, compromised immunity, lower physical capacity and an increased risk of several NCDs [18–21]. The physiopathological mechanisms by which foetal malnutrition can lead to NCDs are better elucidated to date. Gluckman and collaborators have shown that malnutrition is responsible for a modification of gene expression via epigenetic modification by methylation of foetal DNA. They hypothesized that the changed genetic expression may change physiological set points that will eventually change the way individuals respond to environmental exposures later on their lives [22]. The management of CVDs management leads to direct and indirect costs, thus perpetuating the vicious circle of poverty.

Direct costs are related to chronic diseases and these costs entail the direct payment by patients for cardiovascular healthcare services, cardiovascular investigation tests (12-led electrocardiogram, Holter electrocardiogram, stress electrocardiogram, heart ultrasound, transesophageal ultrasound) and medications for CVDs. Patients with CVDs are often confronted with a dilemma: to suffer and possibly die without treatment, or to seek treatment and drag their families into poverty. The situation is particularly serious for people with long-term chronic CVDs such as chronic heart failure, stroke survivals with significant physical disabilities because the costs of medical care is often life-long and relatively expensive. Indirect costs are a reduction in income subject to illness due to loss of productivity resulting from illness or death; the cost of time spent by adult members of the family household caring for those who are ill. There is also the loss of income that will result from the sale of goods necessitated by the need to meet direct costs and unpredictable expenses, and the missed opportunities for children who are forced to give up school to care for sick adults or contribute to the family economy [21]. Hence, CVDs will not only have a detrimental effect on the income of the patients with CVDs, but also on that of the family; subsequently, there will be with a marked pejorative impact on the economy of different African nations resulting in a drop in the economy of the African continent.

6. Prevention of cardiovascular diseases and insurance health system of African countries

6.1 Prevention of cardiovascular diseases

According to the WHO, primary prevention of CVDs is defined as measures put in place to decrease the incidence of cardiovascular events (ischaemic heart disease and strokes) in individuals at risk of CVDs who have not yet developed overt or clinical CVDs. Efforts geared at preventing recurrent clinical cardiovascular events in individuals with CVDs are called secondary prevention [22]. Reports have shown the beneficial impacts of pharmacological interventions in primary and secondary the prevention of CVDs, though with caveats for population-based interventions. The need for economic assessment of these studies to identify those which have best value for money is paramount in inform decision making by health policy makers in designing a health system insurance policy [23]. Furthermore, WHO projects that by 2030, NCDs will overtake all other causes of mortality in all Africa [24]. With the increasing CVDs burden in Africa, the AHN was created in 2001. The AHN is a joint collaboration of various cardiovascular societies and national heart foundations sharing the same agenda: curbing CVDs in Africa, thereby improving the cardiovascular health for all Africans. The vision of the AHN is to play a leading role in the prevention and reduction of the burden related to CVDs, including cerebrovascular accident to halt from no longer being the major etiology of disability and premature death in the African continent. The AHN shares the vision of the World Heart Federation (WHF), the main organization of national and continental cardiovascular societies and foundations globally. The WHF's global target of '25 by 25' represents the objective of decreasing premature deaths caused by CVDs by 25% by the year 2025—an interim goal addressed by the Sousse' Declaration of 2018 [25]. The objective of the AHN held in Tunisia in 2018 was on the prevention of CVDs. The conference was endorsed by the Minister of Health of Tunisia, highlighting the importance of governmental collaborations in attending 'health-for-all'. Themes arising from the conference included the management of various cardiovascular risk factors, legislation of these cardiovascular risk factors, and using the leverage of other local and international organizations to improve cardiovascular health in Africa. Cited cardiovascular risk factors to be urgently cared for in Africa include diabetes mellitus, hypertension and dyslipidaemia. There is therapeutic inertia in the therapeutic algorithms of these conditions especially hypertension. The AHN emphasized on the importance of the timely treatment of resistant hypertension. Obesity was highlighted as the main driver of the diabetes epidemic in Tunisia as well as Africa, with 75% of patients with Type 2 diabetes mellitus dying from CVDs. A 1% improvement in glycosylated hemoglobin was shown to decrease mortality from ischemic heart disease by more than 14% in the Tunisian population although glycemic control is not often achieved in the African continent due to low awareness, treatment and control of diabetic patients who often present late with acute complications of diabetes mellitus such as hyperglycemic comas. Various barriers to control had been identified, namely the inability of clinicians to apply treatment guidelines, inadequate monitoring or surveillance of blood pressure and glycaemia, lack of community education and empowerment, and most importantly, the cost of accessing healthcare. There is also a poor awareness of the cardiovascular risks associated with dyslipidemia in SSA. The South African perspective displayed an increase in the burden of dyslipidemia due to anti-retroviral therapy (ART) induced dyslipidemia in patients living with HIV/AIDS and treated with ART. This needs to be promptly managed in order to prevent CVDs. Previous studies have identified the huge burden of premature ischemic heart disease partly due to dyslipidemia in Africa compared to other regions [26]. This reflects a lack of prevention, early detection and effective management of CVDs in Africa. Preventing CVDs remains a major challenge for development within the region as it results in significant health, financial and social consequences for individuals and government. Likewise, the control of tobacco use, known a risk factor of six of the eight leading causes of CVDs death was highlighted as being important. The role of healthcare providers and health authorities in preventing CVDs due to tobacco use was addressed through a governmental vote on the increment of tobacco taxation as there remains a discrepancy between taxes paid and the treatment cost of tobacco related health disease and death. The WHO 'MPOWER' package was emphasized as a tool to assist countries with tobacco reduction measures. In addition, patients should be motivated by clinicians and family members to quit smoking with both counseling and the early use of pharmacotherapy. In the same vein, the formulation of legislations to control cardiovascular risk factors including the control intervention for the effective implementation of physical exercise and encouraging a low-calorie dense foods to prevent CVDs mortality related to obesity and diabetes mellitus are strongly recommended. This will however, require an involvement from policy makers for the formulation of public health interventions geared at curbing the burden of CVDs in Africa. Moreover, there is a shortage in drugs and equipment for monitoring CVDs between African countries which needs to be addressed for CVDs prevention. This is due to preference in healthcare expenditures for infectious diseases at the detriment of CVDs in Africa. Various partnerships including the WHF, the United Nations the Non-communicable disease alliance (NCD Alliance), Pan African Society of Cardiologists (PASCAR), American Heart Association (AHA), Medtronic Foundation, Heart and Stroke Foundation of South Africa, World Heart Day events, The Kenyan-Heart Talking Walls project are key continental and inter-continental foundations trying to achieve and prevent cardiovascular health for all in Africa. Also, the social media is a crucial platform to increase awareness in communities regarding CVDs awareness and prevention. Successful CVDs preventive interventions such as the RESOLVE and the WHO Global Hearts projects need to be taken by African Stakeholders to improve cardiovascular health by addressing important issues such as improved management of hypertension, decreasing salt intake and tobacco use. It is worth to mention that CVDs prevention in Africa can significantly be achieved by identifying health advocates as well as effective leadership and the coalition of professional groups. Hence, an 'Africa-specific' guidelines for CVDs prevention need to be formulated and adopted. CVD risk factors prevention in Africa cannot be overemphasized as cardiac surgery to amend cardiovascular diseases still remain expensive and scarce in a continent already overburdened with poverty.

The International Forum for Hypertension Control and Prevention in Africa formulated treatment guidelines for CVDs prevention in 2003 [27]. Since then, CVDs preventive interventions to identify cardiovascular risk factors and set guidelines are now under way. Some African countries have conducted epidemiological studies, a few have begun to continually monitor and assess their programmes, and others, Nigeria and South Africa, have their own guidelines for managing hypertension. There is hope though, and some attention has finally been focused on CVDs prevention in Africa. However, challenges such as poor healthcare infrastructure, underfunded and understaffed health systems in Africa, inadequate access to cheap generic drugs and lack of public recognition and acceptance of the importance of CVDs will continue to hinder the effective implementation of both population-based health programmes and those aimed at people at high CVDs risk [28, 29]. The continent's people need education on healthier lifestyles such as weight reduction, smoking cessation, and greater physical activity.

6.2 Insurance health system of African countries

CVDs are very burdensome to manage in Africa due to a lack of a national health insurance policy in most SSA countries [30]. Health systems insurance is primordial for achieving universal healthcare by providing financial protection to patients. It helps protect people from high healthcare costs by pooling funds to allow a cross-subsidization between the rich and poor and between the healthy and the sick [31]. Healthcare insurance coverage is still inexistent or at an embryonic stage in most African countries. This has largely contributed to poverty, poor cardiology service delivery and mortality from CVDs in Africa. Implementing an African health system insurance remains an important goal to improve the health status of individuals in Africa [4]. Reports illustrates that in the several SSA countries, direct out-of-pocket payments as a share of total health expenditure are still above 40%, exorbitantly high above WHO 20% threshold level of the total health expenditure below which financial risk protection can be ensured, and thus leading to poverty in Africa [32]. There is a serious handicapping sparsity of health systems insurance in most African nations where only about 15% of the 55 countries have national comprehensive health insurance schemes [33]. Evidence abounds that in SSA, the poor bear the highest burden of diseases and subsequently, experience very high expenses on healthcare costs [34]. Hence, the development of a health system insurance scheme should be advocated in public health and financial planning within African countries for better healthcare delivery in general. A universal healthcare system with national-level health insurance scheme would probably be more efficacious to avoid the low-socioeconomic class of the population from being marginalized. Strategies such as compulsory taxations from employees, deductions from sales taxes, and an increment on tobacco taxes have been shown to be effective in some countries in SSA [35] .A comparative study of five African countries (Ghana, Tanzania, Kenya, Rwanda and Ethiopia) sought to help fill this gap by looking at how a national health system insurance schemes can cover the poor or not, as the case may be. Selected countries had were national insurance schemes with the intent of providing health insurance for all their inhabitants. Ghana, Kenya and Tanzania had similar health insurance programmes [36–40]. Ghana's National Health Insurance Scheme (NHIS), covers every citizen by law. Tanzania and Kenya had separate insurance schemes for the public and private sectors. Rwanda and Ethiopia operated a Community-Based Health Insurance (CBHI), but Rwanda's CBHI was the only one with wide coverage of the poor. Hence, setting down insurance policies or programmes does not guarantee reaching the poor. Many have questioned whether African countries have been too eager to adopt Western-style policies that are not necessarily appropriate to their context-specific fiscal laws. The selected countries are characterized by large informal sectors, making it difficult for the rolling out of health insurance scheme models that depend on this group. After almost 12 years of introducing national health insurance in Ghana, less than 40% of the population were covered by the health system insurance scheme. In spite of provisions made to cover the poor, health system insurance programmes have faced challenges in enrolling this group. Defining who the poor are is a task that policymakers have grappled with. Many terms have been used to identify the poor—ultrapoor, very poor, indigent and vulnerable. Coining these terms and explaining what they mean and who qualifies to be categorized as such has become not only burdensome but costly—and political [41].

The way forward to establishing a sustainable cost-effective and context specific health system insurance scheme in SSA should take into consideration the following. Firstly, the fact that the educational and socioeconomic status of a family play key roles in the decision of whether to enroll in health insurance should take into consideration that community-based health insurance provides some financial protection by reducing out-of-pocket spending [42]. Secondly, data analysis from micro-level household indicates that community financing improves access by rural and private sector workers to needed heath care and provides them with some financial protection against the cost of illness. Thirdly, analysis from macro-level cross-country gives empirical support to the hypothesis that risk-sharing in health financing matters in terms of its impact on both the level and distribution of health, financial fairness and responsiveness indicators [43].

7. Conclusion

In view of the vicious circle of poverty, lifestyle and cardiovascular disease in Africa, we propose some solutions to break this cycle. Women of childbearing age need to be well nourished, empowered and educated. They are "the most proximal levers" on which we can act to ensure optimal foetal and infant nutrition to break the vicious circle of poverty; malnutrition, underdevelopment and non-communicable disease. Obstacles hampering primary and secondary prevention of CVDs in SSA such as insufficient health care systems and infrastructure, scarcity of cardiologists, skewed budget allocation and disproportionate prioritization away from NCDs, high cost of cardiac treatments and interventions coupled with rarity of health insurance systems in most African countries need to be urgently addressed by the various governments and ministries of health of different African countries.

Author details

Franck Ngowa Nzali[1], Mazou Ngou Temgoua[1], Joel Noutakdie Tochie[2,3]*
and Simeon Pierre Ckoukem[3,4]

1 Department of Internal Medicine and Specialties, Faculty of Medicine and Biomedical Sciences, University of Yaoundé I, Cameroon

2 Department of Anesthesiology and Critical Care Medicine, Faculty of Medicine and Biomedical Sciences, University of Yaoundé I, Cameroon

3 Health and Human Development (2HD) Research Network, Douala, Cameroon

4 Department of Internal Medicine and Specialties, Faculty of Medicine and Pharmaceutical Sciences, University of Dschang, Dschang, Cameroon

*Address all correspondence to: joeltochie@gmail.com

References

[1] Master Environnement et Santé [Internet]. [cité 17 nov 2020]. Disponible sur: http://www.m2-ssents.uvsq.fr/spip.php?article801

[2] Aubry P, Gaüzère B-A. Les maladies non transmissibles dans les pays du sud. Medecine tropicale. 2017;1-6.

[3] ZIPES D, LIBBY P, BONOW R, MANN D, TOMASELL G, BRAUNWALD E. BRAUNWALD'S HEART DISEASE. BRAUNWALD'S HEART DISEASE A TEXTBOOK OF CARDIOVASCULAR MEDICINE [Internet]. ELEVENTH. Elservier; 2019. p. 24-6. Disponible sur: https://t.me/MedicalBooksStore

[4] The Global Burden of Disease: Main Findings for Sub-Saharan Africa [Internet]. World Bank. [cité 18 nov 2020]. Disponible sur: https://www.worldbank.org/en/region/afr/publication/global-burden-of-disease-findings-for-sub-saharan-africa

[5] Maher et Sekajugo - 2010 - Health transition in Africa practical policy prop.pdf [Internet]. [cité 18 nov 2020]. Disponible sur: https://www.who.int/bulletin/volumes/88/12/10.077891.pdf?ua=1

[6] Gouda HN, Charlson F, Sorsdahl K, Ahmadzada S, Ferrari AJ, Erskine H, et al. Burden of non-communicable diseases in sub-Saharan Africa, 1990-2017: results from the Global Burden of Disease Study 2017. The Lancet Global Health [Internet]. Elsevier; 1 oct 2019 [cité 18 nov 2020];7(10):e1375-87. Disponible sur: https://www.thelancet.com/journals/langlo/article/PIIS2214-109X(19)30374-2/abstract

[7] Définitions et approches de la pauvreté [Internet]. [cité 29 nov 2020]. Disponible sur: http://www.bsi-economics.org/416-definitions-approches-pauvrete

[8] Rapport 2018 sur la pauvreté et la prospérité partagée: compléter le puzzle de la pauvreté [Internet]. World Bank. [cité 29 nov 2020]. Disponible sur: https://www.banquemondiale.org/fr/research/brief/poverty-and-shared-prosperity-2018-piecing-together-the-poverty-puzzle-frequently-asked-questions

[9] La santé des populations: le rapport sur la santé dans la Région africaine. La santé des populations: le rapport sur la santé dans la Région africaine. Organisation Mondiale de la Santé; 2006. p. 1-192.

[10] Selon la Banque mondiale, l'extrême pauvreté continue à reculer dans le monde, mais à un rythme ralenti [Internet]. World Bank. [cité 28 déc 2020]. Disponible sur: https://www.banquemondiale.org/fr/news/press-release/2018/09/19/decline-of-global-extreme-poverty-continues-but-has-slowed-world-bank

[11] Ellenga-Mbolla B, TR G, Kaky GS, Dilou-Bassemouka L, Ikama MS. Coût du traitement médicamenteux de l'HTA. Médecine d'Afrique noire. 26 janv 2010;57:9-14.

[12] Yaya SH, Kengne AP. L'hypertension artérielle en Afrique: présent et nouvelles perspectives.: 16.

[13] Comment étendre la couverture de l'assurance santé en Afrique ? [Internet]. ID4D. 2017 [cité 28 déc 2020]. Disponible sur: https://ideas4development.org/couverture-maladie-afrique/

[14] Onyango AW, Jean-Baptiste J, Samburu B, Mahlangu TLM. Regional Overview on the Double Burden of Malnutrition and Examples of Program and Policy Responses: African Region. ANM [Internet]. Karger Publishers; 2019 [cité 27 nov 2020];75(2):127-30.

Disponible sur: https://www.karger.com/Article/FullText/503671

[15] Wachs TD. The nature and nurture of child development. Food and Nutrition Bulletin. SAGE Publications Sage CA: Los Angeles, CA; 1999;20(1):7-22.

[16] Streeten P. Human development: means and ends. the american Economic review. JSTOR; 1994;84(2):232-237.

[17] Yuyun MF, Sliwa K, Kengne AP, Mocumbi AO, Bukhman G. Cardiovascular Diseases in Sub-Saharan Africa Compared to High-Income Countries: An Epidemiological Perspective. Glob Heart [Internet]. [cité 8 oct 2020];15(1). Disponible sur: https://www.ncbi.nlm.nih.gov/pmc/articles/PMC7218780/

[18] Barker DJ. The fetal and infant origins of adult disease. BMJ: British Medical Journal [Internet]. BMJ Publishing Group; 17 nov 1990 [cité 28 nov 2020];301(6761):1111. Disponible sur: https://www.ncbi.nlm.nih.gov/pmc/articles/PMC1664286/

[19] Goedecke JH, Jennings CL, Lambert EV. Obesity in South Africa. Chronic diseases of lifestyle in South Africa. 1995;2005(2006):65.

[20] Levitt NS, Lambert EV, Norris SA. Early life origins of adult chronic disease: a South African perspective. Medical Research Council; 2006;

[21] Shetty PS, McPherson K. Diet, nutrition and chronic disease: lessons from contrasting worlds. John Wiley and Sons; 1997.

[22] World Health Organization (WHO). Prevention of cardiovascular disease: guidelines for assessment and management of cardiovascular risk. Geneva, Switzerland: 2007.

[23] Ortegón M, Lim S, Chisholm D et al. Cost effectiveness of strategies to combat cardiovascular disease, diabetes, and tobacco use in sub-Saharan Africa and South East Asia: mathematical modelling study. BMJ 2012;344:e607 10.1136/bmj.e607

[24] World Health Organization. Global status report on noncommunicable diseases 2010 [Internet]. World Health. 2010. p. 176. Available from: http://whqlibdoc.who.int/publications/2011/9789240686458_eng.pdf

[25] WHO. Global action plan for the prevention and control of noncommunicable diseases 2013-2020. World Heal Organ. 2013;102.

[26] Federation WH. Sousse Declaration 2018 [Internet]. 2018 [cited 2018 Nov 15]. Available from: https://www.world-heart-federation.org/news/sousse-declaration-together-can-combat-premature-mortality-cvd-africa/

[27] Lemogoum D, Seedat YK, Mabadeje AF, Mendis S, Bovet P, Onwubere B, et al; International Forum for Hypertension control and prevention in Africa. Recommendations for prevention, diagnosis and management of hypertension and cardiovascular risk factors in sub-Saharan Africa. J Hypertens 2003;21: 1993-2000.

[28] Agyepong IA, Sewankambo N, Binagwaho A, Coll-Seck AM, Corrah T, Ezeh A, et al. The path to longer and healthier lives for all Africans by 2030: The Lancet Commission on the future of health in sub-Saharan Africa. *Lancet (London, England)*. 2018; 390(10114): 2803-59. DOI: https://doi.org/10.1016/S0140-6736(17)31509-X

[29] Bonny A, Ngantcha M, Jeilan M, Okello E, Kaviraj B, Talle MA, et al. Statistics on the use of cardiac electronic devices and interventional electrophysiological procedures in

Africa from 2011 to 2016: Report of the Pan African Society of Cardiology (PASCAR) Cardiac Arrhythmias and Pacing Task Forces. *Europace: European pacing, arrhythmias, and cardiac electrophysiology: Journal of the working groups on cardiac pacing, arrhythmias, and cardiac cellular electrophysiology of the European Society of Cardiology*. 2018; 20(9): 1513-26. DOI: https://doi.org/10.1093/europace/eux353

[30] Benjamin EJ, Virani SS, Callaway CW, Chamberlain AM, Chang AR, Cheng S, et al. Heart Disease and Stroke Statistics – 2018 Update: A Report From the American Heart Association. *Circulation*. 2018; 137(12): e67–e492. DOI: https://doi.org/10.1161/CIR.0000000000000573

[31] Mathauer I, Schmidt J-O, Wenyaa M. Extending social health insurance to the informal sector in Kenya. An assessment of factors affecting demand. Int J Health Plann Manage 2008; 23(1):51-68

[32] World Health Organization (WHO). State of health financing in the African region. Brazzaville: WHO Africa; 2013. Available at: https://www.afro.who.int/sites/default/files/2017-06/state-of-health-financing-afro.pdf

[33] Agyepong IA, Sewankambo N, Binagwaho A, Coll-Seck AM, Corrah T, Ezeh A, et al. The path to longer and healthier lives for all Africans by 2030: The Lancet Commission on the future of health in sub-Saharan Africa. *Lancet (London, England)*. 2018; 390(10114): 2803-59. DOI: https://doi.org/10.1016/S0140-6736(17)31509-X

[34] World Health Organization. Health systems financing: the path to universal coverage. World Health Report 2010 Geneva: World Health Organization; 2010. http://www.who.int/whr/2010/en.).

[35] World Health Organization (WHO). Public financing for health in Africa: From Abuja to the SDGs. 2016. Available at: https://www.who.int/health_financing/documents/public-financing-africa/en/.

[36] National Health Insurance Authority . National Health Insurance Authority Annual Report Accra: NHIA-Ghana ; 2013 .

[37] Marwa CW . Provision of national health insurance fund services to its members; pain or gain? Unif J Sport Health Sci 2016 ;2 (1):1-6 .

[38] Kunda T . Increasing equity among community based health insurance members in Rwanda through a socioeconomic stratification process. Paper presented at the Third International Conference of the African Health Economics and Policy Association, 2014 .

[39] Feleke S , Workie M , Hailu Z et al. Ethiopia's community-based health insurance: a step on the road to universal health coverage Washington, DC: US Agency for International Development; 2015.

[40] Deolitte CL . A strategic review of NHIF and market assessment of private prepaid health schemes Nairobi: Ministry of Medical Services ; 2011 .

[41] Aryeetey GC, Jehu-Appiah C, Spaan E et al. Costs, equity, efficiency and feasibility of identifying the poor in Ghana's National Health Insurance Scheme: empirical analysis of various strategies. Trop Med Int Health 2012;17(1):43-51.

[42] Ekman B. Community-based health insurance in low-income countries: a systematic review of the evidence. *Health Policy Plan* 2004; 19: 249-71.

[43] Preker AS, Carrin G, Dror D, Jakab M, Hsiao W, Arhin-Tenkorang D. Effectiveness of community health financing in meeting the cost of illness. *Bull World Health Organ* 2002; 80: 143-50.

Chapter 11

Lifestyle and Cardiovascular Risk Factors: Urban Population versus Rural Population in Sub-Saharan Africa

Emmanuel Limbole Bakilo, Dadi-Serge Nkarnkwin, Lucette Womba, Venance Atheno, Mireille Kika, Jean Booto, Reagan Wiyaka, Martine Ekeba and Gilot Ngoma

Abstract

Cardiovascular diseases (CVD) are a major public health problem in Sub-Saharan Africa (SSA), as in the rest of the world, with increasingly increasing morbidity and mortality. We are presenting here, not the results of an epidemiological study, but rather a reflection on the problem of CVD and their risk factors (RFs) in SSA, taking into account the differences in lifestyle between rural and urban areas, the objective being to highlight the differences in the epidemiological profile trends relating to CVDs and their RFs between these two environments on the basis of existing data, to indicate some characteristic features of lifestyle in these two environments and to draw lessons from this in terms of the prospects for combating this new epidemic in this part of the world. We have indicated in this presentation that the prevalence of CVDs as well as that of their RFs show increasing trends in SSA due to new lifestyles linked in particular to urbanization and its numerous economic and social corollaries. However, data on their geographical and sociological distribution, especially in rural and urban areas, are still incomplete. The first existing epidemiological surveys seem to indicate that they are more firmly established in urban areas than in rural areas, probably linked to the difference in lifestyles between these two areas. We concluded by mentioning that it is necessary for SSA states to take the option of launching vast epidemiological and clinical research programs tending to make basic epidemiological data available, taking into account the specific geographic and sociological characteristics of African society. This knowledge, documented in the form of scientific evidence, would make it possible to consider with relevance and effectiveness measures to combat this new epidemic in developing countries.

Keywords: lifestyle, cardiovascular risk factors, rural area, urban area, Sub-Saharan Africa

1. Introduction

Cardiovascular diseases (CVDs), one of the main components of noncommunicable diseases (NCDs), are the first leading cause of mortality worldwide: more people die annually from CVDs than from any other cause.

In 2012, an estimated 17.5 million people died from these diseases, representing 30% of all deaths worldwide. An estimated 7.5 million of these deaths are due to coronary heart disease and 6.7 million to stroke. Low- and middle-income countries are disproportionately affected, accounting for over 80% of CVD deaths. By 2030, nearly 23.6 million people will die from cardiovascular diseases, primarily heart disease and stroke. According to projections, these conditions will remain the leading cause of death in the world [1].

During the 3rd high-level meeting on NCDs, it was reported that seven in 10 people (71%) worldwide die from these diseases, which mainly consist of cardiovascular disease, cancer, diabetes and lung chronic diseases, an average of 41 million people each year. These include 15 million people dying from NCDs between the ages of 30 and 69; over 85% of these "premature" deaths occur in low- and middle-income countries [2].

CVDs, as other NCDs, are favored by factors that are related to genetics, physiology and sociological environment, and are called risk factors (RFs) or specifically cardiovascular risk factors (CVRFs).

The main RF of CVDs or NCDs, are related to the sociological environment, particularly with our lifestyle or our everyday behavior and are thus called behavioral RFs; they are thus deeply influenced by the culture and customs of the environment. It is this link between the sociological environment and the RFs of CVDs or NCDs, which could determine the African disparities between the rural environment, guardian of traditional culture and the urban environment, strongly influenced by Western culture.

1.1 Objective of the presentation

In this chapter, we want to present an overview on CVDs and their RFs in rural and urban areas in Sub-Saharan Africa (SSA), to indicate some characteristic features of lifestyle in these two environments and to draw conclusions from them in terms of prospects for combating this new epidemic in this part of the world.

1.2 Methodology

We conducted a literature review related to the topic of the chapter, based on the available documentation as well as on the international scientific literature accessible through the PUBMED search engine where, after entering the keywords, the most relevant publications were selected. The use of this documentation was carried out taking into account the general situation in the world, the specific situation of the ASS with comparative observation between rural and urban areas.

2. Overview of cardiovascular diseases and risk factors in Sub-Saharan Africa

2.1 Overview

CVDs are a group of disorders of the heart and blood vessels; they include mainly [3]:

- coronary heart disease – disease of the blood vessels supplying the heart muscle;
- cerebrovascular disease – disease of the blood vessels supplying the brain;

- peripheral arterial disease – disease of blood vessels supplying the arms and legs;
- rheumatic heart disease – damage to the heart muscle and heart valves from rheumatic fever, caused by streptococcal bacteria;
- congenital heart disease – malformations of heart structure existing at birth;
- deep vein thrombosis and pulmonary embolism – blood clots in the leg veins, which can dislodge and move to the heart and lungs.

CVDs are promoted by a number of factors called "risk factors" (RFs).The main CVRFs are: poor diet, lack of physical activity, smoking, and harmful use of alcohol. These RFs, related to lifestyle, are called behavioral RFs. They can be the cause of physiological disturbances such as high blood pressure, hyperglycemia, hyperlipidemia and obesity; they are called intermediate risk factors.

CVRFs are also classified into non-modifiable factors and modifiable factors. The unchangeable risk factors are age, sex, race, and inheritance. Modifiable factors correspond to behavioral and biological factors. The **Figure 1** shows the link between CVRFs and CVDs.

STEPS studies carried out on a continental African scale in the 1980s indicated high prevalence of CVRFs and especially hypertension.

The summary of the results of these studies is presented in **Table 1**.

Cardiovascular diseases are become a major public health problem throughout the African Region. The main CVDs are: high blood pressure, stroke,

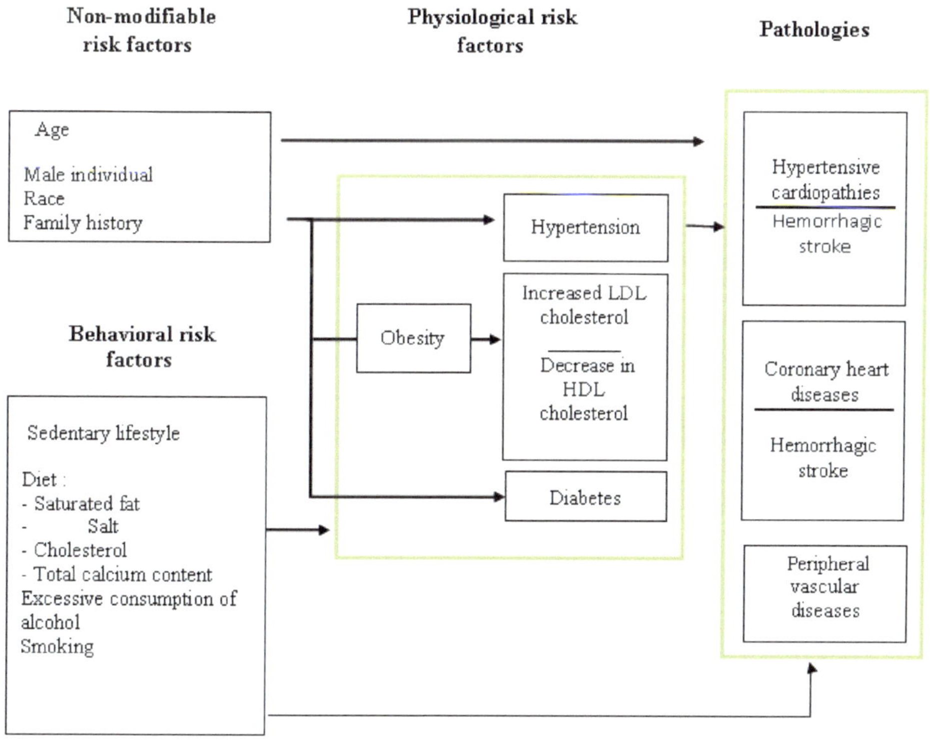

Figure 1.
Relationship between CVRFs and CVDs. Source: Wong ND., Black et Grdin JM., Preventive cardiology: a practical approach, Chicago, Mc Graw Hill, 2005.

Country	Year[1]	%Who Currently Smoke Tobacco	% Who Ate < 5 Servings of F&V Per Day[2]	% Not Engaged in Vigorous Physical Activity	% Who Are Obese[3]	% With Raised Blood Pressure[4]	% With Raised Blood Glucose[5]	% With Raised Total Blood Cholesterol[6]	% With None of the CRFs[7]	% With > 3 of the CRFs, Ages 25–44 Years Old	% With > 3 of the CRFs, Ages 45–64 Years Old	% With > 3 of the CRFs, Ages 24–64 Years Old
Benin	2008	8.8	78.5	58.2	9.4	28.7	3.0	7.9	11.0	9.5	21.8	14.9
Botswana	2007	19.7	96.6	72.7	15.6	33.1	—	—	1.2	25.7	50.4	34.5
Cameroon	2003	6.3	—	84.3	15.9	17.3	13.9	—	—	—	—	—
Cape Verde	2007	9.9	86.1	68.7	10.5	38.7	12.7	13.0	5.0	19.6	41.8	24.8
CAR	2010	14.1	66.1	55.6	7.2	34.5	21.0	—	12.2	12.3	29.4	17.7
Chad	2008	11.2	84.8	74.0	13.7	27.6	—	—	0.3	22.8	37.3	27.8
Comoros	2011	12.9	85.7	61.7	13.5	25.4	4.8	25.9	5.9	18.5	32.3	23.0
Congo, Dem. Rep.	2005	6.4	87.9	96.1	5.8	17.1	—	—	5.3	19.9	34.0	24.1
Congo, Brazzaville	2004	11.1	—	—	8.6	33.3	20.8	—	—	—	—	—
Cote d'Ivoire	2005	14.4	83.5	93.0	8.5	25.9	—	—	4.9	24.5	44.3	30.1
Eritrea	2004	7.8	98.1	83.9	3.4	16.6	—	—	0.8	13.5	26.1	19.4
Ethiopia	2006	4.6	98.9	—	7.1	30.9	—	—	0.3	17.2	34.2	—
Gabon	2009	12.1	93.4	65.0	15.9	20.3	—	—	1.2	30.0	50.0	36.4
Gambia, The	2010	15.6	93.0	58.7	12.1	26.3	—	—	2.1	20.7	39.8	25.8
Guinea	2009	12.8	79.3	52.3	5.1	28.1	5.2	9.8	7.9	15.4	35.2	21.6
Lesotho	2012	24.5	92.7	44.2	19.9	31.0	6.3	4.6	2.2	22.1	41.6	26.7
Liberia	2011	9.9	96.1	59.9	22.0	30.7	19.2	—	1.1	28.7	43.2	33.5
Madagascar	2005	19.6	62.0	75.1	2.2	35.8	—	—	12.8	12.1	17.7	13.8
Malawi	2009	14.1	97.5	17.8	4.6	32.9	5.6	8.7	1.0	13.0	23.7	16.5
Mauritania	2006	18.9	94.8	95.7	20.9	22.4	6.2	24.4	—	—	—	—

DOI: http://dx.doi.org/10.5772/intechopen.96881

Country	Year[1]	%Who Currently Smoke Tobacco	% Who Ate < 5 Servings of F&V Per Day[2]	% Not Engaged in Vigorous Physical Activity	% Who Are Obese[3]	% With Raised Blood Pressure[4]	% With Raised Blood Glucose[5]	% With Raised Total Blood Cholesterol[6]	% With None of the CRFs[7]	% With > 3 of the CRFs, Ages 25–44 Years Old	% With > 3 of the CRFs, Ages 45–64 Years Old	% With > 3 of the CRFs, Ages 24–64 Years Old
Mozambique	2005	18.7	95.0	31.1	7.5	34.9	3.8	2.1	2.4	14.0	28.6	19.0
Niger	2007	4.6	96.4	56.4	3.2	36.3	22.5	—	0.9	17.5	26.8	21.4
Sao Tome and Principe	2008	5.5	83.3	51.6	35.0	38.6	6.5	7.5	6.4	15.6	36.1	22.1
Seychelles	2004	22.2	78.8	73.5	25.1	39.6	9.5	59.7	4.2	29.9	52.1	38.8
Sierra Leone	2009	25.8	90.9	31.0	7.8	34.8	—	—	1.4	22.7	37.2	27.0
Swaziland	2007	7.1	87.4	49.3	24.3	36.0	14.5	5.8	1.9	30.4	47.8	35.5
Tanzania	2012	14.1	97.2	32.4	8.7	26.0	9.1	26.0	0.8	12.2	28.0	16.6
Togo	2010	6.8	94.9	45.7	6.2	19.0	2.6	14.2	2.4	13.1	23.7	16.1
Zambia	2008	6.5	97.0	76.0	14.4	33.3	4.6	23.8	1.0	16.6	46.8	23.7
Zanzibar	2011	7.3	97.9	52.1	14.3	33.0	3.8	24.5	0.6	18.9	38.1	24.2

Source of Data: The World Health Organization. STEPS Country Reports. http://www.who.int/chp/steps/reports/en/. Last accessed on 21 May 2013.
[1]*Year of most recent STEPS survey.*

[2]*Percentage who ate less than 5 combined servings of fruit and/or vegetables on average pet day*

[3]*Percentage who are obese (BMI at least 30 kg/m^2).*

[4]*Percentage with raised BP (SBP at least 140 and/or DBP at least 90 mm Hg or currently on medication for raised BP).*

[5]*Percentage with raised blood glucose as defined below or currently on medication for raised blood glucose:*
- *plasma venous value _7.0 mmol/L or _126 mg/dl;*
- *capillary whole blood value _6.1 mmol/L or _110 mg/dl.*

[6]*Percentage with raised total blood cholesterol.*

[7]*CRFs are the combined risk factors including (a) current daily smokers; (b) consumption of less than 5 servings of fruits and/or vegetables on average per day; (c) low level of activity (<600 MET-minutes); (d) overweight (BMI at least 25 kg/m^2); (e) raised BP (SBP at least 140 and/or DBP at least 90 mm Hg or currently on medication for raised BP).*
*This table (**Table 1**) shows across the continent a very high rate of insufficient physical activity, a high rate of arterial hypertension with nevertheless disparities between the countries, a relatively low rate of obesity compared to the rates observed in Western countries and a higher rate of a combination of RFs from 45 years.*

Table 1.
Prevalence of behavioral RFs and classical biological CVRFs according to STEPS studies [4].

cardiomyopathy and coronary heart disease. In addition, rheumatic heart disease remains a worrying problem [5].

The **Tables 1** and 2 and **Figures 1** and 2 below relating to cardiovascular morbidity and mortality in SSA clearly illustrate the current place occupied by CVDs in this region of the world.

There are also a number of underlying determinants of CVDs. They stem from major social, economic and cultural developments - globalization, urbanization, aging populations, poverty, stress and hereditary factors [3]. It is these socio-cultural and economic disturbances that could partly determine the differences observed between rural and urban areas in Africa.

2.2 Cardiovascular risk factors: rural versus urban environment

Several African studies have indicated a higher prevalence of FDRCV in urban areas than in rural areas and attributed this disparity to lifestyle change in urban areas. The most documented RFs are hypertension, diabetes, obesity, and high cholesterol.

The prevalence of hypertension is very high in SSA. It varies according to the studies and according to the regions globally between 19 and 43% in the general population and can exceed 70% beyond 65 years; it is higher in urban areas than in rural areas [7–9]. Studies carried out across a few African countries have shown

CVDs	**Morbidity**		**Mortality**	
	n	**%**	**n**	**%**
Stroke	**10367**	16,57	**2124**	19,68
Heart failure	**5477**	8,76	**876**	8,12
Ischemic cardiopathy	**501**	0,80	**86**	0,80
Pulmonary embolism	**278**	0,44	**103**	0,95
Deep vein thrombosis	**246**	0,39	—	—
Pericarditis	**81**	0,13	**13**	0,12
Valvular heart diseases	**79**	0,13	**12**	0,11
Bacterial endocarditis	**6**	0,01	**2**	0,02
Acute articular rhumatism	**13**	0,02	**1**	0,01
Other	**2432**	3,89	**597**	5,53
All CVDs.	**19480**	**31,14**	**3814**	35,35
All internal medicine diseases	**62553**	**100,00**	**10790**	100,00

Source: Statistics from the National Cardiovascular Disease Control Program, PNMCV / DR. Congo, 2018.
This table shows that CVDs represent 31.1% of all hospitalizations in the medical sector in Kinshasa hospitals between 2007 and 2016; Stroke is the leading cause of morbidity in hospitalization in the medicine sector with 53% of cardiovascular morbidity and 16.6% of overall morbidity, followed far behind by heart failure and ischemic heart disease. We can also observe the low frequency of heart valve disease (including rheumatic valve disease), probably due to the easier access to antibiotics and other preventive measures, mainly in urban areas.
The table indicates also that CVDs represent in Kinshasa hospitals, between 2007 and 2016, 35.4% of overall mortality in the medicine sector; stroke accounts for 55.7% of cardiovascular mortality and 19.7% of overall mortality, followed by pulmonary embolism and ischemic heart disease.
These results on hospital morbidity and mortality in Kinshasa join those of a hospital survey carried out more than twenty years ago in a hospital establishment in Kinshasa, where stroke represented 31% of cardiovascular morbidity, 6% of morbidity overall, 57% of cardiovascular mortality and 12% of overall mortality [6].

Table 2.
Cardiovascular morbidity and mortality from 2007 to 2016 in eight hospitals in Kinshasa, DR Congo.

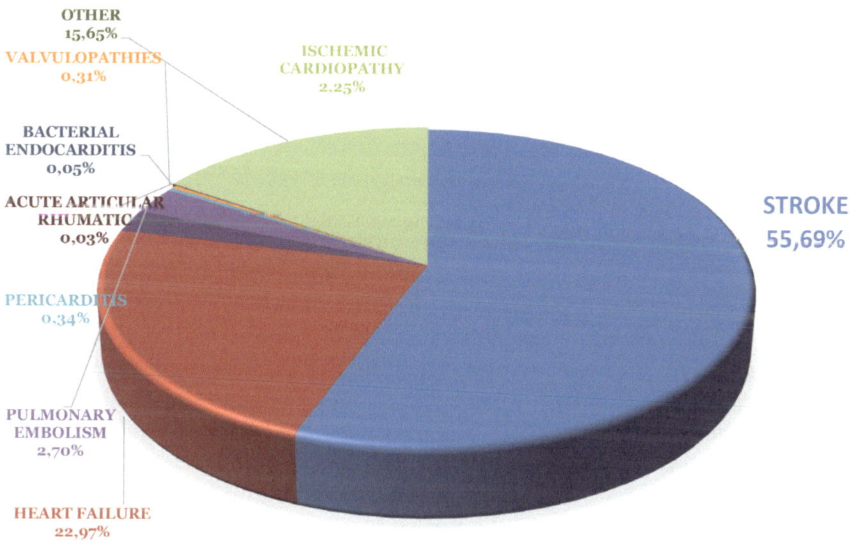

Figure 2.
Proportions of Death from Different CVDs. Source: Statistics from the National Cardiovascular Disease Control Program, PNMCV / DR Congo, 2018. This figure indicates that stroke and all-cause heart failure were the two leading causes of cardiovascular mortality in Kinshasa hospitals between 2007 and 2016, with 55.7% and 23% respectively, followed by pulmonary embolism (2,7%) and ischemic cardiopathy (2,25%).

some prevalence figures: 19.3% and 21.4% respectively in Nigeria and Kenya in rural areas, 23.7% and 38% in Tanzania and Namibia in urban areas [10]. In South Africa, 43% in rural areas, 77.3% in subjects aged over 50 in urban areas [10]. In Benin, the prevalence of high blood pressure, obesity and diabetes has been higher in urban than in rural areas, while, exceptionally, that of smoking has been higher in rural areas [11].

The disparity in hypertension prevalence rates between the different SSA countries is probably linked, beyond the methodology and the conditions for carrying out each study, to the socio-cultural characteristics of each society, including in particular the dietary habits with different salt intake levels.

At the African level, a meta-analysis of SSA carried out in 2007 [12] indicated that diabetes was the second cardiovascular risk factor. Its prevalence is higher in urban areas than in rural areas. This is the case in the Democratic Republic of Congo, where prevalences of 4.8% and 25% were observed in rural and urban areas respectively [13].

The prevalence of obesity is steadily increasing in large cities in SSA, mainly due to the new lifestyle imposed by urbanization. Thereby, the prevalence of obesity is higher in urban than in rural areas and is estimated at over 60% in some regions [10].

In SSA, hypercholesterolemia follows the same geographic distribution as obesity, ie more prevalent in urban areas than in rural areas [7].

In DR Congo, there has been a gradual increase in the prevalence of hypertension over the years, in view of certain surveys carried out mainly in the capital, from 9.9% in 1986 to 26% in 2018 [14–16]; Unfortunately, there is no large-scale survey, in the general population, comparing the burden of CVRFs in rural versus urban areas.

2.3 Lifestyle in rural versus urban areas

According to World Bank data, more than 50% of the population in SSA lives in rural areas, which is characterized by the predominance of traditional economic and social survival activities: agriculture, animal husbandry and fishing. As these activities have not been modernized, they are essentially carried out by hand and thus require their providers to have a high, regular and permanent level of physical activity. In addition, the diet contains fewer processed products than in urban areas. All this could explain the low prevalence of CVRFs in comparison to the urban environment where we find the following characteristics: tendency to sedentary lifestyle, insufficient physical activity, diet high in sugar, fat and salt, stress psychosocial etc.

Hence the interest of general measures among populations as recommended by the WHO, including reducing salt consumption. In fact, in the 2013–2020 global action plan to combat NCDs [17] adopted in 2013, one of the targets to be achieved by 2025 was the 30% reduction in average salt consumption by populations to reduce the prevalence of hypertension. The effective implementation of this recommendation requires general measures, among the populations, aimed at reducing salt consumption, in particular by discouraging the use of added salt during food preparation or at the table.

It is also useful to mention that locking rural populations in an environment dominated by traditional mores and mentalities can constitute a handicap to understanding and adopting new behaviors necessary for the fight against NCDs. This can make rural populations fragile once they are exposed to NCD RFs. This is precisely what is observed among populations from rural areas and living in peri-urban areas, mentally close to their traditional areas but confronted with a Western-type society that exposes them to the RFs of NCDs. An awareness-raising effort for the fight against NCDs, adapted to each environment and each social category, deserves to be encouraged.

3. Discussion

The difference in lifestyle between rural and urban areas in SSA is a sociological reality known to all; however, the impact on the burden of CVRFs in these two settings has not yet been sufficiently studied. This is mainly due to the high cost of epidemiological surveys in the general population. Nevertheless, the few studies carried out in these two environments and mentioned in this chapter, although small in scope, have been able to provide some information tending to confirm the difference between these two environments.

The rural environment is characterized by its still strong attachment to the customs and mores of traditional African society where individuals are physically active, most often consuming natural foods and less exposed to stress related to the vagaries of modern society. There is therefore a low exposure to CVDFs and hence to CVDs. Conversely, progress in the fight against infections is less noticeable there, which would explain an infectious mortality even more marked than in urban areas, a residue of the era of major pandemics. All of this deserves to be documented by solid epidemiological investigations that can inform health and policy decisions. On the basis of current plot data related to CVDs and CVRFs in rural areas, it could be said that rural areas in SSA are still between the 1st and 2nd stage of the epidemiological transition following the subdivision described by Meslé and Vallin in 2007 [18], while the urban environment could be considered to be already in the middle of the 2nd stage, in view of the real decline of the infectious risk to the benefit of NCDs and their RFs.

As a reminder, the concept of epidemiological transition was launched by Omran in 1971 [19] and subdivided into three stages below by Meslé and Vallin in 2007:

- the stage of high infectious morbidity and mortality, with low life expectancy;

- the stage of decline in pandemics, leading to an improvement in life expectancy;
- the stage of the reign of chronic diseases or NCDs, a consequence of the increase in life expectancy.

This concept was supplemented by that of health transition [20], which is more global, encompassing not only the epidemiological situation but also the different responses from society to health issues.

Conversely, the urban and peri-urban environment in SSA are characterized by a tendency to sedentary lifestyle, a diet rich in sodium and calories, excessive alcohol consumption, socio-professional stress, all this in a context of poverty or social insecurity. Linked in particular to an uncontrolled rural exodus. This results in an increase in biological or physiological RFs [15, 21, 22] and a vicious circle between NCDs which exacerbate poverty and vice versa, poverty which promotes NCDs [23], poverty understood in the classic World Bank sense, namely an income of less than $ 1.9 per day per person or the inability to afford basic minimum services.

There is growing evidence that poverty promotes NCDs, particularly through poor accessibility to treatment [24] and other health services; in low-income countries, the high prevalence of RDF of NCDs, the early onset of their complications [25–29] as well as the excess mortality associated with these diseases constitute strong arguments in favor of this link between poverty and NCDs. The following statement by Ambassador Taonga Mushayavanhu, Permanent Representative of the Republic of Zimbabwe to the United Nations Office at Geneva, within the framework of the "Dialogue on NCDs, Poverty and Development Cooperation" forum is sufficiently enlightening on the question:

"In developed countries, the population often takes advantage of multisectoral policies and plans put in place by the government to reduce exposure to risk factors and empower health systems", explains the Ambassador, who adds: "Developing countries have little capacity to fight NCDs, which leads to premature death, reduces productivity, slows economic growth and locks the most destitute in chronic poverty. In a report published in April 2013, the African Union pointed out that the exorbitant costs associated with NCDs push 100 million people into poverty each year, hampering development. Yet the tools, knowledge and strategies available today can prevent most of these diseases" [23].

It should be recalled that NCDs have already been the subject of three high-level meetings at the United Nations, in 2011, 2014 and 2018, each time bringing together the various member states of the world organization at the highest level of representation. World leaders have recognized that NCDs pose the greatest threat to health and development worldwide, especially in the developing countries. To this end, a political declaration on NCDs was adopted at the first high-level meeting.

At the Sixty-sixth World Health Assembly held in May 2013 and as part of the follow-up to the Political Declaration of the First High-Level Meeting of the United Nations General Assembly on the Prevention and Control of Noncommunicable Diseases, States approved the Global Plan of Action for the Control of Noncommunicable Diseases for 2013–2020 [17], whose objectives and voluntary global targets are as follows.

3.1 Objectives

1. To raise the priority accorded to the prevention and control of noncommunicable diseases in global, regional and national agendas and

internationally agreed development goals, through strengthened international cooperation and advocacy;

2. To strengthen national capacity, leadership, governance, multisectoral action and partnerships to accelerate country response for the prevention and control of noncommunicable diseases;

3. To reduce modifiable risk factors for noncommunicable diseases and underlying social determinants through creation of health-promoting environments;

4. To strengthen and orient health systems to address the prevention and control of noncommunicable diseases and the underlying social determinants through people-centred primary health care and universal health coverage;

5. To promote and support national capacity for high-quality research and development for the prevention and control of noncommunicable diseases;

6. To monitor the trends and determinants of noncommunicable diseases and evaluate progressin their prevention and control.

3.2 Voluntary global targets

1. A 25% relative reduction in the overall mortality from cardiovascular diseases, cancer, diabetes, or chronic respiratory diseases;

2. At least 10% relative reduction in the harmful use of alcohol, as appropriate, within the national context;

3. A 10% relative reduction in prevalence of insufficient physical activity;

4. A 30% relative reduction in mean population intake of salt/sodium;

5. A 30% relative reduction in prevalence of current tobacco use in persons aged 15+ years;

6. A 25% relative reduction in the prevalence of raised blood pressure or contain the prevalence of raised blood pressure, according to national circumstances;

7. Halt the rise in diabetes and obesity;

8. At least 50% of eligible people receive drug therapy and counselling (including glycaemic control) to prevent heart attacks and strokes;

9. An 80% availability of the affordable basic technologies and essential medicines, including generics, required to treat major noncommunicable diseases in both public and private facilities.

Unfortunately, during various evaluations of the progress made in the implementation of the commitments made by the States, the observation was disappointing: most of them had not reached the desired level in the process of implementation of the States commitments [30].

To this end, seven main obstacles to the implementation of these commitments have been identified, namely:

1. lack of political will, mobilization, capacity and action;

2. lack of policies and plans for NCDs;

3. difficulties in setting priorities;

4. impact of economic, business and market factors;

5. insufficient technical and operational capacities;

6. Insufficient funding (internal and international) to transpose scaling up measures to combat NCDs; and.

7. lack of accountability.

This explains, in most states in SSA, a situation of inertia in the implementation of the recommendations and commitments made by the leaders of these states, with multiple consequences: absence of administrative and legal reforms to support the fight against NCDs, lack of support for national programs, where they exist, scarcity of basic epidemiological data on NCDs, lack of support for healthcare establishments for the management of NCDs, etc.

In this context, it is understandable why in SSA states, there are no national registers of NCDs, nor large-scale general population data on NCDRFs or CVRFs, and even less on CVDs; healthcare establishments are not equipped for the correct management of NCDs or CVDs. These states for the most part do not have structures for universal health coverage to promote accessibility for all to quality care. Comparative information on NCDs and their RFs between rural and urban areas is not sufficiently documented, apart from a few small series.

In view of this gloomy picture of CVDs in SSA, one of the priority actions should concern the carrying out of large national surveys of the prevalence of CVRFs so as to make basic epidemiological data available. This would make it possible to identify evidence on the possible differences between the different environments, urban and rural, and to draw the necessary consequences in terms of prospects for the control of CVDs.

4. Conclusion

CVDs are one of the major current public health problems in SSA and globally. They are among the main causes of morbidity and mortality in SSA, but data on their geographical and sociological distribution, especially in rural and urban areas, are still incomplete. The first existing epidemiological surveys seem to indicate that they are more firmly established in urban areas than in rural areas, probably linked to the difference in lifestyles between these two areas. SSA states need to take the option of launching vast epidemiological and clinical research programs aimed at making basic epidemiological data available, taking into account the sociological specificities of African society. This knowledge, documented in the form of scientific evidence, would make it possible to consider with relevance and effectiveness measures to combat this new epidemic in developing countries.

Author details

Emmanuel Limbole Bakilo[1,2,3,4*], Dadi-Serge Nkarnkwin[1,3,4], Lucette Womba[4], Venance Atheno[3,4], Mireille Kika[4], Jean Booto[4], Reagan Wiyaka[3,4], Martine Ekeba[4] and Gilot Ngoma[4]

1 Cardiology Service, Kinshasa University Clinics, Faculty of Medicine, University of Kinshasa, Kinshasa, DR, Congo

2 Internal Medicine Service, Ngaliema Clinic, Kinshasa, DR, Congo

3 Gombe Center of Internal Medicine and Cardiology (CMCG), DR, Congo

4 National Cardiovascular Diseases Control Program, DR, Congo

*Address all correspondence to: drlimbole@gmail.com

References

[1] About cardiovascular diseases, WHO, 2020.

[2] Third high-level meeting on NCDs, UN, 2018.

[3] Cardiovascular diseases, WHO, 2017.

[4] Mensah, G.A., 2008. Ischaemic heart disease in Africa. Heart, 94(7), p.836–843.

[5] Regional Committee for Africa, 55. (2005). Cardiovascular Diseases in the African Region: Current Situation and Prospects: Report of the Regional Director. WHO. Regional Office for Africa.

[6] Mbala Mukendi M., Tambwe M.J., Lizwa B.B., Dikasa N.L., J.R M'Buyamba Kabangu. Morbidity and mortality in Zairian adults; Panorama med. 1994; 5: 234–237.

[7] Onen CL. Epidemiology of ischaemic heart disease in sub-Saharan Africa. Cardiovasc J Afr. 2013;24(2): 34–42.

[8] Hendriks ME, Wit FWNM, Roos MTL, Brewster LM, Akande TM, de Beer IH, et al. Hypertension in sub-Saharan Africa: cross-sectional surveys in four rural and urban communities. PloS One. 2012;7(3):e32638.

[9] Addo J, Smeeth L, Leon DA. Hypertension in sub-saharan Africa: a systematic review. Hypertension. 2007; 50(6):1012–1018.

[10] Steyn K, Gaziano TA, Bradshaw D, Laubscher R, Fourie J, South African Demographic and Health Coordinating Team. Hypertension in South African adults: results from the Demographic and Health Survey, 1998. J Hypertens.

[11] Houehanou, Y.C.N. et al., 2015. Magnitude of cardiovascular risk factors in rural and urbanareas in Benin: findings from a nationwide steps survey. *PloS One*, 10(5), p.e0126441.

[12] Sagui E. [Stroke in sub-Saharan Africa]. Médecine Trop Rev Corps Santé Colon. 2007;67(6):596–600.

[13] Kasiam LOJB, Longo-Mbenza B, Nge OA, Kangola KN, Mbungu FS, Milongo DG. Classification and dramatic epidemic of diabetes mellitus in Kinshasa Hinterland: the prominent role of type 2 diabetes and lifestyle changes among Africans. Niger J Med J Natl Assoc Resid Dr Niger. 2009;18(3): 311–320.

[14] J R M'Buyamba-Kabangu, R Fagard, P Lijnen, J Staessen, M S Ditu, K A Tshiani, A Amery. Epidemiological study of blood pressure and hypertension in a sample of urban Bantu of Zaïre. J Hypertens. 1986 Aug;4(4):485-91.

[15] Benjamin Longo-Mbenza [1], Dieudonné Vangu Ngoma, Damien Nahimana, Dominique Mupepe Mayuku, Simon Mbungu Fuele, Florent Ekwanzala, Christian Beya. Screen detection and the WHO stepwise approach to the prevalence and risk factors of arterial hypertension in Kinshasa. Eur J Cardiovasc Prev Rehabil. 2008 Oct;15(5):503–8.

[16] Buila NB, Ngoyi GN, Bayauli PM, Katamba FK, Lubenga YN, Kazadi SM, Kiadi GD, Lepira FB, Kabanda GK, Kika ML, Beaney T, Ster AC, Poulter NR, M'Buyamba-Kabangu JR. Analysis of blood pressure and selected cardiovascular risk factors in the Democratic Republic of the Congo: the May Measurement Month 2018 results. Eur Heart J Suppl. 2020 Aug; 22(Suppl H): H50–H52.

[17] WHO 2013. Global action plan for the prevention and control of NCDs 2013–2020.

[18] Meslé, F. & Vallin, J., 2007. [From epidemiological transition to health transition]. Médecine Tropicale, 67(6), p.545–551.

[19] Omran AR. The epidemiologic transition: a theory of the epidemiology of population change. 1971. Milbank Q. 2005;83(4):731–757.

[20] Frenk J, Bobadilla JL, Stern C *et Coll* - Elements for a theory of the health transition. Health Transition Review 1991 ; 1 : 21–38.

[21] Aspray, T.J. et al., 2000. Rural and urban differences in diabetes prevalence in Tanzania: the role of obesity, physical inactivity and urban living. Transactions of the Royal Society of Tropical Medicine and Hygiene, 94(6), p.637–644.

[22] Poulter, N.R. et al., 1985. Determinants of blood pressure changes due to urbanization: a longitudinal study. *Journal of Hypertension.* Supplement, 3(3), p.S375–S377.

[23] WHO, 2015. Dialogue on NCDs, Poverty and Development Cooperation.

[24] Diane Macquart et al. Factors associated with poor adherence to medication among hypertensive patients in twelve low and middle income Sub-Saharan countries. PLoS One. 2019; 14(7): e0219266.

[25] Limbole EB, Magne J, Lacroix P. Stroke characterization in Sun-saharan Africa: Congolese population. Int J Cardiol. 2017 Aug 1;240:392–397.

[26] Damasceno A, Gomes J, Azevedo A, Carrilho C, Lobo V, Lopes H, et al. An epidemiological study of stroke hospitalizations in Maputo, Mozambique: a high burden of disease in a resource-poor country. Stroke J Cereb Circ. 2010; 41(11):2463–2469.

[27] Longo-Mbenza B, Lelo Tshinkwela M, Mbuilu Pukuta J. Rates and predictors of stroke-associated case fatality in black Central African patients. Cardiovasc J Afr. 2008;19(2): 72–76.

[28] Longo-Mbenza B, Phanzu-Mbete LB, M'Buyamba-Kabangu JR, Tonduangu K, Mvunzu M, Muvova D, et al. Hematocrit and stroke in black Africans under tropical climate and meteorological influence. Ann Med Int. 1999;150(3):171–177.

[29] Damorou F, Yayehd K, Pessinaba S, Tcherou T, Amonu J. Mortality associated with cardiovascular diseases in three hospitals of Lomé-city. Pan Afr Med J. 2011;10:40.

[30] UN, 2018. High Level Meeting on NCDs.

Chapter 12

Alcohol Consumption Practice and Associated Risk Factors among University of Limpopo Students

Mbelege Rosina Nkwana, Gift Makaleng, Mafoloa Suzan Monyeki, Hlengani James Siweya and Kotsedi Daniel Monyeki

Abstract

In South Africa, substance rehabilitation centers found alcohol as the primary substance abuse in eight out of the nine provinces. This study aimed to investigate the prevalence of alcohol use and associated risk factors among University of Limpopo students with mean age of 21.5 years. This was a cross-sectional study and constituted a total of 500 female students and 417 male students from the University of Limpopo. Logistic regression was used to calculate the association between alcohol consumption and its predictors. Information about their alcohol consumption, the type of alcohol and the practice related to alcohol consumption was collected using a validated questionnaire. Tobacco and marijuana product use were significantly ($P < 0.05$) associated with alcohol use among University of Limpopo students for unadjusted (OR ranges 4.31 95%CI 2.71 6.87 to 4.92 95%CI 3.16 7.70) and after adjusting for age gender and amount of money deposited into the student account by the bursary scheme (OR ranges from 4.14 95%CI 2.59 6.62 to 4.50 95%CI 2.87 7.06). Tobacco product use, marijuana use and enhancing interpersonal relationships are major risk factors associated to current alcohol use. Future studies are required to investigate the development of lifestyle and cardiovascular disease over time among University of Limpopo students.

Keywords: alcohol, tobacco, marijuana, students, university of Limpopo

1. Introduction

A university living setting provides a unique opportunity for students who enter this environment for the first time. Yet, living in a new environment is associated with stress and changes of lifestyle [1]. At the university level, students adjust to a certain level of being an adult and experiencing freedom. These students create a social and cultural environment by drinking alcohol to obtain a positive outcome (e.g. enhancement, coping) or to avoid a negative outcome (like peer rejection) [2]. This environment could further create unhealthy lifestyles such that students are more involved in risky behaviour and serious drinking problems than their peers who are not enrolled in the University [2–4] . Unhealthy behaviour such as tobacco product use, marijuana use, injuries and interpersonal problems are the vital risk factors associated with excessive alcohol consumption. Besides, alcohol use among university students has been associated with poor academic performance, personal injuries, loss of memory, temporary illness (such as nausea, vomiting, and hangover), unprotected sexual activity, acquaintance rape, sexual violence and other problems like suicide,, impaired driving skills,, vandalism or fights [5].

The high percentage of alcohol use and abuse in the university environment by students is viewed as representing the prime drinking years for individuals [6]. For example, Young and De Klerk. [7] reported that more than 50% of Rhodes University student respondents who participated in their study were dependent on alcohol. The prevalent of alcohol use in a university in the South-East of Nigeria was reported to be 78.4% [8].

The prevalence of alcohol use by university students in South Africa has been found to range from 20% to 80% in 2009 by Peltzer & Ramlagan [9]. The prevalence of alcohol drinking at the University of Venda, South Africa was reported to be 65% of the current drinkers [10]. In South Africa, substance rehabilitation centers found alcohol as the primary substance abuse in eight out of the nine provinces [9]. Excessive alcohol consumption during University year's impacts negatively on student lifestyles even on post-University level, leading to accidents, health problems, and personal problems [11].

Alcohol drinking may be responsive to internal rewards such as the manipulation of management of one's own internal emotional state and external reward such as social acceptance [2]. Various factors affect the alcohol drinking patterns of students in the university environment. Some university student prefer beer and other drugs for economic reasons, Regardless of the various alcoholic beverages like cider, wine, spirits, champagne, whisky, gin or brandy [12]. Gender differences in alcohol use was reported among university students in the USA with a significantly high number of males compared to females drinking alcohol [13]. Furthermore, staying on-campus has been linked with excessive alcohol drinking than staying off-campus [14]. Little is known about the prevalence of alcohol use and associated risk factors among the University of Limpopo. This study aimed to investigate the prevalence of alcohol use and associated risk factors among University of Limpopo students aged 17 to 43 years.

2. Method

2.1 Geographical area

The study was conducted at the University of Limpopo, that was previously known as the University of The North (Sovenga). The University of Limpopo is situated at the foothill of Hwiti (Wolkberg range) in Mankweng, midway between Polokwane and Makgoebaskloof in Limpopo province, South Africa. The research was approved by the University of Limpopo research ethics committee (TREC/61/2019: IR).

2.2 Sampling and sample size

All the participants of the study were full-time students enrolled for the academic year 2019 in University of Limpopo. The participants represented the four available faculties (Science and Agriculture, Humanities, Management and Law, and Health Sciences). The total number of participants was n = 917 of which 45.5%

(n = 417) were males and 54.5% (n = 500) were females (mean age of 21.5 years). A convenient sampling method was used to have easy access to the participants.

2.3 Instruments

The questionnaire used in this study was based on questions, which have been used in the Ellisras Longitudinal Study and other studies [15, 16]. The questionnaire was shared with experts to ensure content, face and construct validity. The questionnaire was then revised and piloted with a sample of students to make sure it was valid, reliable, acceptable and accurately understood.

The questionnaire comprised of three sections. The first section of the questionnaire included of participants's age,gender, marital status and place of residence, field of study, year of entering the university and the level of study. The academic level was categorised as lower level (first and second year), moderate high (third-year level) and high level (postgraduate level).

Current alcohol drinkers were defined as anyone who drinks alcohol regularly for the past 30 days. The following question was asked: "During the past 30 days, have you had at least one drink of any alcoholic beverage such as beer, wine, a malt beverage, or liquor regularly?" The number of days in the past month where you had a drink between 07:30 and 16:00 and the frequency of drinking alcohol regularly the past 30 days were classified into: Less than four times in the past 30 days, 2 to 3 days a week in the past 30 days and more than four days a week the past 30 days. This was classified into the less than four times in 30 days. The onset (initiation age) age for alcohol drinker use was determined by the question "If yes, indicate how old you were when you first tried this ____. How old were you when you first drank alcohol regularly ______." Onset age was grouped as less than 15 years, between 15 and 19 years and over 20 years.

2.4 Other associated factors

All studied characteristics together with peer relation, personal enjoyment and tension reduction were chosen based upon literature that had identified associations between these variables and binge drinking [17, 18]. The selection questions included: I drink alcohol because it will boost my creativity (Yes/NO)? I drink alcohol because I want to be popular (Yes/NO)? I drink alcohol because it helps me to face difficulties with confidence (Yes/NO)? I drink alcohol because it would comfort me when I get blamed (Yes/NO)?

Tobacco and marijuana products use was assessed using the following questions: Does anyone you live with use tobacco products (Yes/No)? Does anyone you live with smoke hubbly bubbly (Yes/No)? Does anyone you live with smoke weed/marijuana (Yes/No)? Does anyone you live with drink alcohol (Yes/No)?

2.5 Statistical analysis

Descriptive statistics including frequency distribution and percentage frequencies were used to determine the prevalence of current alcohol use among University of Limpopo students. A chi-squared test was used to compare sets of nominal data that had larger frequency counts while the Fisher's exact test was used when frequency cells were small (less than five or ten) between genders [19, 20]. Logistic regression was used to determine the associated risk factors for current alcohol use among the University of Limpopo students. All statistical analyses were performed using SPSS version 25. The statistical significance was set at $P < 0.05$.

3. Results

Table 1 shows the descriptive statistics for positive response on alcohol consumption of the University of Limpopo students aged 17 to 43 years. The prevalence of current regular alcohol use was significantly ($p < 0.021$) higher for males (61.9%) compared to females (47.8%). Students who first consumed alcohol at age of less than 15 years were 24.7% males and 8.8% females, the difference was

	Males		Females	
	%	(n)	%	(n)
Faculties of the University of Limpopo				
Science and Agriculture	33.8	(141)	19.6	(98)
Humanities	26.9	(112)	23.8	(119)
Management and Law	17.0	(71)	13.0	(65)
Health Sciences	22.3	(93)	43.6	(218)
Bursaries Received				
Receiving funding from other bursaries	11.0	(46)	9.2	(46)
Receiving funding from NSFAS	70.3	(293)	80.4	(402)
Students Study level				
Lower level (First and Second year)	56.8	(237)	53.8	(269)
Moderate high level (third-year level)	23.0	(96)	25.6	(128)
High level (post graduate level)	20.1	(84)	20.6	(103)
Alcohol consumption				
Have you ever drunk alcohol?	74.3	(310)	62.8	(314)
Age when you had first drink of alcohol				
Less than 15 years	31.4	(131)	14.2	(71)
15 to 19 years	35.7	(149)	40.0	(200)
20 years and above	7.2	(30)	8.6	(43)
Are you currently drinking alcohol regularly during the past 30 days	61.9*	(258)	47.8*	(239)
Age when you first started drinking alcohol regularly during the past 30 days				
Less than 15 years	24.7*	(103)	8.8*	(44)
15 to 19 years	30.0	(125)	30.8	(154)
20 years and above	7.2	(30)	8.2	(41)
Types of alcoholic drinks you drink regularly in the past 30 days				
Beer	44.4*	(185)	9.6*	(48)
Cider	35	(146)	30.2	(151)
Wine	24.9	(104)	29.2	(146)
Spirit	29.3*	(122)	12.8*	(64)
Home made	8.4*	(35)	3.0*	(15)
Champagne	15.8	(66)	12.4	(62)

**≥0.05; **≥0.001.*

Table 1.
Descriptive statistics for positive response on alcohol consumption of the University of Limpopo students aged 17 to 43 years.

significant (P < 0.05). Many males (44.4% and 29.3%) in the current study significantly (P < 0.05) prefer beer and spirits compared to females (9.6% and 12.8%), respectively. Females preferred wine than males (29.2% and 24,9%) respectively. Though, the difference was not significant. The use of homemade alcohol was significantly (p < 0.05) higher for males (8.4%) compared to females (3.0%).

Table 2 presents the prevalence of positive response on the frequency of drinking and reasons for drinking alcohol among University of Limpopo students aged 17 to 43 years. A significantly high number of females (27.6%) drink alcohol fewer than 4 times in the past 30 days than males (21.6%). There was a significant (P < 0.05) number of males (13.4%) who drink alcohol regularly between the period of 07:30 and 16:00 2 to 3 days a week in the past month compared to females (7.4%). The prevalence of students who drink alcohol for popularity and bosting confidence is also higher in males (34.8% and 23.5%) than in females (1.8%, and 7.8%), respectively. The prevalence of tobacco and marijuana products use among relatives/friends who live with males students were significantly higher (ranges from 16.8 to 42.2%) compared to those who live with females students (prevalence ranges from 10.6 to 27.4%).

Table 3 shows the logistic regression (Odds ratio and 95% confidence interval and p-value) for the association of current regular alcohol drinking use and the associated risk factors for University of Limpopo students aged 17 to 43 years. Tobacco and marijuana product use of relatives/friends living with students were

	Males		**Females**	
	%	**(n)**	**%**	**(n)**
Rate of drinking alcohol regularly the past 30 days				
< than 4 times in 30 days	21.6*	(90)	27.6*	(138)
2 to 3 days a week in the past 30 days	11.8	(49)	6.8	(34)
> than 4 days a week in the past 30 days	28.5*	(119)	13.4*	(67)
Number of days in the past month where you had a drink between 07:30 and 16:00				
< than 4 times in the past 30 days	29.0	(121)	22.4	(112)
2 to 3 days a week in the past 30 days	13.4*	(56)	7.4*	(37)
> than 4 days a week the past 30 days	7.2	(30)	4.0	(20)
Reasons for drinking alcohol				
I drink alcohol because it will enhance my creative ability	6.7	(28)	6.6	(33)
I drink alcohol because I want to be popular	34.8*	(145)	1.8*	(9)
I drink alcohol because it helps me to face difficulties with confidence	23.5*	(99)	7.8*	(39)
I drink alcohol because it would ease me when I get blamed	18*	(75)	4.6*	(23)
Tobacco and marijuana product use				
Does anyone you live with use tobacco product?	25.2*	(105)	14.2*	(71)
Does anyone you live with smoke hubbly bubbly?	16.8*	(70)	11.4*	(57)
Does anyone you live with smoke weed/marijuana?	22.8*	(95)	10.6*	(53)
Does anyone you live with drink alcohol?	42.2*	(178)	27.4*	(137)

*≥0.05; **≥0.001.

Table 2.
Positive response on frequency of drinking and reasons for drinking alcohol among University of Limpopo students aged 17 to 43 years.

	Unadjusted				Adjusted for age, gender and receiving money into own Bank account			
	OR	P-value	(95%CI)		OR	P-value	95 %CI	
Educational level								
Lower level	0.96	0.765	(0.74	1.25)	0.98	0.900	(0.74	1.31)
Moderate high	0.84	0.254	(0.62	1.13)	0.84	0.264	(0.62	1.14)
High level	1.30	0.113	(0.94	1.80)	1.28	0.161	(0.91	1.82)
Tobacco and marijuana product use of relatives/friend living with participated students								
Smoking hubbly bubbly	4.31	0.000**	(2.71	(6.87)	4.14	0.000**	(2.59	6.62)
Smoke Marijuana	4.93	0.000**	(3.16	(7.70)	4.50	0.000**	(2.87	7.06)
Tobacco smoking	4.54	0.000**	(3.04	(6.78)	4.24	0.000**.	(2.82	6.35)
Student residence								
On campus	0.86	0.322	(0.64	(1.16)	1.07	0.650	(0.79	1.45)
Off Campus	1.16	0.322	(0/86	(1.57)	0.93	0.650	(0.69	1.26)
Reasons for drinking alcohol								
I drink alcohol because it will enhance my creative ability	4.52	0.000*	(3.73	(8.21)	3.65	0.000**	(2.74	6.66)
I drink alcohol because I want to be popular	1.86	0.001**	(0.07	(3.71)	2.31	0.005*	(1.87	7.86)
I drink alcohol because it helps me to face difficulties with confidence	1.10	0.321	(0.31	(4.42)	0.24	0.371	(0.15	3.34)
I drink alcohol because it would ease me when I get blamed	3.41	0.561	(2.45	(4.73)	2.21	0.461	(1.57	4.63)

**≥0.05; **≥0.001.*

Table 3.
Odds ratio and 95% confidence interval and p-value for the association of current regular alcohol drinking use and the associated risk factors for University of Limpopo students aged 17 to 43 years.

significantly ($P < 0.05$) associated with the current regular alcohol use among University of Limpopo students for unadjusted (OR ranges 4.31 95%CI 2.71 6.87 to 4.92 95%CI 3.16 7.70) and after adjusted for age, gender, and amount of money deposited into the student account by the bursary scheme (OR ranges from 4.14 95%CI 2.59 6.62 to 4.50 95%CI 2.87 7.06). Place of residence and educational level of students were not significantly associated with current regular alcohol use among students. Current regular alcohol use among students was significantly ($P < 0.05$) associated with enhancing creativity (OR = 4.52 95%CI 3.73 8.210) and popularity (OR = 1.86 95%CI 0.07 3.71) motive among University of Limpopo students before adjusting the cofounders, even after adjusting cofounders, creativity (OR = 3.65 95%CI 2.74 6.66) popularity (OR = 2.31 95%CI 1.87 7.86)).

4. Discussions

This study aimed to investigate the prevalence of alcohol use and related risk factors among University of Limpopo students aged 17 to 43 years. The prevalence of current alcohol drinkers was significantly higher for males compared to females in a University of Limpopo. Similar patterns were reported earlier in South African Universities [7, 9, 10]. Among students in South Africa, Lategan *et al*, [12] found significant differences in drinking behaviour between males and females, with male students drinking frequently more alcohol than female students. Kypri, et al., [21] reported similar results among students in a university in New Zealand and further indicated that these students drank over the legal limit.

In the current study, a significant number of males compared to females ($P < 0.05$) preferred drinking beer and spirits. Weschler et al., [22] reported that several students (both genders) chose spirits (43.8%), beer (19.2%) cider (17.4%) and very few chose wine (3.7%).

Students who preferred spirits and beer showed risky drinking behaviour such as driving while drunk and smoking [12]. Alcohol use at university tends to reach a peak among students aged between 18 and 25 years and are also at the risk of increasing their alcohol consumption later [23]. These university students may develop drinking patterns early in life and it will eventually affect their health and reduce their life expectancy later in their lifestyle.

In the current study alcohol use among students is associated with the use of tobacco and alcohol among friends and family they are staying with. Taremian et al., [24] showed a relatively high incidence of alcohol (17%) abuse among University students in Tehran, however drugs abuse was also high with 34% water-pipe smoking, 24% cigarette, and 2.2% marijuana. Patterns of alcohol consumption and use of drugs vary depending on drinking motives. Cox and Klinger, [25] reported that alcohol drinking and drug use motives could be characterised into two underlying dimensions reflecting the valence (positive or negative) and source (internal or external) of the outcome an individual hopes to achieve. These drinking and drug problems of university students affect their academic achievement badly, emotional adaptableness, and the ability to get jobs after obtaining their career qualification [26].

In our current study alcohol use was not significantly associated with the students residents (off campus/on campus). Dawson et al., [27] found the similar results were there was no differences in amount of alcohol drinking among students living on and off-campus. Similar results were found in the current study. Contrary, Simons-Morton et al., [14] reported that independency and peer pressure increases the risk of alcohol consumptions among students living off-campus.

In the present study, most students drank alcohol to improve interpersonal relationships. The greatest motive for drinking was to be popular followed by difficulties with confidence among males in the current study. Yoo et al., [28], reported a similar response among Korean Medical Students. The high prevalence of drinking among university students not only undermines academic performance, it also places student at risk of injuries, mortality, crime, and sexual assault [29]. It is necessary and essential to identify the significance of alcohol consumption complications in the institutional environment and system that can launch a healthy drinking culture. The problem of university student alcohol consumption can be solved by Policy-based tactics. A healthy drinking culture should be advocated by both the university authority, staff, students and parents such that skilled graduates of the University of Limpopo could pursue his/her career with dignity and vision.

This study has some limitations. We did not randomly select the students to participate in the study but have invited them to take part in the study. There is a possibility that our sample may not be generalizable to the University of Limpopo students. This study forms the base; ever since the higher education sector decided to deposit the bursary money into the student account every month to cover their essentials. Given the cross-sectional nature of the current study, a causal relationship could not be achieved. This was based on interviewing students by well-trained field workers hence recall bias should not be ruled out as an interview was conducted between lecture classes.

5. Conclusions

The prevalence of the current alcohol consumption is high among University of Limpopo male students compared to female students. Living with a person using Tobacco product, marijuana and alcohol are major associated risk factors for current alcohol use in the University of Limpopo students. Drinking problems should not be handled in isolation by the university authority in policy formulation for the culture of healthy drinking but also educate the students on the use of drugs and the motives for drinking. Future studies are required to investigate the development of lifestyle and cardiovascular disease over time among University of Limpopo students.

Acknowledgements

The authors are obligated to the participants (University of Limpopo students) for taking part in the study, resident manager for granting us permission to enter student resident to interview student. Ellisras longitudinal study team for helping with data collection.

Conflict of interest

Authors declare no conflict of interest.

Author details

Mbelege Rosina Nkwana[1], Gift Makaleng[1], Mafoloa Suzan Monyeki[1], Hlengani James Siweya[2] and Kotsedi Daniel Monyeki[1*]

1 Department of Physiology and Environmental Health, University of Limpopo, South Africa

2 Executive Dean Faculty of Science and Agriculture, University of Limpopo, Sovenga, South Africa

*Address all correspondence to: kotsedi.monyeki@ul.ac.za

References

[1] Lapsley DK, Edgerton J. Separation-Individuation, Adult Attachment Style, and College Adjustment. *Counseling & Development J.* 2011; 80(4): 484-492.

[2] Cooper ML. Motives for alcohol use among adolescent: Development and validation of a four factor model. Psycological Assessment 1994; 6 (2):117-128

[3] Lorant V, Nicaise P, Soto VE, d'Hoore W. Alcohol drinking among college students: College responsibility for personal troubles. BMC Public Health, 2013; 13: 615

[4] Lukács A, Simon N, Demeter JS, Kissné Dányi É, Kiss-Tóth E. Alcohol consumption among university students. EGÉSZSÉGTUDOMÁNYI KÖZLEMÉNYEK: A MISKOLCI EGYETEM KÖZLEMÉNYE. 2013;3(2):57-61.

[5] Perkins HW. Surveying the damage: a review of research on consequences of alcohol misuse in college populations. Journal of Studies on Alcohol, supplement. 2002 Mar(14):91-100.

[6] Schulenberg JE, Maggs JL. A developmental perspective on alcohol use and heavy drinking during adolescence and the transition to young adulthood. Journal of Studies on Alcohol, Supplement. 2002 Mar(14):54-70.

[7] Young C, de Klerk V. Patterns of alcohol use on a South African university campus: The findings of two annual drinking surveys. African Journal of Drug and Alcohol Studies. 2008;7(2).

[8] Chikere EI, Mayowa MO. Prevalence and perceived health effect of alcohol use among male undergraduate students in Owerri, South-East Nigeria: a descriptive cross-sectional study. BMC Public health. 2011 Dec 1;11(1):118.

[9] Peltzer K, Ramlagan S. Alcohol use trends in South Africa. Journal of Social Sciences. 2009 Jan 1;18(1):1-2.

[10] Kyei, K.A. and Ramagoma, M. 2013. Alcohol consumption in South African universities: Prevalence and factors at the University of Venda, Limpopo province. *Journal of Social Sciences*, 36: 77-86.

[11] Arria AM, Caldeira KM, Allen HK, Vincent KB, Bugbee BA, O'Grady KE. Drinking like an adult? Trajectories of alcohol use patterns before and after college graduation. Alcoholism: clinical and experimental research. 2016 Mar;40(3):583-90.

[12] Lategan BW, Du Preez R, Pentz CD. Socio-demographic insights into South African student drinking behaviour. South African Journal of Higher Education. 2017 Nov;31(5):90-115.

[13] Harrell ZA, Karim NM. Is gender relevant only for problem alcohol behaviors? An examination of correlates of alcohol use among college students. Addictive behaviors. 2008 Feb 1;33(2):359-65.

[14] Simons-Morton B, Haynie D, Liu D, Chaurasia A, Li K, Hingson R. The effect of residence, school status, work status, and social influence on the prevalence of alcohol use among emerging adults. Journal of studies on alcohol and drugs. 2016 Jan;77(1):121-32.

[15] Matshipi M, Monyeki KD, Mafumo N, Monyeki SM, Siweya HJ, Kemper HC. The use of alcohol and knowledge of cardiovascular diseases among Ellisras rural children aged 14-22 years: Ellisras longitudinal study. International journal of environmental

research and public health. 2019 Jan;16(15):2650.

[16] Benz MB, DiBello AM, Balestrieri SG, Miller MB, Merrill JE, Lowery AD, Mastroleo NR, Carey KB. Off campus residence as a risk factor for heavy drinking among college students. Substance use & misuse. 2017 Jul 29;52(9):1236-41.

[17] Bedendo A, Andrade AL, Opaleye ES, Noto AR. Binge drinking: a pattern associated with a risk of problems of alcohol use among university students. Revista Latino-Americana de Enfermagem. 2017;25.

[18] Suchy W, Gaczkowska A, Pawelczyk A, Pukacki P, Chudzik R. Alcohol use among medicine and law students in Poland. Journal of Medical Science. 2015;84(3):183-8.

[19] Lauer RM, Lee JU, Clarke WR. Predicting adult cholesterol levels from measurements in childhood and adolescence: the Muscatine Study. Bulletin of the New York Academy of Medicine. 1989 Dec;65(10):1127.

[20] Altman RD. Criteria for classification of clinical osteoarthritis. Journal of Rheumatology. 1991 Jan 1;18(SUPPL. 27):10-2.

[21] Kypri K, Langley JD, McGee R, Saunders JB, Williams S. High prevalence, persistent hazardous drinking among New Zealand tertiary students. Alcohol and Alcoholism. 2002 Sep 1;37(5):457-64.

[22] Wechsler H, Nelson TF. What we have learned from the Harvard School of Public Health College Alcohol Study: Focusing attention on college student alcohol consumption and the environmental conditions that promote it. Journal of Studies on alcohol and Drugs. 2008 Jul;69(4):481-90.

[23] Nkambule NR, Bhayat A, Madiba TK. Knowledge, attitude and practices of alcohol and smoking among undergraduate oral health students at a South African University. South African Dental Journal. 2018 Feb;73(1):27-30.

[24] Taremian F, Bolhari J, Pairavi H, Ghazi Tabatabaeii M. The prevalence of drug abuse among university students in Tehran. *Iranian J psychiatry and clinical psychology.* 2008; 13(4):335-42.

[25] Cox WM, Klinger E. Incentive motivation, affective change, and alcohol use: A model. Why people drink: Parameters of alcohol as a reinforcer. 1990:291-314.

[26] Zvauya R, Oyebode F, Day EJ, Thomas CP, Jones LA. A comparison of stress levels, coping styles and psychological morbidity between graduate-entry and traditional undergraduate medical students during the first 2 years at a UK medical school. BMC research notes. 2017 Dec 1;10(1):93.

[27] Dawson DA, Grant BF, Stinson FS, Chou PS. Another look at heavy episodic drinking and alcohol use disorders among college and noncollege youth. Journal of studies on alcohol. 2004 Jul;65(4):477-88.

[28] Yoo HH, Cha SW, Lee SY. Patterns of Alcohol Consumption and Drinking Motives Among Korean Medical Students. Medical Science Monitor: International Medical Journal of Experimental and Clinical Research. 2020;26:e921613-1.

[29] Hingson RW, Zha W, Weitzman ER. Magnitude of and trends in alcohol-related mortality and morbidity among US college students ages 18-24, 1998-2005. Journal of Studies on Alcohol and Drugs, Supplement. 2009 Jul(16):12-20.

Section 4

Metabolic Syndrome and Reproductive Health

Chapter 13

Metabolic Syndrome in Reproductive Health: Urgent Call for Screening

Shisana M. Baloyi and Kebogile Mokwena

Abstract

Metabolic syndrome (MetSy) is a compilation of interrelated pathologic conditions characterized by central obesity, hypertension, insulin resistance and atherogenic dyslipidaemia. The prevalence of MetSy is rising globally. There is growing evidence which linked the individual components of MetSy to the increasing prevalence of poor reproductive health in both the male and female community. This text reviews the recent evidence associating MetSy to poor reproductive health as well as the underlying pathophysiology. The aims to study the relationship between MetSy and reproductive health. The effects of MetSy on fertility were examined and supporting evidence explaining the pathophysiology of dysfunction with each MetSy component extracted from the following medical databases, including CINAHL, MED- LINE, EMBASE, PubMed, and ERIC were described. Noncommunicable disease is rising at an alarming rate globally. Metabolic disorders like hyperlipidaemia, obesity, and insulin resistance can directly or indirectly affect the reproductive health and fertility in both men and women through the interruption of hypothalamic – pituitary – gonadal axis functions. Metabolic syndrome's adverse effects are likely transgenerational (Barker hypothesis), where children born to obese mothers are at increased risk for obesity, diabetes and cardiovascular disease later in life. Therefore MetSy deserves attention and screening should be upscaled at all contacts for all age group of patients to save the future generations.

Keywords: body mass index, diabetes, fertility, metabolic disorders, obesity, male and female reproductive health, screening

1. Introduction

Metabolic Syndrome (MetSy) is one of the fastest-growing non-communicable disorders globally [1, 2]. Metabolic syndrome (MetSy) is a precursor to Non-communicable Diseases (NCDs) and is responsible for the high prevalence of chronic diseases like diabetes, hypertension, heart conditions and cerebrovascular incidents. The burden of NCDs is rising globally and is becoming worse in developing countries, where more women than men are at risk. Women also bear the greatest morbidity and mortality in almost all countries [2]. By the year 2030, studies project that NCDs and related diseases will be the cause of more than 75% of deaths globally [3]. Cardiovascular diseases (CVDs) are predicted to be the future major cause of deaths in low-income countries, more than all the infectious diseases, maternal and perinatal conditions, and nutritional disorders combined [2, 3]. The risk factors associated with NCDs include smoking, high blood pressure, unhealthy diet, inactivity, overweight and obesity, hypercholesterolemia, elevated blood sugar and alcohol consumption [4].

In 2016, the WHO recorded 39% of adults aged 18 years and over (39% of men and 40% of women) to be overweight and on the whole about 13% of the world's adult population (11% of men and 15% of women) were obese in 2016 [5]. Obesity and overweight). The worldwide prevalence of obesity nearly tripled between 1975 and 2016 [5]. Obesity in men in reproductive age is increasing worldwide, impacting negatively on reproductive potential, sperm function and assisted reproduction outcomes. Changes in modern eating behaviors are needed to invert the negative correlation between lifestyle and sperm quality [6]. Current studies predict that approximately 25% of children less than 16 years old will be obese by the year 2050. This is of serious concern as childhood obesity predisposes individuals to adult obesity and the associated obesity related medical sequelae. One such sequela is the impact on reproductive health in both the male and females population [7].

2. Defining the metabolic syndrome (MetSy)

Metabolic syndrome (MetSy) presents as a group of interrelated factors that increases the risk of acquiring cardiovascular disease (CVD) such as coronary heart disease (CHD), arterial atherosclerotic vascular disease and type-2 diabetes mellitus (T2DM), which was described as "Syndrome X" by Reaven in 1988. "Syndrome X" was characterized by impaired glucose tolerance (IGT), hyperinsulinemia, elevated triglycerides (TG), and reduced high-density lipoprotein cholesterol (HDLc) [8]. To date, several definitions of MetSy have been proposed by various international organizations and expert groups by incorporating its different components. These include definitions by the National Cholesterol Education Program Adult Treatment Panel III (NCEP:ATPIII), American Association of Clinical Endocrinology (AACE), International Diabetes Federation (IDF), American Heart Association (AHA) in collaboration with National Heart, Lung and Blood Institute (NHLBI), and World Health Organization (WHO) [9]. A summary of these definitions is presented in **Tables 1** and **2**.

In an effort to provide more consistency in both clinical care and research of patients with MetSy, these various international organizations and expert groups published a consensus joint statement in 2009 on uniform diagnostic criteria, The Harmonized Definition of Metabolic Syndrome [10]. The Harmonized Definition of Metabolic Syndrome (MetSy) includes the presence of 3 of the 5 risk factors, these being enlarged waist circumference (WC) with population-specific and country-specific criteria (WC > 102 cm in men and WC > 88 cm in women), serum triglycerides ≥150 mg/dL or 1.69 mol/l, high density lipoprotein (HDL-c) < 40 mg/dL or 1.03 mmol/l in men and < 50 mg/dL or 1.29 mmol/l in women, systolic blood pressure ≥ 130 mm Hg or diastolic blood pressure ≥ 85 mm Hg, as well as fasting glucose ≥100 mg/dL or 5.6 mmol/l. Also included are patients taking medication to manage hypertriglyceridemia, low high-density lipoproteins (HDL-c), hypertension and hyperglycaemia.

MetSy predicts that the development of type 2 diabetes mellitus (T2DM) leads, in addition, to increased cardiovascular morbidity [9]. Thus, the main components of MetSy are: dyslipidaemia, characterized by elevated triglycerides and low High-Density Lipoproteins (HDL cholesterol), elevated blood pressure (BP), hyperglycaemia, abdominal obesity and/or insulin resistance (IR). Metabolic syndrome is not a disease per se, but a combination of metabolic abnormalities which can present in different ways in accordance with the various components that constitute the syndrome.

National Cholesterol Education Program Adult Treatment Panel III (NCEP:ATPIII): Any three or more of the following:

- Waist circumference > 102 cm in men and > 88 cm in women;
- TG ≥ 150 mg/dl (1.69 mmol/l);
- HDL-cholesterol <40 mg/dl (1.03 mmol/l) in men and < 50 mg/dl (1.29 mmol/l) in women;
- BP ≥ 130/85 mmHg;
- Fasting glucose ≥100 mg/dl (5.56 mmol/l).

American Association of Clinical Endocrinology (AACE): Impaired glucose tolerance plus two or more of the following:

- BMI ≥ 25 kg/m2;
- TG ≥ 150 mg/dl (1.69 mmol/l) and/or HDL-cholesterol <40 mg/dl (1.03 mmol/l) in men and < 50 mg/dl (1.29 mmol/l) in women;
- BP ≥ 130/85 mmHg.

International Diabetes Federation (IDF): Central obesity (defined by waist circumference with ethnicity-specific values#, but can be assumed if BMI > 30 kg/m2), plus two of the following:

- TG ≥ 150 mg/dl (1.69 mmol/l);
- HDL-cholesterol <40 mg/dl (1.03 mmol/l) in men and < 50 mg/dl (1.29 mmol/l) in women;
- BP ≥ 130/85 mmHg;
- Fasting glucose ≥100 mg/dl (5.56 mmol/l).

American Heart Association in collaboration with National Heart, Lung and Blood Institute (AHA/NHLBI): Any three of the following:

- Waist circumference ≥ 102 cm in men, and ≥ 88 cm or greater in women;
- TG ≥ 150 mg/dl (1.69 mmol/l);
- HDL-cholesterol <40 mg/dl (1.03 mmol/l) in men and < 50 mg/dl (1.29 mmol/l) in women;
- BP ≥ 130/85 mmHg;
- Fasting glucose ≥100 mg/dl (5.56 mmol/l). TG: Triglyceride; HDL: High density lipoprotein; BP: blood pressure: BMI: body mass index #See **Table 2.1**.

WHO clinical criteria for defining MetS:

- Resistance to insulin by one of the following:

Type 2 Diabetes

- Impaired fasting glucose
- Impaired Glucose Tolerance
- Insulin resistance defined euglycemic hyperinsulinemic

More any two of the following:

- Antihypertensive and/or high blood pressure (systolic or diastolic ≥140 ≥ 90 mm/Hg)
- Plasma triglycerides ≥150 mg/dl ˂HDL cholesterol 39 mg/dl (in women)˃BMI 30 kg/m^2 and/or the waist/hip ˃ 0.85 (in women)
- Urinary albumin excretion rate ≥ 20 g/min or albumin creatinine ratio ≥ 30 mg/g

---

Table 1.
Metabolic syndrome definitions [9].

3. Pathophysiological development of metabolic syndrome

Many different factors such as genetics, lifestyle (diet and physical activity), obesity and insulin resistance have been hypothesized to play a role in the development of MetSy [8, 11, 12]. Visceral adiposity as a result of a high caloric intake has been demonstrated to be a primary trigger and a major causative factor for the pathogenesis in MetSy [13–15]. A metanalysis conducted by Ryckman et al. [16]

Analyte	Range	Classification
Total Cholesterol[1] (mmol/L)	< 5.2	Desirable
	5.2–6.1	Borderline high
	> 6.1	High
HDL[1,2] (mmol/L)	> 1.53	Less than average risk
	1.03–1.53	Average risk (male)
	1.29–1.53	Average risk (female)
	< 1.03	Increased risk (male)
	< 1.29	Increased risk (female)
LDL[1] (mmol/L)	< 2.6	Optimal
	2.6–3.3	Near optimal
	3.4–4.1	Borderline high
	4.2–4.9	High
	> 4.9	Very high
CHOL/HDL[3,4] (mmol/L)	< 3.5	Optimal (male)
	< 3.4	Optimal (female)
	> 5.0	Above average risk (male)
	> 4.4	Above average risk (female)
VLDL5[5]	0.1-1.7	Normal / near optimal
	> 0.77	High
Non-HDL[1,2] (mmol/L)	< 3.4	Optimal
	3.4–4.1	Near optimal
	4.2–4.9	Borderline high
	5.0–5.7	High
	> 5.7	Very high
Triglycerides[1] (mmol/L)	< 1.69	Desirable
	1.69–2.25	Borderline high
	2.26–5.63	High
	> 5.63	Very high
Glucose[6,7,8] (mmol/L)	< 5.6	Normal (fasting)
	< 7.8	Normal (non-fasting)
	4.1–6.6	Reference interval (fasting)
	< 2, > 30	Critical

[1]*National Cholesterol Education Program ATP III.*
[2]*Lab Tests Online - Lipid Panel.*
[3]*Harvard Medical Health Guide.*
[4]*American Heart Association.*
[5]*Lab Tests Online – VLDL.*
[6]*Abaxis – Piccolo® Lipid Panel Plus Reagent Disc.*
[7]*American Diabetes Association.*
[8]*Mayo Clinic.*

Table 2.
Reference ranges for clinical and biochemical measurements.

found that the presence of a single element of metabolic syndrome could contribute to the development of metabolic syndrome, and that diabetes alone will later contribute to the development of hypertension. Obesity appears more common in females and this is attributed to the fact that most women gain weight outside the recommended levels during pregnancy [17].

4. Global epidemiology of metabolic syndrome

Due to the aging population, global increase in obesity and sedentary lifestyles, the prevalence of MetSy is increasing throughout the world and it has become an epidemic of the 21st century [18]. Prevalence rates vary widely due to the criteria used, age of the population, gender, ethnic group, prevalence of obesity in the background population, and environment. The incidence of MetSY often parallels the incidence of obesity and incidence of T2DM. The global prevalence of MetSy has be estimated to be about one quarter of the World population [19]. The prevalence of MetSy is 0–50% or more in African populations, commoner in females and increases with age and urban housing (Okafor, 2012) [20].

5. Screening for MetSy in the general public

Screening can include individuals with pre-symptomatic or unrecognized symptomatic disease [21]. Several studies have shown the importance of screening [22–24].

Health-screening programmes have been effectively used to pinpoint public-health challenges [25–40], and many countries have implemented nationwide health screening and intervention programmes that specifically target MetSy [41]. The first Framingham Risk Score is a gender-specific score that identifies patients at risk of developing cardiovascular complications within a 10-year period. It factors in age, sex, LDL cholesterol, HDL cholesterol, smoking, blood pressure and also whether the patient is on treatment or not for hypertension, lipidaemia and diabetes, and smoking [42]. Artigao-Rodenas et al. [42] applied the Framingham Risk Score in a prospective cohort study of four years in Spain and found that the model had a good predictive value, with negative predictive values in both sexes, a specificity of 85.6% in women and sensitivity of 79.1% in men in a population with high risk of cardiovascular disease. The model had a significant cumulative probability of individual survival by tertiles in both sexes with a p value <0.001.

6. Obesity screening anthropometric indices: body mass index (BMI) and mid-upper arm circumference(MUA)

BMI is currently the metric measure used to determine categories of bodyweight in adults (**Table 3**). Other methods and techniques of estimating body fat and body-fat distribution includes measurements of the waist circumference (WC), waist-hip ratio, underwater weighing, bioelectrical impedance analysis, skin-fold thickness and imaging techniques such as ultrasound, computed tomography, and magnetic resonance imaging with the later giving the most accurate estimates of body composition [44]. The problem of using MUAC is that there is no consensus on its cut-offs internationally [45]. Waist circumference has likewise been shown to estimate body fat, but is a fairly better guide to cardiometabolic disease risks as it identifies people with relatively low BMI but with increased intra-abdominal fat accumulation [46].

In most studies which have measured estimated total body fat by a reference method, BMI was found not to be a strong predictor of body fat [47] and therefore other methods should be developed to better classify individuals at risk of

	BMI (kg/m2)	Obesity Class	Disease Risk* (Relative to Normal Weight and Waist Circumference)	
			Men ≤40 in (≤.102 cm) Women ≤.35 in (≤.88 cm)	> 40 in (> 102 cm) > 35 in (> 88 cm)
Underweight	< 18.5		—	—
Normal†	18.5–24.9		—	—
Overweight	25.0–29.9		Increased	High
Obesity	30.0–34.9 35.0–39.9	I II	High Very High	Very High Very High
Extreme Obesity	≥.40	III	Extremely High	Extremely High

Disease risk for type 2 diabetes, hypertension, and CVD.
†*Increased waist circumference can also be a marker for increased risk even in persons of normal weight.*

Table 3.
Body mass index and obesity [43].

developing MetSy [48]. This is important because there are established ethnic differences in the relationship between abdominal adiposity and metabolic disease risk [49, 50]. Baloyi and Mokwena [51] conducted a prospective cross-sectional study among the pregnant women attending antenatal care at Regional Hospital in Bloemfontein, South Africa in which they excluded BMI and WC in defining MetSy but considered the presence of 3 of the 5 risk factors based on the Harmonized Definition of Metabolic Syndrome. The prevalence of MetSy in this sample was 15.46% and the screening tool enables the screening of pregnant women for metabolic syndrome in all trimesters.

Adapted from "Preventing and Managing the Global Epidemic of Obesity. Report of the World Health Organization Consultation of Obesity." WHO, Geneva, June 1997.

7. Gender as risk factors for metabolic syndrome

Studies have demonstrated that there are sex differences concerning risk factor predictors of MetSy, suggesting that levels of sex steroids hormones, estrogen/androgen, balance potentially play a vital role in determining MetSy [52–56]. In women, raised BMI, low HDL cholesterol, increased WC and hyperglycaemia were significantly greater contributors to the MetSy, whereas in men hypertension and elevated triglycerides were the main factors [55]. Case and Menendez [57] found two factors in SA that contributed to the gender prevalence disparity, nutritionally deprived during childhood and a higher socio-economic status than males. They identified women to have been nutritionally deprived during childhood; and having a higher socio-economic status. The contributing risk factors prevalent in women are abdominal obesity and insulin resistance, as well as physical inactivity, aging and polycystic ovarian syndrome in some [58]. Other factors contributing to the higher prevalence of MetSy in women is that women live longer than men, and it is reported that women develop cardiovascular disease (CVD) at an older age compared to men [59, 60]. There is a wide disparity in economic status among the black population compared to the other ethnic groups, and this correlates with the wide gap in the prevalence of obesity and disease between these ethnic groups that may be partly attributed to or mediated by these social inequalities [61].

8. Lifestyle habits as risk factors for metabolic syndrome in women

There is an inverse relationship between socio-economic status and obesity in high-income countries but consistent positive association between obesity and socio-economic status in low- resource countries [62]. The transition towards Western lifestyle and urbanization which is accompanied by access to clean water and electricity, reduced housing density, more money available to spend on food, higher energy intake, commuting by taxi/vehicle and reduced physical activity or increased sedentary behavior have positively associated with obesity [56, 63]. The risk of developing specific components of MetSy such as obesity, hyperlipidaemia, hypertension, and elevated fasting blood sugar, has been largely attributed to environmental stressors including poor nutrition with consumption of high-calorie diets which are cheaper and fill the stomach at a cheaper price than healthy food, lack of exercise, and smoking [4]. There is a growing trends among the youths and young adult engaging in alcohol binge drinking, this conduct was found to be significantly associated with lower levels of high-density lipoprotein cholesterol (HDL-C). The low HDL-C increases the risk of developing cardiovascular diseases among these participants [64].

9. Consequences of the metabolic syndrome

Available data support the theory of "developmental origins of adult disease" hypothesis, the "Barker Hypothesis", which posits that a significant portion of the risk for adult metabolic conditions is determined by exposure occurring in the perinatal period [65]. The "Barker Hypothesis" proposes that a poor in-utero environment produced by maternal dietary or placental insufficiency may "program" susceptibility in the foetus to later development of cardiovascular and metabolic disease. The "Barker Hypothesis" further proposes that maternal MetSy has an epigenetic effect, making the next generation unwell and leading to an increase in T2DM and cardiovascular disease in juvenile age and in later life from obesity [65, 66]. The MetSy is further associated with polycystic ovary syndrome in girls, obstructive sleep apnoea, hypogonadism and some form of gynecological cancers especially endometrial cancer [67].

10. Metabolic syndrome and reproductive health

10.1 The physiology of the hypothalamic – pituitary – gonadal axis

Under normal conditions in both males and females, gonadotropin-releasing hormone is produced and released from the hypothalamus, which stimulates the production and release of the gonadotropins, follicle-stimulating hormone (FSH) and luteinizing hormone (LH) from the anterior pituitary. FSH and LH act on the respective gonads, testicles in men and ovaries in women, to stimulate spermatogenesis and steroidogenesis, and folliculogenesis and steroidogenesis respectively [68].

10.1.1 Luteinizing hormone

In both sexes, LH stimulates secretion of sex steroids from the gonads. In the testes, LH binds to receptors on Leydig cells, stimulating synthesis and secretion of testosterone. Theca cells in the ovary respond to LH stimulation by secretion of testosterone, which is converted into estrogen by adjacent granulosa cells. In females, the LH surge leads to ovulation of mature follicles on the ovary and later to form corpus luteum, which secrete the steroid hormones progesterone and oestradiol. In the event of pregnancy progesterone is necessary for the maintenance of that pregnancy.

10.1.2 Follicle-stimulating hormone

The FSH is responsible for the maturation of ovarian follicles. Administration of FSH to humans and animals induces "superovulation", an increased number of mature gametes. FSH is also critical for spermatogenesis and sperm cell maturation at the Sertoli cells.

10.1.3 Control of gonadotropin secretion

LH and FSH secretion is under the influence of gonadotropin-releasing hormone (GnRH, also known as LH-releasing hormone). GnRH is a ten amino acid peptide that is synthesized and secreted from hypothalamic neurons and binds to receptors on gonadotrophs.

As depicted in **Figure 1** below, GnRH stimulates secretion of LH, which in turn stimulates gonadal secretion of the sex steroids testosterone, estrogen and progesterone. In a classical negative feedback loop sex steroids(oestrogens, progesterone, testosterone) inhibit secretion of GnRH and also appear to have direct negative effects on gonadotrophs.

This regulatory loop leads to pulsatile secretion of LH and, to a much lesser extent, FSH. The number of pulses of GnRH and LH varies from a few per day to one or more per hour. In females, pulse frequency is clearly related to stage of the cycle.

Several hormonal substances such as inhibin and activin from the gonads, which selectively inhibit and activate FSH secretion from the pituitary, influence GnRH secretion, and positive and negative control over GnRH [69]. Thus gonadotropin secretion is actually considerably more complex than depicted in **Figure 1** below.

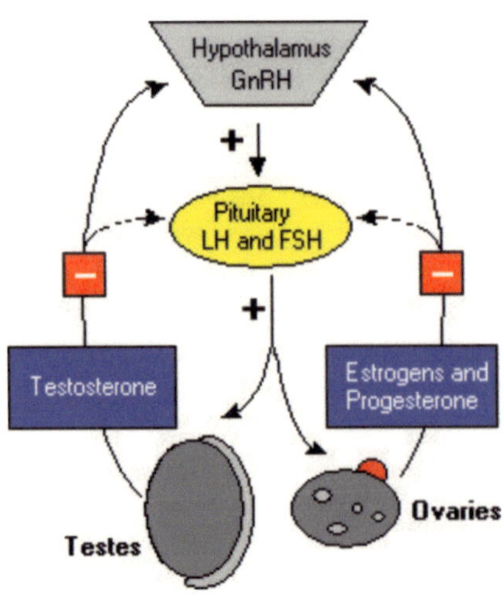

Figure 1.
(vivo.colostate.edu).

10.2 Metabolic syndrome and impact on reproductive health

Obesity is a cardinal feature of MetSy and has been increasing in [70]. The effect of obesity on reproduction and as a cause of female infertility has been more extensively studied in females [70]. Obesity has been recently associated with an increased incidence of male factor infertility. A study from Norway looked at planned pregnancies and the time to achieving pregnancy, after adjusting for female BMI and smoking habits, the results showed that overweight and obese men had an odds ratio of infertility of 1.19 and 1.36, respectively [71]. Ramlau-hansen et al. [72] conducted a similar study comprising nearly 48,000 couples for six years assessing the effects of both male and female obesity on infertility and found that overweight and obese men coupled with normal- weight females had an odds ratio for reduced fertility of 1.18 and 1.53, respectively. A further observation was that couples where both parents were overweight or obese, the odds ratios for reduced fertility were 1.41 and 2.74, respectively [73]. Obese people have decreased gonadotropin levels, and increased circulating estrogen levels [74]. The increase in estrogen is likely secondary to peripheral aromatization of androgens from cholesterol in the adipose tissue. A hypogonadotropic hypogonadism state is created due to estrogen negative feedback onto the hypothalamus [74].

10.3 Metabolic syndrome and female reproductive health

Metabolic disorders, including diabetes, obesity, and hyperlipidaemia plays a significant role in the development of female-specific reproductive health issues, which have a significant impact on public health. MetSy also increases the risk of reproductive cancers such as, breast, endometrial, bladder and cervical cancers [73]. Obesity particularly impacts women of reproductive age, as it is associated with an increased risk of infertility and adverse obstetric outcome such as miscarriage, stillbirth, birth defects and cesarean section [70, 75, 76]. MetSy can affect women's reproductive health and fertility directly or indirectly by interfering with the hypothalamic – pituitary – gonadal (HPG) axis function. MetSy creates conditions of negative energy balance and metabolic stress which cause hypogonadism by suppressing the expression of the hypothalamic KiSS/kisspeptin [77, 78].

In addition to the effect of peripheral aromatization which create the hypogonadotropic hypogonadism state in obese women, a lack of residual insulin secretion in diabetes is also associated with the status quo [79]. The hypothalamic origin of the decreased levels of gonadotropin in amenorrhoeic and diabetic patients are related to a toxic effect of hyperglycaemia on the neurons of the hypothalamus leading to reduced LH response to GnRH stimuli [80].

10.3.1 Premature adrenarche in girls

Adrenarche is the puberty of the adrenal gland. Pubarche is denoted by the appearance of pubic hair and or axillary hair. Premature adrenarche in girls is when pubarche occurs before age 8 years in girls and 9 years in boys. The chief hormonal products of adrenarche are DHEA and DHEAS produced from zona reticularis. Premature adrenarche represents an early clinical feature of MetSy (obesity, hypertension, dyslipidaemia, insulin resistance) for some girls. Conceivably the early recognition of these children will permit allow early intervention, such as lifestyle modifications, including dietary, activity level intervention with possibility of using insulin-sensitizing agents in some individuals. Premature pubarche due to premature adrenarche and hyperinsulinemia may precede the development of ovarian hyperandrogenism [81].

Interference with the hypothalamic – pituitary – gonadal axis function may affect follicular recruitment and impact subsequent oocyte quality and affecting overall subfertility in obese women. Studies of women undergoing assisted reproductive technologies (ART) have demonstrated that obesity also has direct effects on the quality oocytes and embryos and on the status of the endometrium. Audit data from retrospective studies demonstrated obesity to be associated with increased risk for miscarriage in spontaneous conceptions [82] as well in pregnancy achieved through donor oocytes after IVF [83]. The pathophysiology underlying this association is complex and likely multifactorial, involving the oocyte, embryonic development, and the endometrium. Apart from fertility and pregnancy problems, female adiposity may influence the timing of onset of puberty, associated with irregular menses, ovulatory dysfunction and ovarian aging [77].

10.3.2 PCOS and obesity

Polycystic ovary syndrome (PCOS) is a hormonal disorder common, among women of reproductive age affecting 5 to 10 percent, often complicated by chronic anovulatory infertility and hyperandrogenism with the clinical manifestations of oligomenorrhoea, hirsutism and acne [84, 85]. The link between PCOS and obesity is complicated. Signs and symptoms of polycystic ovarian syndrome begin for some females soon after menarche. Women with PCOS have insulin resistance (IR) [86]. This insulin resistance is one reason why women with PCOS tend to gain weight or experiences challenges in losing weight. In some females, PCOS develops later on, following substantial weight gain. Women affected by obesity are also more likely to face reproductive problems like polycystic ovarian syndrome (PCOS) and women with PCOS have a greater risk for obesity. Obesity and PCOS share some common features, anovulation and hyperandrogenism although simple or non-syndromic obesity is much more prevalent than PCOS and seems to have a different pathophysiology with respect to the obesity-related reproductive impairment [87]. The difference in the two is that PCOS is characterized by increased serum LH whereas obese women typically have in general lower serum LH. Obesity may modify some aspects hypothalamic – pituitary – gonadal axis function [88]. Although obesity can affect many facet of PCOS, it is a cause of this syndrome and without doubt have an effect on reproduction regardless of PCOS symptomatology [87]. In this review, we will focus on how obesity in the absence of PCOS affects the HPO axis.

10.4 Metabolic syndrome and male reproductive health

Obesity, as a cardinal feature of MetS, has been associated with an increased incidence of male factor infertility. Although the effect of excess body fat on reproduction has been more extensively studied in females, there has been a recent increase in literature assessing the relationship between obesity and semen characteristics, male endocrine changes, male sexual function and male factor infertility. Over the past decade, numerous studies have found an inverse correlation between increased obesity and semen quality that negatively affects male fertility, with an increased chance of subfertility among couples in which the male partner is obese. Various mechanisms for this relationship have been proposed and can be broadly divided into direct negative effects on spermatogenesis and sperm function (lower sperm counts, poorer sperm quality), hormonal factors and, and increased rates of erectile dysfunction [89, 90]. In males, a state of primary hypogonadism is also well defined as an underlying feature associated with MetS [89].

10.4.1 Pathophysiology of obese male factor infertility

Obesity in men contribute to the poor reproductive function through numerous postulated mechanisms. First, hormonal perturbations that involves peripheral conversion of testosterone to estrogen in excess peripheral adipose tissue may lead to secondary hypogonadism through HPG axis inhibition. Second, elevated levels of inflammatory mediators and reactive oxygen species (ROS), generating oxidative stress at the level of the testicular micro environment may result in decreased spermatogenesis and sperm DNA fragmentation. Lastly, the accumulation of supra pubic and inner thigh fat may result in increased testicular heat, which cumulatively can have substantial, detrimental effects on spermatogenesis [74, 90–92].

Men with obesity, the metabolic syndrome and type 2 diabetes have low total and free testosterone and low sex hormone-binding globulin SHBG. On the other hand, the presence of low testosterone and/or SHBG predicts the future development of metabolic syndrome and T2DM [93]. Thus, the observed decrease in testosterone levels in obese males is likely due to several factors, including decreased synthesis of testosterone, inhibition of SHBG synthesis, and decreased gonadotropin secretion [93]. In summary, total testosterone, free testosterone and SHBG are all commonly decreased in obese males. Obesity is also characterized by higher insulin levels and insulin resistance this is suggested to impair steroidogenesis at the Leydig cells which may negatively impact the male reproductive function in the case of obesity [94, 95]. Derby et al. [96] conducted a longitudinal trial of 942 men ages 40–70 years enrolled in the Massachusetts Male Aging Study, demonstrated that BMI was negatively associated with total testosterone, free testosterone, and SHBG, as well as that these levels decline more rapidly with age in obese men.

Adipose tissue behaves like an endocrine gland, it produces hormonally active proteins involved in satiety and metabolism as well as HPG axis regulation [97]. The white adipose tissue produces leptin [74, 97] which has been found to stimulate gonadotropin-releasing hormone secretion in the hypothalamus and FSH and LH secretion in the anterior pituitary in the rat animal studies [98, 99]. Leptin is also believed to have a direct effect on regulation of testosterone production in the testicle taking into account the presence of leptin receptors in Leydig cells [100]. Obesity generates a leptin resistant state, given that high circulating leptin levels are linked with increased adiposity and lower testosterone levels [101].

Obesity creates a proinflammatory state with production of adipokines and cytokines by adiopocytes that result in an increase in systemic inflammation [102] Any form of Inflammation of the reproductive tract has been shown to be associated with infertility in male patients. The cytokines tumor necrosis factor (TNF-a) and interleukin-1(IL-1) have been implicated as the main mediators of the inflammatory process [103]. Inflammation increases levels of reactive oxygen species generating oxidative stress at the level of the testicular that can negatively impact normal reproductive pathways [104]. Elevated oxidative stress leads to increased DNA damage of spermatozoa and is negatively correlated with normal sperm morphology [105–107]. Tunc et al. [108] compared reactive oxygen levels in semen samples from both overweight/obese men and men of normal BMI and found that there was a weak but statistically significant positive correlation between increasing BMI and reactive oxygen species levels.

Spermatogenesis is also adversely effected by elevated testicular temperature. Increased adiposity in the legs and pannus overlying the scrotum may lead to increased testicular temperatures. Shafik and Olfat [109] performed lipectomy to remove the excess scrotal lipoma from a series of infertile men and later observed improvements in their semen parameters in 64.7% of study participants and pregnancies in 19.6% [109]. Prolonged inactivity in obese men has also been associated with increased scrotal temperatures [110].

11. Intervention approaches to reduce the burden of MetSy

11.1 Health promotion (Ottawa charter)

Health promotion is 'the process of enabling people to increase control over and to improve their health' Introduced into public health in Ottawa in 1986 [111]. Health promotion strategies can be achieved by developing and changing lifestyles, to impact on the social, economic and environmental conditions that determine health.

The Ottawa Charter for Health Promotion set out five strategies that are essential for the success for any health promotion strategy: Build healthy policy; Create supportive environments; Strengthen community actions; Develop personal skills; and Reorient health services. Health promotion actions should target the population at risk, early in life to stop the metabolic storm, by increasing their knowledge and warning them about the dangers of MetSy, enforcing bans on alcohol and tobacco advertising, promotion and sponsorship, raising taxes on alcohol and tobacco and reducing the price of healthy diet food. It is of vital importance to note that the ideal time for intervention is pre-conception. Health-care workers who attend to women of reproductive age and diagnose obesity, have a duty to counsel and refer these patients to high-risk obstetric specialists for consultation to discuss the many risks associated with obesity in pregnancy [112].

These obese patients should be encouraged strongly to undertake nonsurgical interventions to achieve weight reduction to achieve ideal body weight (BMI, 18.5–24.9 kg/m2) before conception. These include, among others, behavioral modification, dietary changes, exercise, and pharmacotherapy [113]. Dietician consultation is recommended for diet advice that is high in fiber, fresh fruit, vegetables, lean protein, and complex carbohydrates, while avoiding foods that contain large amounts of sugar, saturated fats, and cholesterol. Regular fitness exercises based on available facilities such as brisk walking, stair climbing, jogging, or swimming that use the larger skeletal muscles should be incorporated into weight reduction programs. Once the diagnosis of MetSy in Pregnancy or elements of it is made, it's possible to provide intervention to prevent progression of the condition and complications in pregnancy and the associated adverse perinatal outcomes [114].

Insulin resistance and central obesity are regarded as the main underlying causes of metabolic syndrome. Therefore, reduction in body weight will lead to fatty acid mobilization and should be the key focus in management of the MetSy [115]. Stinson et al. [116] showed that overconsumption of poor diet is an important component of the MetSy, and thus needs to be targeted for its reduction and treatment. A literature review on randomized control trials has shown improvement in MetSy following intervention focusing on diet and lifestyle modification, either in certain components or taken as a whole syndrome within a period of 2 weeks–1 year [117]. Informing and educating the public should include nutrition, promotion of regular physical activity, reduction of substance abuse as well as prevention or management of central adiposity, diabetes, atheromatosis and hypertension, and setting a national agenda to motivate all population groups to change stereotype perceptions and behaviors aimed at health and quality-of-life promotion.

Literature provides evidence of efficacy in adhering to the Mediterranean diet (MeD) in reducing body weight [118]. The Mediterranean Dietary pattern is comprised of fruit, cooked vegetables and legumes, grains (whole, not refined) and, in moderation, wine, nuts, fish and dairy products, particularly yogurt and cheese. It is a food pattern that has the potential of improving health and quality of life in people who adhere to it appropriately, characterizing a way of life and culture [119]. These interventions to alter diet and lifestyle have the potential to succeed only if they are executed early, and thus, offer enough evidence to develop appropriate public policies.

11.2 Bariatric surgery and pregnancy

Obese women with overtly high BMI of more than 40 kg/m^2 or BMI of 35 kg/m^2 with the presence of comorbid NCD conditions (such as diabetes mellitus, coronary artery disease, or severe sleep apnea), should be referred to a specialist surgeon for possible bariatric surgery [120]. Great success has been reported with women who have undergone Bariatric surgery followed by healthy lifestyle modifications [121], by generally demonstrating overall recovery in quality-of-life measures and resolution of their medical comorbidities [122, 123].

Patients who have undergone bariatric surgery should be counseled to avoid pregnancy for a period of 12–18 months after the procedure. Falling pregnant during this interval has been associated with higher risk of surgical complications and exposure of the foetus to rapid weight change [124].

12. Summary

MetSy is not only as a predictor of cardiovascular disease but also as a potential contributing factor to poor reproductive health and interfere with fertility in both male and female affected across her lifespan. Perhaps the most concerning information presented in this chapter is the Barker hypothesis, that the metabolic syndrome's adverse effects are likely transgenerational where children born to obese mothers are at increased risk for obesity, diabetes and cardiovascular disease later in life. There is also increasing and worrying evidence that lifestyle factors such as alcohol binge consumption increases the incidence of metabolic syndrome. Obesity exerts it detrimental effect in the human body by generating a physiological resistant state in the such as a leptin resistant state, insulin resistant.

Noncommunicable disease is rising globally at an alarming rate, future studies focus should be on the strategies needed to improve public health programs and policies aimed at reducing the prevalence of metabolic syndrome through screening at all contacts for all types of patients to save the future generations. Instituting early and targeted lifestyle interventions such as balanced diet and frequent physical activity for metabolic syndrome is a medical exigency.

Conflict of interest

The authors declare that there is no conflict of interest that could be perceived as prejudicing the impartiality of the review.

Author details

Shisana M. Baloyi[1,2]* and Kebogile Mokwena[1]

1 Department of Public Health, Sefako Makgatho Health Sciences University, South Africa

2 Department of Obstetrics and Gynaecology, University of the Free State, South Africa

*Address all correspondence to: baloyism@ufs.ac.za

References

[1] Shalini M, Suresh BK, Srinivasa MA, Girish B, Mounika K, Vaishnavi B. Metabolic syndrome among urban and rural women population – a cross sectional study. J Clin Diagn Res. 2013;7(9):1938-1940. doi:10.7860/JCDR/2013/6467.3363)

[2] Bentley-Lewis R, Aguilar D, Riddle MC, Claggett B, Diaz R, Dickstein K, Gerstein HC, Johnston P, Køber LV, Lawson F, Lewis EF, Maggioni AP, McMurray JJ, Ping L, Probstfield JL, Solomon SD, Tardif JC, Wu Y, Pfeffer MA; ELIXA Investigators. (2015). Rationale, design, and baseline characteristics in Evaluation of lixisenatide in Acute Coronary Syndrome, a long-term cardiovascular end point trial of lixisenatide versus placebo. American Heart Association Journal. 169(5):631-638.

[3] Beaglehole, R., and R. Bonita.(2008). Global public health: A scorecard. Lancet 372(9654): 1988-1996.

[4] Boutayeb A (2006). The double burden of communicable and non-communicable diseases in developing countries. Transactions of the Royal Society of Tropical Medicine and Hygiene, 100 (3): 191-9.

[5] World Health Organization. (2016). World health statistics 2016: monitoring health for the SDGs sustainable development goals. World Health Organization.

[6] Ferramosca, A., Di Giacomo, M., Moscatelli, N., & Zara, V. (2018). Obesity and male infertility: role of fatty acids in the modulation of sperm energetic metabolism. European Journal of Lipid Science and Technology, 120(4), 1700451.

[7] Johnson M.D., Sanfilippo J.S. (2015). Childhood and Adolescent Obesity: Implications for Reproductive Health and Function. In: Jungheim E. (eds) Obesity and Fertility. Springer, New York, NY. https://doi.org/10.1007/978-1-4939-2611-4_3

[8] Reaven, G. M. (1988). Banting lecture 1988. Role of insulin resistance in human disease. Diabetes.37, 1595-1607.

[9] Kassi E, Pervanidou P, Kaltsas G, Chrousos G. 2011. Metabolic syndrome: definitions and controversies. BioMed Central (BMC) Medicine, 9(48):1-13.

[10] Alberti KGMM, Eckel RH, Grundy SM, Zimmet PZ, Cleeman JI, Donato KA, Fruchart J, W. James WPT, Loria CM, Smith SC. (2009). Harmonizing the Metabolic Syndrome. A Joint Interim Statement of the International Diabetes Federation Task Force on Epidemiology and Prevention; National Heart, Lung, and Blood Institute; American Heart Association; World Heart Federation; International Atherosclerosis Society; and International Association for the Study of Obesity. Circulation. American Heart Association journal.120:1640-1645.

[11] Reaven GM. (1993).Role of insulin resistance in human disease (syndrome X): an expanded definition. Annual Review Medicine .44:121-31.

[12] Smith DO, LeRoith D.(2004). Insulin resistance syndrome, pre-diabetes, and the prevention of type 2 diabetes mellitus. Clinical Cornerstone ; 6:7-6

[13] Matsuzawa Y, Funahashi T and Nakamura T. (2011). The concept of metabolic syndrome: contribution of visceral fat accumulation and its molecular mechanism. Journal of Atherosclerotic Thrombosis 2011; 18(8): 629-639.

[14] Gallagher EJ, Leroith D, Karnieli E.(2011). The metabolic

syndrome from insulin resistance to obesity and diabetes. Medical Clinical North America; 95:855-873

[15] Roberts CK, Hevener AL, and Barnard RJ. (2013). Metabolic Syndrome and Insulin Resistance: Underlying Causes and Modification by Exercise Training. Comprehensive Physiology. 3(1): 1-58.

[16] Ryckman KK, Spracklen CN, Smith CJ, Robinson JG, Saftlas AF. (2015). Maternal lipid levels during pregnancy and gestational diabetes: a systematic review and meta-analysis. British Journal of Obstetrics and Gynaecology. 122(5):643-51.

[17] Nicholas P, Sharma AJ, Kim SY, and Hinkle SN. (2015). Prevalence and Characteristics Associated With Gestational Weight Gain Adequacy. Obstetrics and Gynecology.125:773-81.

[18] Tavares, H.P., Arantes, M.A., Tavares, S.B.M.P., Abbade, J.F., dos Santos, D.C.D.M., de Mattos Paranhos Calderon, I. and Rudge, M.V.C. (2015) Metabolic Syndrome and Pregnancy, Its Prevalence, Obstetrical and New-borns Complications. Open Journal of Obstetrics and Gynecology, 5, 618-625. http://dx.doi.org/10.4236/ojog.2015.511087

[19] Saklayen M. G. (2018). The Global Epidemic of the Metabolic Syndrome. Current hypertension reports, 20(2), 12. https://doi.org/10.1007/s11906-018-0812-z)

[20] Okafor CI. (2012). The metabolic syndrome in Africa: Current trends. Indian Journal of Endocrinology and Metabolism. 16(1): 56-66.

[21] Madras, B. K., Compton, W. M., Avula, D., Stegbauer, T., Stein, J. B., & Clark, H. W. (2009). Screening, brief interventions, referral to treatment (SBIRT) for illicit drug and alcohol use at multiple healthcare sites: comparison at intake and 6 months later. Drug and alcohol dependence, 99(1), 280-295.

[22] Tuomilehto, J., Lindström, J., Eriksson, J. G., Valle, T. T., Hämäläinen, H., Ilanne-Parikka, P. & Salminen, V. (2001). Prevention of type 2 diabetes mellitus by changes in lifestyle among subjects with impaired glucose tolerance. New England Journal of Medicine, 344(18), 1343-1350.

[23] Satterfield, D. W., Volansky, M., Caspersen, C. J., Engelgau, M. M., Bowman, B. A., Gregg, E. W. & Vinicor, F. (2003). Community-based lifestyle interventions to prevent type 2 diabetes. Diabetes Care, 26(9), 2643-2652.

[24] Klein, S., Sheard, N. F., Pi-Sunyer, X., Daly, A., Wylie-Rosett, J., Kulkarni, K., & Clark, N.G. (2004). Weight Management Through Lifestyle Modification for the Prevention and Management of Type 2 Diabetes: Rationale and Strategies: A statement of the American Diabetes Association, the North American Association for the Study of Obesity, and the American Society for Clinical Nutrition. Diabetes care, 27(8), 2067-2073.

[25] Heckman, B. D., Fisher, E. B., Monsees, B., Merbaum, M., Ristvedt, S., & Bishop, C. (2004). Coping and anxiety in women recalled for additional diagnostic procedures following an abnormal screening mammogram. Health Psychology, 23(1), 42.

[26] Pua, Y. H., & Ong, P. H. (2005). Anthropometric indices as screening tools for cardiovascular risk factors in Singaporean women. Asia Pacific journal of clinical nutrition, 14(1), 74.

[27] Cuzick, J., Clavel, C., Petry, K. U., Meijer, C. J., Hoyer, H., Ratnam, S. & Iftner, T. (2006). Overview of the European and North American studies on HPV testing in primary cervical cancer screening. International Journal of Cancer, 119(5), 1095-1101.

[28] Partridge, E. E., Abu-Rustum, N. R., Campos, S. M., Fahey, P. J., Farmer, M., Garcia, R. L & Massad, S. L. (2010). Cervical cancer screening. Journal of the National Comprehensive Cancer Network, 8(12), 1358-1386.

[29] Hacker, K. A., Myagmarjav, E., Harris, V., Suglia, S. F., Weidner, D., & Link, D. (2006). Mental health screening in pediatric practice: factors related to positive screens and the contribution of parental/personal concern. Pediatrics, 118(5), 1896-1906.

[30] Krowka, M. J., Swanson, K. L., Frantz, R. P., McGoon, M. D., & Wiesner, R. H. (2006). Portopulmonary hypertension: Results from a 10-year screening algorithm. Hepatology, 44(6), 1502-1510.

[31] Weist, M. D., Rubin, M., Moore, E., Adelsheim, S., & Wrobel, G. (2007). Mental health screening in schools. Journal of School Health, 77(2), 53-58.

[32] Grisso, T., Vincent, G., & Seagrave, D. (Eds.). (2005). Mental health screening and assessment in juvenile justice. Guilford Press.

[33] Neelemaat, F., Kruizenga, H. M., De Vet, H. C. W., Seidell, J. C., & Butterman, M. (2008). Screening malnutrition in hospital outpatients. Can the SNAQ malnutrition screening tool also be applied to this population? Clinical Nutrition, 27(3), 439-446.

[34] Hu, Yaomin, Wei Liu, Yawen Chen, Ming Zhang, Lihua Wang, Huan Zhou, Peihong Wu et al. "Combined use of fasting plasma glucose and glycated hemoglobin A1c in the screening of diabetes and impaired glucose tolerance." Acta diabetologica 47, no. 3 (2010): 231-236.

[35] Sheehy, A. M., Flood, G. E., Tuan, W. J., Liou, J. I., Coursin, D. B., & Smith, M. A. (2010, January). Analysis of guidelines for screening diabetes mellitus in an ambulatory population. In Mayo Clinic Proceedings (Vol. 85, No. 1, pp. 27-35). Elsevier.

[36] Pialoux, T., Goyard, J., & Lesourd, B. (2012). Screening tools for frailty in primary health care: a systematic review. Geriatrics & gerontology international, 12(2), 189-197.

[37] Cooper, S. A., Morrison, J., Melville, C., Finlayson, J., Allan, L., Martin, G., & Robinson, N. (2006). Improving the health of people with intellectual disabilities: outcomes of a health screening programme after 1 year. Journal of Intellectual Disability Research, 50(9), 667-677.

[38] Mokwena, K., & Shiba, D. (2014). Prevalence of postnatal depression symptoms in a primary health care clinic in Pretoria, South Africa: management of health care services. African Journal for Physical Health Education, Recreation and Dance: Public Health Research as a cornerstone of health services reform: Supplement 1, 20, 116-127.

[39] Coker, A. L., Pope, B. O., Smith, P. H., Sanderson, M., & Hussey, J. R. (2001). Assessment of clinical partner violence screening tools.

[40] Quigley, H. A., Park, C. K., Tracey, P. A., & Pollack, I. P. (2002). Community screening for eye disease by laypersons: the Hoffberger program. American journal of ophthalmology, 133(3), 386-392.

[41] Kohro, T., Furui, Y., Mitsutake, N., Fujii, R., Morita, H., Oku, S.& Nagai, R. (2008). The Japanese national health screening and intervention program aimed at preventing worsening of the metabolic syndrome. International heart journal, 49(2), 193-203.

[42] Artigao-Rodenas LM, Carbayo-Herencia JA, Divisón-Garrote JA, Gil-Guillén VF,

Massó-Orozco J. (2013) Framingham Risk Score for Prediction of Cardiovascular Diseases: A Population-Based Study from Southern Europe. PLoS ONE 8(9): e73529. doi:10.1371/journal.pone.0073529

[43] WHO.(2000). Obesity: Preventing and Managing the Global Epidemic: Report of a WHO Consultation on Obesity.

[44] Pereira, P. F., Serrano, H. M., Carvalho, G. Q., Ribeiro, S. M., Peluzio, M., Franceini, S., & Priore, S. E. (2015). Measurements of location of body fat distribution: an assessment of colinearity with body mass, adiposity and stature in female adolescents]. Revista paulista de pediatria : orgao oficial da Sociedade de Pediatria de Sao Paulo, 33(1), 63-71.

[45] Ververs M, Antierens A, Sackl A, Staderini N, Captier V.(2013). Which anthropometric indicators identify a pregnant woman as acutely malnourished and predict adverse birth outcomes in a humanitarian context? PLoS Curr .5. https://dx.doi.org/10.1371/currents.dis.54a8b618c1bc031ea140e3f2934599c8

[46] Seidell JC, Han TS, Feskens EJ, Lean ME. (1997). Narrow hips and broad waist circumferences independently contribute to increased risk of non-insulin-dependent diabetes mellitus. J Intern Med. 242: 401-406.

[47] Han, Thang S, and Mike Ej Lean. "A clinical perspective of obesity, metabolic syndrome and cardiovascular disease." JRSM cardiovascular disease vol. 5 2048004016633371. 25 Feb. 2016, doi:10.1177/2048004016633371

[48] Almeda-Valdes, P., Aguilar-Salinas, C. A., Uribe, M., Canizales-Quinteros, S., & Méndez-Sánchez, N. (2016). Impact of anthropometric cut-off values in determining the prevalence of metabolic alterations. European journal of clinical investigation, 46(11), 940-946.

[49] Leslie, W. D., Weiler, H. A., & Nyomba, B. G. (2007). Ethnic differences in adiposity and body composition: the First Nations bone health study. Applied Physiology, Nutrition, and Metabolism, 32(6), 1065-1072.

[50] Whincup, P. H., Nightingale, C. M., Owen, C. G., Rudnicka, A. R., Gibb, I., McKay, C. M., ... & Cook, D. G. (2010). Early emergence of ethnic differences in type 2 diabetes precursors in the UK: the Child Heart and Health Study in England (CHASE Study). PLoS medicine, 7(4), e1000263.

[51] Baloyi, S. M., & Mokwena, K. (2020). Metabolic syndrome among pregnant women attending an antenatal care clinic at a tertiary hospital in the Free State province, South Africa. In Obstetrics and Gynaecology Forum (Vol. 30, No. 1, pp. 14-18). In House Publications.

[52] Agirbasli M, Agaoglu NB, Orak N, et al. Sex hormones and metabolic syndrome in children and adolescents. Metabolism. 2009;58:1256-1262. DOI:10.1016/j. metabol.2009.03.024.

[53] Kim HA, Lee SY, Kwon HS, et al. Gender differences in the association of insulin resistance with metabolic risk factors among Korean adolescents: Korea National Health and Nutrition Examination Survey 2008-2010. Diabetes Res Clin Pract. 2013;99: 54-62. doi:10.1016/j.diabres.2012.10.011.

[54] Lee, S., Ko, Y., Kwak, C., & Yim, E. S. (2016). Gender differences in metabolic syndrome components among the Korean 66-year-old population with metabolic syndrome. BMC geriatrics, 16(1), 27.

[55] Beigh, S. H., & Jain, S. (2012). Prevalence of metabolic syndrome and

gender differences. Bioinformation, 8(13), 613-6.

[56] Micklesfield, L. K., Lambert, E. V., Hume, D. J., Chantler, S., Pienaar, P. R., Dickie, K., Puoane, T., Goedecke, J. H. (2013). Socio-cultural, environmental and behavioural determinants of obesity in black South African women. Cardiovascular journal of Africa, 24(9-10), 369-75.

[57] Case, A., & Menendez, A. (2009). Sex differences in obesity rates in poor countries: evidence from South Africa. Economics & Human Biology, 7(3), 271-282.

[58] Fezeu, L., Balkau, B., Kengne, A. P., Sobngwi, E., & Mbanya, J. C. (2006). Metabolic syndrome in a sub-Saharan African setting: central obesity may be the key determinant. Atherosclerosis, 193(1), 70-6.

[59] Regitz-Zagrosek, V., Lehmkuhl, E. & Weickert, M.O. (2006). Gender differences in the metabolic syndrome and their role for cardiovascular disease. Clinical Research in Cardiology 95: 136. https://doi.org/10.1007/s00392-006-0351-5

[60] Njelekela, M. A., Mpembeni, R., Muhihi, A., Mligiliche, N. L., Spiegelman, D., Hertzmark, E., Liu, E., Finkelstein, J. L., Fawzi, W. W., Willett, W. C., ... Mtabaji, J. (2009). Gender-related differences in the prevalence of cardiovascular disease risk factors and their correlates in urban Tanzania. BMC cardiovascular disorders, 9, 30. doi:10.1186/1471-2261-9-30

[61] Piccolo, R. S., Yang, M., Bliwise, D. L., Yaggi, H. K., & Araujo, A. B. (2013). Racial and socioeconomic disparities in sleep and chronic disease: results of a longitudinal investigation. Ethnicity & disease, 23(4), 499-507.

[62] Dinsa, G. D., Goryakin, Y., Fumagalli, E., & Suhrcke, M. (2012). Obesity and socioeconomic status in developing countries: a systematic review. Obesity reviews : an official journal of the International Association for the Study of Obesity, 13(11), 1067-79.

[63] Katulanda P, Ranasinghe P, Jayawardana R, Sheriff R, Matthews DR. (2012). Metabolic syndrome among Sri Lankan adults: prevalence patterns and correlates. Diabetol Metabolic Syndrome. 4(1):24.

[64] Monyeki, K. D., Siweya, H. J., Kemper, H., Kengne, A. P., Musinguzi, G., Nkwana, M. R., Mothiba, T., Malatji, T., Baloyi, S. M., Malema, R., Leach, L., Matshipi, M., Sebati, R. B., Seloka, M. A., Sibuyi, E., & Monyeki, S. M. (2020). The Relationship between Binge Drinking and Metabolic Syndrome Components amongst Young Adults Aged 21 to 31 Years: Ellisras Longitudinal Study. International journal of environmental research and public health, 17(20), 7484. https://doi.org/10.3390/ijerph17207484

[65] Barker, D. J. (1990). The fetal and infant origins of adult disease. BMJ: British Medical Journal, 301(6761), 1111.

[66] Nathan BM, Moran A. (2008). Metabolic complications of obesity in childhood and adolescence: more than just diabetes. Current opinion in endocrinology, diabetes, and obesity. 15(1):21-9.

[67] Cornier MA, Dabelea D, Hernandez TL, Lindstrom RC, Steig AJ, Stob NR.(2008). The metabolic syndrome. Endocrine reviews. 29(7):777-822.

[68] Grover A, Smith CE, Gregory M, et al. Effects of FSH receptor deletion on epididymal tubules and sperm morphology, numbers, and motility. Mol Reprod Dev. 2005 Oct. 72(2):135-44. [Medline]

[69] Frances J. Hayes, Janet E. Hall, Paul A. Boepple, William F. Crowley, Jr., Differential Control of Gonadotropin Secretion in the Human: Endocrine Role of Inhibin, The Journal of Clinical Endocrinology & Metabolism, Volume 83, Issue 6, 1 June 1998, Pages 1835-1841, https://doi.org/10.1210/jcem.83.6.4884

[70] Jungheim ES, Travieso JL, Carson KR, et al. Obesity and reproductive function. Obstet Gynecol Clin North Am 2012;39(4):

[71] Nguyen, R. H., Wilcox, A. J., Skjærven, R., & Baird, D. D. (2007). Men's body mass index and infertility. *Human Reproduction*, *22*(9), 2488-2493.

[72] Ramlau-hansen CH, Thulstrup AM, Nohr EA, et al. Subfecundity in overweight and obese couples. Hum Reprod 2007; 22(6):1634e7.

[73] Cardozo, E. R., Dune, T. J., Neff, L. M., Brocks, M. E., Ekpo, G. E., Barnes, R. B., & Marsh, E. E. (2013). Knowledge of obesity and its impact on reproductive health outcomes among urban women. Journal of community health, 38(2), 261-267.

[74] Hammoud AO, Gibson M, Peterson CM, Meikle AW, Carrell DT. Impact of male obesity on infertility: a critical review of the current literature. Fertil Steril. 2008;90(4):897-904.

[75] Ford ES.(2005). Risks for all-cause mortality, cardiovascular disease, and diabetes associated with the metabolic syndrome: a summary of the evidence. Diabetes care. 28(7):1769-78.

[76] Ford ES, Giles WH, Mokdad AH. (2004). Increasing prevalence of the metabolic syndrome among u.s. Adults. Diabetes care.:2444-9.

[77] Codner E, Eyzaguirre FC, Iñiguez G, et al. Chilean group for the study of ovarian function in type, D. Ovulation rate in adolescents with type 1 diabetes mellitus.Fertil Steril. 2011;95(1):197-202. doi:10.1016/j.fertnstert.2010.10.041.

[78] Roa J, Garcia-Galiano D, Varela L, Sanchez-Garrido MA, Pineda R, Castellano JM. The mammalian target of rapamycin as novel central regulator of puberty onset via modulation of hypothalamic Kiss1 system. Endocrinology. 2009;150:5016-5026.

[79] Iniguez G, Torrealba IM, Avila A, Cassorla F, Codner, E. Adiponectin serum levels and their relationships to androgen concentrations and ovarian volume during puberty in girls with type 1 diabetes mellitus. Hormone Res. 2008;70:112-117. 799.

[80] Codner E, Merino PM, Tena-Sempere M. Female reproduction and type 1 diabetes: from mechanisms to clinical findings. Hum Reprod. 2010;18(5):568-585.

[81] Saenger, P., DiMartino-Nardi, J. Premature adrenarche. J Endocrinol Invest 24, 724-733 (2001). https://doi.org/10.1007/BF03343917

[82] Fedorcsák, P., Dale, P. O., Storeng, R., Ertzeid, G., Bjercke, S., Oldereid, N., ... & Tanbo, T. (2004). Impact of overweight and underweight on assisted reproduction treatment. Human Reproduction, 19(11), 2523-2528.

[83] Bellver, J., Melo, M. A., Bosch, E., Serra, V., Remohí, J., & Pellicer, A. (2007). Obesity and poor reproductive outcome: the potential role of the endometrium. Fertility and sterility, 88(2), 446-451.

[84] Norman RJ, Dewailly D, Legro RS, Hickey TE. Polycystic ovary syndrome. Lancet 2007;370:685-97.

[85] Ehrmann DA. Polycystic ovary syndrome. N Engl J Med 2005;352:1223-36.

[86] Rojas, J., Chávez, M., Olivar, L., Rojas, M., Morillo, J., Mejías, J., ... & Bermúdez, V. (2014). Polycystic ovary syndrome, insulin resistance, and obesity: navigating the pathophysiologic labyrinth. International journal of reproductive medicine, 2014.

[87] Legro RS. Obesity and PCOS: implications for diagnosis and treatment. Semin Reprod Med. 2012;30:496-506.

[88] Pagán YL et al. Inverse relationship between luteinizing hormone and body mass index in polycystic ovarian syndrome: investigation of hypothalamic and pituitary contributions. J Clin Endocrinol Metab. 2006;91:1309-16.

[89] Kasturi SS, Tannir J, Brannigan R. The metabolic syndrome and male infertility. J Androl. 2008;29:251-259).

[90] Hammoud AO, Gibson M, Peterson CM, Hamilton BD, Carrell DT (2006) Obesity and male reproductive potential. J Androl 27: 619-626.

[91] MacDonald AA, Herbison GP, Showell M, Farquhar CM (2010) The impact of body mass index on semen parameters and reproductive hormones in human males: a systematic review with meta-analysis. Hum Reprod Update 16: 293-311.

[92] Stokes VJ, Anderson RA, George JT (2014) How does obesity affect fertility in men - and what are the treatment options? Clin Endocrinol (Oxf).

[93] Pasquali R, Casimirri F, De Iasio R, Mesini P, Boschi S, et al. (1995) Insulin regulates testosterone and sex hormone-binding globulin concentrations in adult normal weight and obese men. J Clin Endocrinol Metab 80: 654-658

[94] Pitteloud N, Hardin M, Dwyer A a, Valassi E, Yialamas M, Elahi D, et al. Increasing insulin resistance is associated with a decrease in Leydig cell testosterone secretion in men. J Clin Endocrinol Metab. 2005; 90(5):2636-41. https://doi.org/10.1210/jc.2004-2190 PMID: 15713702

[95] Leisegang K, Udodong A, Bouic PJD, Henkel RR. Effect of the metabolic syndrome on male reproductive function: A case-controlled pilot study. Andrologia. 2014; 46(2):167-76. https://doi.org/10.1111/ and.12060 PMID: 23278477

[96] Derby CA, Zilber S, Brambilla D, et al. Body mass index, waist circumference and waist to hip ratio and change in sex steroid hormones: the Massachusetts Male Ageing Study. Clin Endocrinol (Oxf) 2006;65(1):125e31.

[97] Eisenberg ML, Kim S, Chen Z, et al. The relationship between male BMI and waist circumference on semen quality: data from the LIFE study. Hum Reprod 2014;29(2):193e200.

[98] Kort HI, Massey JB, Elsner CW, et al. Impact of body mass index values on sperm quantity and quality. J Androl 2006; 27(3):450e2.

[99] Jensen TK, Andersson AM, Jørgensen N, et al. Body mass index in relation to semen quality and reproductive hormones among 1,558 Danish men. Fertil Steril 2004;82(4):863e70.

[100] Sermondade N, Faure C, Fezeu L, et al. BMI in relation to sperm count: an updated systematic review and collaborative meta-analysis. Hum Reprod Update 2013;19(3):221e31.

[101] Chavarro JE, Toth TL, Wright DL, et al. Body mass index in relation to semen quality, sperm DNA integrity, and serum reproductive hormone levels among men attending an infertility clinic. Fertil Steril 2010;93(7):2222e31.

[102] Tsatsanis C, Dermitzaki E, Avgoustinaki P, et al. The impact of

adipose tissue- & derived factors on the hypothalamic-pituitary-gonadal (HPG) axis. Hormones (Athens) 2015; 14:549-562.

[103] Bachir BG, Jarvi K. Infectious, inflammatory, and immunologic conditions resulting in male infertility. Urol Clin North Am 2014;41(1):67e81.

[104] Doshi SB, Khullar K, Sharma RK, etal. Role of reactive nitrogen species in male infertility. Reprod Biol Endocrinol 2012;10: 109.

[105] Kodama H, Yamaguchi R, Fukuda J, et al. Increased oxidative deoxyribonucleic acid damage in the spermatozoa of infertile male patients. Fertil Steril 1997;68(3):519e24.

[106] Aziz N, Saleh RA, Sharma RK, et al. Novel association between sperm reactive oxygen species production, sperm morphological defects, and the sperm deformity index. Fertil Steril 2004;81(2):349e54.

[107] Aitken RJ, Baker MA. Oxidative stress, sperm survival and fertility control. Mol Cell Endocrinol 2006;250(1e2):66e9.

[108] Tunc O, Bakos HW, Tremellen K. Impact of body mass index on seminal oxidative stress. Andrologia 2011;43(2):121e8.

[109] Shafik A, Olfat S. Lipectomy in the treatment of scrotal lipomatosis. Br J Urol 1981; 53:55-61.

[110] Hjollund NH, Storgaard L, Ernst E, et al. The relation between daily activities and scrotal temperature. Reprod Toxicol 2002; 16:209-214.

[111] World Health Organization. (1986). Ottawa charter for health promotion. Health promotion, 1, iii-v.

[112] Gunatilake, R. P. and Perlow J.H. (2011). Obesity and pregnancy: clinical management of the obese gravida. American Journal of Obstetrics & Gynecology ,.Volume 204 , Issue 2 , 106-119

[113] American College of Obstetricians and Gynaecologists (ACOG). (2005).ACOG committee opinion no. 319: the role of the obstetrician gynaecologist in the assessment and management of obesity. Obstetrics and Gynecology.106:895-9.

[114] Liu, J., Laditka, J.N., Mayer-Davis, E.J. and Pate, E.R. (2008) Does Physical Activity during Pregnancy Reduce the Risk Gestacional Diabetes among Previously Inactive Women? Birth, 35, 188-195. (17) (PDF) Metabolic Syndrome and Pregnancy, Its Prevalence, Obstetrical and Newborns Complications. Available from: https://www.researchgate.net/publication/283870248_Metabolic_Syndrome_and_Pregnancy_Its_Prevalence_Obstetrical_and_Newborns_Complications [accessed Dec 10 2018].

[115] Schenk S, Harber MP, Shrivastava CR, Burant CF, Horowitz JF. 2009. Improved insulin sensitivity after weight loss and exercise training is mediated by a reduction in plasma fatty acid mobilization, not enhanced oxidative capacity. Journal of Physiology, 587(20):4949-4961.

[116] Stinson, E. J., Piaggi, P., Ibrahim, M., Venti, C., Krakoff, J., & Votruba, S. B. (2018). High Fat and Sugar Consumption During Ad Libitum Intake Predicts Weight Gain. Obesity (Silver Spring, Md.), 26(4), 689-695.

[117] Kataria I, Chadha R, Pathak R. (2013). Dietary and lifestyle modification in metabolic syndrome: a review of randomized control trials in different population groups. Reviews in Health Care, [S.l.], v. 4, n. 4, p. 209-230. ISSN 2038-6702.

[118] Landaeta-Díaz, L., Fernández, J., Silva-Grigoletto, M. D., Rosado-Alvarez, D., Gómez-Garduño, A., Gómez-Delgado, F., ... Fuentes-Jiménez, F. (2013). Mediterranean diet, moderate-to-high intensity training, and health-related quality of life in adults with metabolic syndrome. European Journal of Preventive Cardiology, 20(4), 555-564. https://doi.org/10.1177/2047487312445000

[119] Serra-Majem LI, Ngo de la Cruz L, Ribas L, Tur JA.(2003). Olive oil and the Mediterranean diet: beyond the rhetoric. European Journal of Clinical Nutrition volume 57, pages S2–S7 (2003)

[120] American College of Obstetricians and Gynaecologists (ACOG). (2009). ACOG practice bulletin no. 105: bariatric surgery and pregnancy. Obstetrics and Gynaecology .113:1405-13.

[121] Chevallier JM, Paita M, Rodde-Dunet MH, et al. Predictive factors of outcome after gastric banding: a nationwide survey on the role of center activity and patients' behavior. Ann Surg 2007;246:1034-9.

[122] Maggard MA, Yermilov I, Li Z.(2008). Pregnancy and fertility following bariatric surgery: a systematic review. Journal for American Medical Academy .300:2286-96.

[123] Weintraub AY, Levy A, Levi I, Mazor M, Wiz- nitzer A, Sheiner E. (2008).Effect of bariatric surgery on pregnancy outcome. International Journal of Gynaecology and Obstetrics 103:246-51.

[124] Wax JR, Cartin A, Wolff R, Lepich S, Pinette MG, Blackstone J. (2008). Pregnancy following gastric bypass surgery for morbid obesity: maternal and neonatal outcomes. Obesity Surgery 2008; 18:540-4.

Section 5

Type 2 Diabetes

Chapter 14

Type 2 Diabetes and Dysautonomy

Ahmed Anas Guerboub and Ghizlaine Belmejdoub

Abstract

Responsibility for the dysfunction of the autonomic nervous system in the genesis or aggravation of cardiovascular and/or metabolic disorders is currently held. Indeed, a significant correlation between sympathetic overactivity and the pathophysiological mechanisms responsible for type 2 diabetes has been proven. Therefore, the treatment of this dysautonomia could improve the management of type 2 diabetes.

Keywords: the autonomic nervous system, dysautonomia, type 2 diabetes, insulino-resistance, insulino-secretion

1. Introduction

The autonomic nervous system (ANS), the dysregulation of which, called dysautonomia, is a frequent and often unrecognized condition which is accompanied by polymorphic functional manifestations [1]. The exploration of the ANS has gained renewed interest in recent years, due to the demonstration of the major role of its alterations in the genesis and aggravation of several diseases [2]. The importance of type 2 diabetes (T2DM) comes not only from its growing prevalence around the world leading the World Health Organization (WHO) to consider it a significantly expanding epidemic; but also given its human and economic consequences, making it a major public health problem.

2. The autonomic nervous system (ANS)

- ANS controls the body's unconscious, vegetative activities. It ensures the normal functioning of vegetative functions (breathing, heart rate, blood pressure, digestion, secretions, body temperature, water balance, etc.), and responds instantly to all physical and emotional demands. It is a system of adaptation of the body to its environment [2].

- The autonomic nervous system consists of two functionally and, in large part, morphologically distinct parts [3]:

  - The orthosympathetic (or sympathetic) system which intervenes in the involuntary activities of the stressful and arousal situations. It is preponderant in the conflicts of the organism with its external environment, when life is threatened. The sympathetic system stimulates all the organs that play a role in the defense response. The sympathetic nerve centers are essentially bulbospinal and their organization is segmental. The preganglionic fibers exit through the ventral root of the corresponding spinal nerve. They separate to form the white communicating branch which joins the corresponding para-vertebral ganglion. These paravertebral ganglia are united in a chain by inter-ganglionic fibers. The fibers which exit from the paravertebral ganglia join the corresponding spinal nerve by the gray communicating branch to go to the target organ.

- o The parasympathetic system which takes care of the involuntary activities of the situations of relaxation and rest. Its nerve centers are located in the brainstem and the sacral marrow. The preganglionic fibers follow the path of the corresponding nerves. They synapse into a pre-visceral or intra-visceral ganglion. The parasympathetic system therefore does not have a structure equivalent to the chain of sympathetic paravertebral ganglia.

- The autonomic or vegetative nervous system is made up of several levels:

  a. Nervous centers located within the central nervous system (medulla oblongata, thalamus and hypothalamus.) and in the spinal cord, constitute the "motor" of the autonomic nervous system.

  b. Peripheral ganglia located on three floors:

    - o The first ganglionic stage comprises the para- vertebral sympathetic chain. This chain is located laterally in the spine and extends from the end of the cervical segment to the coccygeal segment. It includes 3 cervical ganglia, superior, middle and inferior through which the sympathetic fibers of the cervical segment pass.

    - o A second ganglionic stage consists of the pre-visceral ganglia or plexus. They are less numerous than the paravertebral ganglia. They are more ganglion plexuses than ganglia. They are paired and lateral in the neck (carotid plexus, pharyngeal, ...) and pelvis but single and medial in the thorax (cardiac, pulmonary plexus) and abdomen (solar plexus, lumbo-aortic). At the cervical level, this second stage is associated with the 1st stage.

    - o A third lymph node stage includes the visceral or terminal lymph nodes located on the surface or in the thickness of the target organ.

  c. Fibers that connect these levels to each other and to the viscera:

  Between the nerve center and the target organ, the autonomic nervous path is always interrupted by at least one synapse located in a ganglion.

  An autonomous nerve pathway is therefore made up of at least two fibers: the pre-ganglionic fiber and the post-ganglionic fiber.

  The nerve fibers of the autonomic system travel either alongside the fibers of the somatic system (mixed nerves) or independently, along the blood vessels. Norepinephrine is the neurotransmitter at all levels of the sympathetic system, except the ganglionic (acetylcholine) level, while acetylcholine mediates the parasympathetic or vagal system.

- There is a strong interaction between the autonomic nervous system and the endocrine system, especially the hypothalamic–pituitary–adrenal axis. Also, sympathetic hyperactivity is implicated in various symptoms or pathologies such as essential hypertension [4], obesity [4, 5], permanent resting tachycardia, hyperlipidemia, type 2 diabetes [5], sleep apnea [5] or sedentary lifestyle.

3. The ANS measurement methods

- Considered difficult, the assessment of ANS activity has been greatly facilitated by the development of systems allowing non-invasive clinical exploration based mainly on the continuous recording of blood pressure and heart rate by a Holter ECG [6].

- Sympathetic activity can be measured directly by the technique of microneurography which measures muscle sympathetic nerve activity (ANSM) by inserting electrodes into a nerve (usually the peroneal nerve). This technique is very precise and minimally invasive.

- On the other hand, the measurement of the "spill over" of catecholamines is reliable but is not easily applicable due to its very invasive nature. We can also measure catecholamines and their metabolites (metanephrines) in peripheral blood or 24 hours urine, but studies show that plasma catecholamine levels are not sensitive markers of sympathetic activity. Also, they objectify that the urinary catecholamines are not sufficiently sensitive to estimate the sympathetic [6].

4. Epidemiological data

- The importance of the type 2 diabetes (T2DM) stems from:

    - Its increasing prevalence throughout the world, around 463 million diabetics in 2019 according to IDF, and to increase to 700 million in 2045.

    - Its association with a remarkable increase in cardiovascular morbidity and mortality.

- The 2000 World Diabetes Congress in Mexico City placed particular emphasis on the metabolic syndrome by sounding the alarm on the impact of such a prevalence on the population. This puts the metabolic syndrome and diabetes far ahead of HIV-AIDS in terms of morbidity and mortality.

5. Relationship between type 2 diabetes and ANS

A global approach of the responsibility of a dysfunction of the ANS in the genesis or the aggravation of the 3 main pathophysiological mechanisms of type 2 diabetes, which are insulin resistance, decrease in insulin secretion and hyperglucagonemia, has been attempted, by several studies all over the world especially during the last decades.

a. ANS and insulinoresistance

- Currently there is evidence that sympathetic hyperactivity is responsible for resistance to the action of insulin. Indeed, it can even precede the installation of this insulin resistance [7]. Activation of adrenergic receptors, in particular β-adrenergic receptors, has been shown to transform the phenotype of muscle cells into insulin-resistant cells [8].

- Variation of adrenaline and noradrenaline may also reduce insulin-induced glucose uptake. The aforementioned metabolic abnormalities are associated with a depletion of capillaries which reduces the supply of nutrients to the muscles which are therefore largely involved in insulin resistance [9, 10].

- In a recent longitudinal study, Flaa A. et al. studied the relationship between sympathetic activity and future insulin resistance in healthy Caucasian subjects with 18 years of follow-up [11]. They found that sympathetic activity was a predictor of insulin resistance as measured by HOMA-IR (Homeostasis model assessement- Insulin resistance: is a method for **assessing** β-cell function and **insulin resistance** (IR) from basal (fasting) glucose and **insulin** or C-peptide concentrations).

- In addition, there is a strong inflammatory activity in abdominal obesity with macrophage infiltration of visceral adipose tissue. These macrophages will be responsible for the secretion of pro-inflammatory factors such as interleukin 6 (IL6) or tumor necrosis factor alpha (TNF alpha) [12]. The secretion of these two cytokines by the visceral adipose tissue in obesity may play a specific role in the development of insulin resistance. Indeed, these factors can activate inhibitory pathways of the insulin cascade which will therefore have less effect on sensitive peripheral tissues (skeletal muscle and liver for example) and therefore induce insulin resistance [13].

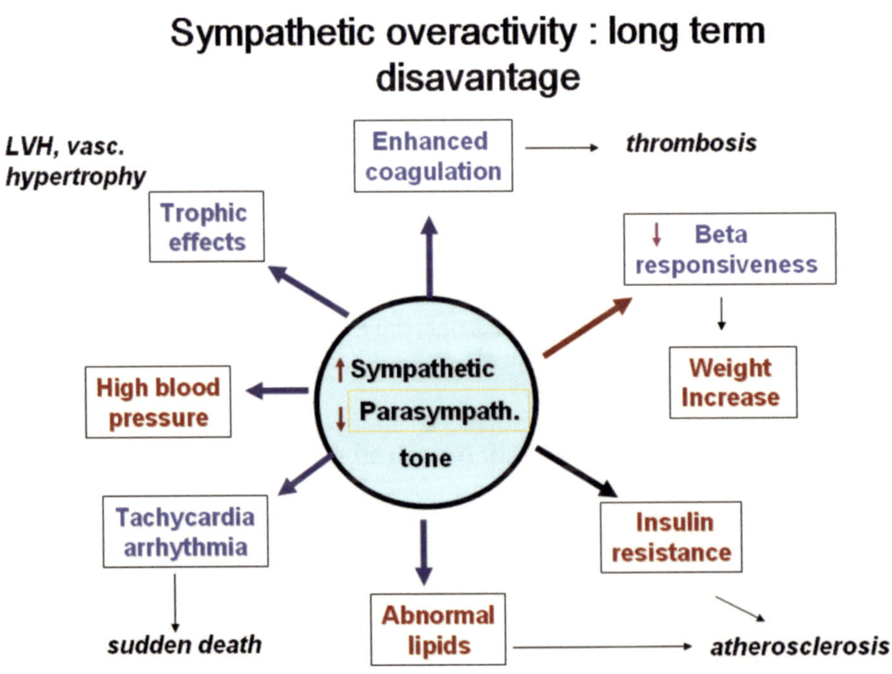

Figure 1.
Schematic representation of the association between sympathic hyperactivity and the different metabolic and cardiovascular pathologies [8]. Sympathetic overactivity is implicated in various symptoms or pathologies such as essential hypertension, obesity, permanent resting tachycardia, hyperlipidemia, type 2 diabetes, sleep apnea.

- These results provide new information on the pathophysiological mechanisms of insulin resistance, suggesting that sympathetic overactivity may be a predisposing factor for future insulin resistance (**Figure 1**).

b. ANS and insulinosecretion:

There are hormones that are part of the metabolic extension of the sympathetic while others are the metabolic extension of the parasympathetic. Insulin is part of the parasympathetic-vagal tendency.

The vagal deficiency secondary to T2DM is added to the depletion of the beta cells of the islets of Langerhans in the pancreas, thus exacerbating the insulin deficiency of type 2 diabetics [14].

c. ANS and hyperglucagonemia:

There is a microcirculation within the islets of Langerhans. Arterial blood first passes through "β" cells and "δ" cells (somatostatin) before reaching "α" cells which therefore do not respond directly to hyperglycemia. Hyperglucagonemia is secondary on the one hand to a direct stimulatory sympathetic action on "α" cells; and on the other hand, to a vagal deficiency responsible for the lifting of the inhibition on the "α" cells and a decrease in the stimulation of the "β" cells responsible for a decrease in GABA and molecules contained in the granules (Zinc) [15].

6. Outlook

To date, little therapeutic benefit has been gained from this information, since centrally acting sympatho-inhibitory drugs and alpha and beta blockers are used in the treatment of arterial hypertension.

Beta blockers are known to make diabetes worse. On the other hand, quite interestingly, drugs having a central sympatho-inhibitory action, such as clonidine and rilmenidine, are neutral or even slightly beneficial in diabetes and the metabolic syndrome.

Antidepressants, especially selective serotonin reuptake inhibitors (SSRIs) can be extremely effective in regulating the autonomic nervous system and blood pressure. At the same time, some studies indicate that serotonin-norepinephrine reuptake inhibitors (a SNRI) are even more effective.

These data may also lead to the proposal of sympathetically inhibiting drugs of central action in patients with metabolic syndrome in order to reduce the cardiovascular and metabolic consequences and perhaps even better in the unincorporated phases of the MS hoping to reduce the probability of evolution towards the constituted SM.

7. Conclusion

The responsibility of sympathetic dysfunction in the genesis or aggravation of cardiovascular and/or metabolic disorders is currently confirmed.

The consequences could vary depending on the genotypic and phenotypic characteristics of individuals and their environment, this encourages us to always explore the autonomic nervous system as part of the etiological assessment of the metabolic syndrome in general or of arterial hypertension and T2DM in particular.

The metabolic and functional consequences of ANS dysfunction could have a role not only in the genesis of T2DM but also in the development of complications and in its management.

A predominance of the sympathetic over the parasympathetic is responsible for insulin resistance, impaired insulin secretion and hyperglucagonemia, hence the importance of the exploration of the S.N.A both for screening and for management.

Author details

Ahmed Anas Guerboub* and Ghizlaine Belmejdoub
Endocrinology Diabetology Department of the Mohammed V Military Hospital, Rabat, Morocco

*Address all correspondence to: docteur.guerboub@gmail.com

References

[1] Low PA, Suarez GA, Benarroch EE. Clinical autonomic disorders: classification and clinical evaluation. In: Low PA, editor. Clinical autonomic disorders. 2nd ed. Philadelphia: Lippincott-Raven; 1997

[2] Low PA. Laboratory evaluation of autonomic function. In: Low PA, editor. Clinical Autonomic Disorders. 2nd Ed. Philadelphia. P: Lippincott-Raven; 1997. pp. 179-208

[3] Grubb BP, Karas B. Clinical disorders of the autonomic nervous system associated with orthostatic intolerance: An overview of classification, clinical evaluation, and management. Pacing and Clinical Electrophysiology. 1999;**22**(5):798-810

[4] Bannister R, Mathias CJ, editors. Autonomic Failure: A Textbook of Clinical Disorders of the Autonomic Nervous System. 3rd Edition. ISBN 0-19-2622196. Oxford: Oxford University Press; 1992

[5] Grassi.G. Differential sympathetic activation in muscle and skin neural districts in the metabolic syndrome. Metabolism. 2009 oct 58(10): 1446-51.

[6] Assessment: clinical autonomic testing report of the therapeutic and technology assessment subcommittee of the american academy of neurology. Neurology 1996; 46: 873-80.

[7] Masuo K. al. Sympathetic nerve hyperactivity precedes hyperinsulinemia and blood pressure elevation in a young, non-obese Japanese population. American Journal of Hypertension. 1997

[8] Palatini P, Julius S. The role of cardiac autonomic function in hypertension and cardiovascular disease. Curr Hypertens Rep. 2009;11:199-205.

[9] Grassi G. al. Differential sympathetic activation in muscle and skin neural districts in the metabolic syndrome. Metabolism. 2009

[10] Lee ZSK. al. Urinary epinephrine and norepinephrine interrelations with obesity, insulin, and the metabolic syndrome in Hong Kong Chinese. Metabolism. 2001

[11] Flaa A. al. Increased sympathetic reactivity may predict insulin resistance: An 18-year follow-up study. Metabolism. 2008

[12] Gutierrez and al. Impact of increased adipose tissue mass on inflammation, insulin resistance, and dyslipidemia. Current Diabetes Reports. 2009

[13] Luca C, Olefsky JM. Inflammation and insulin resistance. FEBS Letters. 2008

[14] Landsberg L. Insulin-mediated sympathetic stimulation: Role in the pathogenesis of obesity-related hypertension (or, how insulin affects blood pressure, and why). Journal of Hypertension. 2001

[15] Girard J, J-F Gautier. Rôle du glucagon dans la physiopathologie et le traitement du diabète. Médecine des maladies métaboliques. 2016.

Section 6

Care and Treatment of Cardiovascular Diseases and Diabetes

Chapter 15

Assessment of Follow-Up Care Received by Patients with Hypertension at Primary Health Care Facilities in Tshwane District of Gauteng Province, South Africa

Julia Manyelo and Debbie Habedi

Abstract

To extend the life expectancy of all South Africans to at least 70 years by 2030, hypertension follow-up care needs to be strengthened so that patients do not develop complications while in care. The aim of this study was to evaluate the follow-up care received by patients with hypertension at primary health care (PHC) facilities in Tshwane district. The study setting was ten PHC facilities in the aforesaid district. Quantitative, descriptive and retrospective methods were adopted, and simple random sampling was used to select ten PHC facilities from which ten files were conveniently sampled. Data were captured in Microsoft Excel 2010 and exported to IBM Statistical Package for the Social Sciences (SPSS) software version 21 in which data coding, outlier detection, missing value analysis and statistical data analysis were performed. In line with the study aim, frequency tables in SPSS were used to produce frequency statistics, and the chi-square test was used to test for the presence of association between compliance by nurses to clinical guidelines and categories of attributes, and further determine if there was a significant difference between adherence and non-adherence. The study found a significant proportion (93.4%) of non-adherence to hypertension guidelines among consulting nurses at selected PHC facilities.

Keywords: assessment, follow-up care, hypertension, primary health care

1. Introduction

Hypertension is a global health condition of developed and developing countries including South Africa. South Africa has the highest prevalence of people with hypertension (between 42% and 54%) compared with the eastern (15%) and western (25%) parts of Southern Africa. Sadly, the condition of these patients is still not controlled even while on treatment [1]. A recommendation of this study is that a regionally tailored intervention is implemented to prevent disastrous consequences relating to hypertension mortality and morbidity. While hypertension is a chronic, lifelong condition that needs regular and continued follow-up care, it also requires skilled health care providers who are supported by the treatment guidelines of the National Department of Health (NDoH), South Africa.

Approximately 17-million patients diagnosed with hypertension, a chronic, non-communicable and preventable disease, visit South PHC clinics for consultation. Hypertensive patients are initially encouraged to follow lifestyle modifications to promote control and management of the disease as part of its non-treatment management. Thereafter, if condition remains uncontrolled, hypertensive patients are informed to use daily treatment for the rest of their lives [2]. The NDoH of South Africa recommends that health professionals who are practicing in PHC clinics provide health education to enhance compliance with the management and control of hypertension [3].

Before 2006 parallel guidelines were developed by the Southern African Hypertension Society and the South African Department of Health, but the 2006 guideline is the combination task of the two bodies [4]. The guideline outlines dissimilar broad steps that health professionals should adhere on to achieve controlled blood pressure effectively, beginning from the patient risk screening/profiling, the measurements and investigations, the classification and complete treatment of hypertensive patients with or without co-morbidities, to their repeat and continuous plan [5]. A research conducted in Pretoria (Tshwane) on adherence to the hypertension guidelines among private practitioners and PHC physicians found that overall adherence to the hypertension practice guidelines used by generalists in private practice was 55%, while among PHC doctors in public-service, it was 56.4% [6].

Although two guidelines, Adult Primary Care (APC)/ Standard Treatment Guidelines (STG) and Essential Medicines List (EML), are available for use in PHC facilities when consulting patients with hypertension, the challenge is whether these guidelines are adhered to or not. To this end, the study sought to assess adherence or non-adherence to these guidelines and to describe the follow-up care received by patients in the Tshwane district of the Gauteng province, South Africa.

As far as the workshop on Diabetes Mellitus was concerned, the former Deputy Minister of Health in South Africa Dr. Joe Phaahla reported concerns about the quality of records in some clinics during auditing of patients' records. Hypertensive patients' medical history was recorded in two sentences, for example *"For follow up. Medication issued"*. The researchers noted this trend with seriousness since students following the R48 are taught comprehensive health assessment, which includes correct history taking and physical examination plus treatment of illnesses. Truly, if health assessment and treatment are done correctly, medical history could not be recorded in two sentences, which proves that if it is not recorded, it was undone. Adherence to the guidelines is stipulated throughout the R48 training programme to prove that there is standardisation regarding how hypertensive patients are treated at PHC level. During clinical practical of students, the researchers also realised that chronic services are regarded as fast track and sometimes, very incompetent nurses are assigned to that because they are considered mainly treatment collection. The South African' health care system is predominantly nurse-based and requires nurses to have the appropriate competence and expertise to manage the country's quadruple burden of diseases, of which hypertension forms a significant part [7]. To achieve this requirement, nursing education and training must produce safe and competent nursing professionals who are capable of making a meaningful contribution [8]. This prompted the researcher's interest in assessing the follow-up care received by the patients with hypertension at PHC facilities in the Tshwane district.

2. Research design and methods

2.1 Patient's history

Detailed history, physical examination and interpretation of investigations should form an integral part of the routine care of patients with hypertension. Regarding measurements, it is important to ensure that PHC nurses who take blood pressure measurements have adequate initial training and their performance periodically reviewed. Equipment for measuring blood pressure must be correctly checked, serviced and adequately recalibrated according to the companies' instructors' manuals. When checking blood pressure, PHC nurses in the clinics should calm the setting and provide a relaxed, temperate atmosphere, with the patients quiet and seated, and arms outstretched and supported. Use of a correct machine for the patient's arm is important [9]. A community-based study to estimate the prevalence of hypertension and its associated factors in municipalities of Kathmandu, Nepal [10], found that factors associated with hypertension were smoking, Body Mass Index (BMI), alcohol use, poor physical activity and diabetes.

The guidelines [9] emphasise the importance of the following lifestyle modifications:

- Administer continuous lifestyle advice to patients
- Promote a healthy diet and regular exercise
- Offer guidance and written or audiovisual materials to promote life-style changes
- Encourage reduced alcohol consumption
- Discourage excessive consumption of coffee and other caffeine-rich products
- Encourage patients to keep their dietary sodium intake low
- Offer advice and help smokers to stop smoking
- Inform patients about support groups such as local initiatives, health care teams or patient organisations that provide support and promote life-style change [9].

In South Africa, the following lifestyle modification is also recommended [11]:

- Educate patients about adequate dietary fibre intake (fruits, vegetables and unrefined carbohydrate).

2.2 Study design

The research is quantitative because it sought to measure the phenomenon by attaching numerical values to express quantity [12]. The observation was carried out in the PHC facilities whereby entries of patients' files were evaluated. Perusal of patients' files and documentation using checklist was also done. Furthermore, quantitative research is described as a formal, objective, systematic methodology to describe variables, to test relationships, and to examine cause and effect [13]. However, for this study, only the former is applicable. The patients whose files were perused had experienced an event that is a "follow-up consultation for hypertension". Moreover, the patients were mostly pensioners and depending on old age grant and even the unemployed ones without the medical aids. They resided around the townships and villages of Tshwane.

2.3 Setting

The study setting was guided by the research questions and the type of data that were required to answer the following questions [14].

- How is the follow-up care received by patients with hypertension at PHC facilities in the Tshwane district?
- What is the adherence or non-adherence to the National Guidelines by nurses about hypertension follow-up care?

A multi-site approach was used whereby ten different PHC facilities were selected. Using multiple sites offers a larger and more diverse sample [12], which improves external validity. Both provincial and municipal facilities were included. Data collection took place at two community health centres (CHCs) and eight clinics. The total number of PHC facilities was ten. The real-life settings were natural, and uncontrolled; the researcher did not attempt to manipulate them in any way.

2.4 Units of analysis

The units of analysis were the files of male and female patients above 30-years old, who were diagnosed with hypertension at PHC facilities in the Tshwane district of Gauteng Province. As recommended [12], this was the entire aggregation of cases in which the researcher was interested.

2.5 Sampling strategy

Ten of the 74 PHC facilities in the Tshwane district were randomly selected from the list on the National Health Research Database (NHRD). All clinics in the Tshwane district appear on the NHRD. The names of the facilities were written on pieces of paper that were placed in a bowl, and jumbled. From this, the first facility was chosen. The names were jumbled again, and the second facility was chosen. The process was repeated until all ten facilities had been chosen. According to the monthly statistics, at the time of the study, an average of 300 hypertensive patients were seen in each of the ten facilities per month. Hence, a proportional sample of ten files was conveniently chosen per facility.

2.6 Pilot study

The pilot study was done a month prior data collection when the research instrument was tested with ten files which were not utilised in the actual study. This was done to check if it could yield required information. The instrument was then revised and refined after the statistician checked it for validity and reliability.

Reliability of an instrument is a major criterion for assessing quality [12]. It is defined as the consistency and accuracy with which an instrument measures what is intended to measure. When used on repeated trials, an instrument with high reliability will produce the similar results [15]. To determine usefulness reliability of the instrument, the researchers utilised South African NDoH hypertension management guidelines. The guidelines support for a consistent standard of care across all PHC facilities in the country. Thus, the measuring instrument was considered reliable because it entailed attributes that are nationally recommended as the standard of care that hypertensive patients should receive during their follow-up visits.

Content validity was proofed by aligning concepts with the hypertension management guidelines of the country's NDoH. Prior the actual real research study was conducted, a clinic that was excluded in the final study sample was piloted to test the data collection process. Inputs from clinicians were used to amend the data collection tool where necessary. Piloting was conducted between the first two months of the year 2018.

The ethics approval certificate (HSHDC/839/2018) was granted by the University of South Africa (UNISA).

2.7 Data collection

Data were collected by auditing the files of patients who were consulted for hypertension follow-up using a checklist. A checklist itemises task descriptions in one column and provides a space besides each item to check off items that are done or not done [16]. The checklist contains activities that must be performed on a follow-up visit for hypertension according to the National Guidelines, the APC and the EML. The checklist was distributed by the researcher herself at the chosen PHC facilities. Some amendments and modifications were made to the checklist following the pilot study. Data were collected over a period of two months (June and July 2018), and all 100 checklists were completed.

The managers of the selected PHC clinics were contacted in advance to inform them of the data collection date. Ten files were chosen per PHC clinic, and from these, the data were gathered. Files were physically collected from the filing room with the help of the administrative staff of the PHC facility. The researchers examined each file to check that it belonged to hypertensive adult patient, who was non-diabetic and not pregnant in order to adhere with the inclusion criteria. Once ten files that adhered with the criteria were found, the data gathering started. All 54 questions on the checklist were ticked/not ticked in accordance with either attribute was recorded or not recorded.

2.8 Data analysis

Data were coded and checked for correctness before being entered into a Microsoft Excel codebook. The data were analysed according to the following steps:

- the last year in which patient was seen at the clinic;
- characteristics of the sample;
- patient's history
- physical examination;
- vital signs;
- side room investigations;
- routine blood tests;
- life style assessment;

- management of the patients; and
- knowledge and skills of health worker.

2.9 Results

Table 1 below indicates whether the attributes listed were assessed, as evidenced by records.

	Frequencies	Percentages (%)
Attributes of physical examination		
Dyspnoea		
Yes	1	1.0
No	0	0.0
Not recorded	98	98.0
Missing/Incomplete	1	1.0
Total	**100**	**100.0**
Jugular venous pressure		
Yes	1	1.0
No	0	0.0
Not recorded	99	99.0
Total	**100**	**100**
Apex beat recorded		
Yes	0	0.0
No	0	0.0
Not recorded	100	100.0
Total	**100**	**100.0**
Oedema		
Yes	64	64.0
No	0	0.0
Not recorded	36	36.0
Total	**100**	**100.0**
Crepitations		
Yes	17	17.0
No	0	0.0
Not recorded	83	83.0
Total	**100**	**100.0**
Heart sounds		
Yes	53	53.0
No	0	0.0
Not recorded	47	47.0

	Frequencies	Percentages (%)
Total	**100**	**100.0**
Cyanosis		
Yes	28	28.0
No	0	0.0
Not recorded	72	72.0
Total	**100**	**100.0**
Clubbing		
Yes	28	28.0
No	0	0.0
Not recorded	72	72.0
Total	**100**	**100**
Attributes of physical measurements		
Blood pressure		
Yes	100	100.0
No	0	0.0
Not recorded	0	0.0
Total	**100**	**100.0**
Pulse rate, rhythm and character		
Pulse rate		
Yes	96	96.0
No	0	0.0
Not recorded	4	4.0
Total	**100**	**100.0**
Pulse rhythm		
Yes	0	0.0
No	0	0.0
Not recorded	100	100
Total	**100**	**100**
Pulse volume		
Yes	0	0.0
No	0	0.0
Not recorded	100	100.
Total	**100**	**100.0**
Waist circumference recorded		
Yes	0	**0.0**
No	0	0.0
Not recorded	100	100.0
Total	**100**	**100.0**
Blood glucose measured		
Yes	23	23.0

	Frequencies	Percentages (%)
No	77	77.0
Total	**100**	**100.0**
Urine tests		
Yes	32	32.0
No	0	0.0
Not recorded	68	68.0
Total	**100**	**100.0**
Eye test done or recorded		
Yes	0	0.0
No	0	0.0
Not recorded	100	100.0
Total	**100**	**100.0**
Attributes of routine blood tests		
eGFR		
Yes	70	70.0
No	0	0.0
Not recorded	30	30.0
Total	**100**	**100.0**
Cholesterol		
Yes	66	66.0
No	0	0
Not recorded	34	34.0
Total	**100**	**100**
Attributes of life-style modification		
Smoking		
Yes	2	2.0
No	8	8.0
Not recorded	90	90.0
Total	**100**	**100.0**
Alcohol use		
Yes	1	1.0
No	8	8.0
Not recorded	91	91.0
Total	**100**	**100.0**
Exercise		
Yes	1	1.0
No	0	0.0
Not recorded	99	99.0
Total	**100**	**100.0**
Salt reduction		
Yes	0	0.0

	Frequencies	Percentages (%)
No	0	0.0
Not recorded	100	100.0
Total	**100**	**100.0**
Fat reduction		
Yes	0	0.0
No	0	0.0
Not recorded	100	100.0
Total	**100**	**100.0**
Non-adherent attributes		
Attributes	**No (%)**	**Yes (%)**
Dyspnoea	99.0	1.0
Jugular venous pressure	99.0	1.0
Apex beat recorded	100.0	0.0
Crepitations	83.0	17.0
No. of pillows used	100.0	0.0
Cyanosis	72.0	28.0
Clubbing	72.0	28.0
Chest pain recorded	100.0	0.0
Walk/climb	100.0	0.0
Pulse rhythm	100.0	0.0
Pulse volume	100.0	0.0
BMI	82.0	18.0
Waist circumference recorded	100.0	0.0
Blood glucose measured	77.0	23.0
Urine tests	68.0	32.0
Eye test done or recorded	100.0	0.0
Smoking	98.0	2.0
Alcohol Use	99.0	1.0
Exercise	99.0	1.0
Salt reduction	100.0	0.0
Fat reduction	100.0	0.0
Adherence to medication recorded	100.0	0.0
Side effects of treatment	100.0	0.0
Heart sounds recorded	47.0	53.0

Table 1.
Attributes of physical examination, measurements, routine blood tests and non-adherent attributes.

2.10 Antihypertensive medications

Antihypertensive drugs are mainly prescribed to reduce blood pressure and the complications associated with the disease. According to a study conducted among South African adult residents of Mkhondo Municipality, clinical guidelines recommend the use of multiple drugs to control blood pressure effectively and reduce the possibility of hypertension related complications [17]. The authors of this study determined that a high prevalence of uncontrolled hypertension was noted irrespective of the number of drugs and the combinations administered [17]. A plausible explanation could be non-adherence to treatment by patients. Hence, it is important for clinicians to follow evidence-based guidelines in prescribing antihypertensive drugs for patients. According to a registry-based observational study in two municipalities in Cuba on assessment of hypertension management and control [18], it found that almost half of the patients receiving treatment were taking two or more antihypertensive drugs. **Figure 1** below indicates the commonly used antihypertensive medications at PHC facilities in the Tshwane district of Gauteng Province, South Africa as hydrochlorothiazide, enalapril and amlodipine.

2.11 Adherent and non-adherent attributes

In this study, the determination of adherence and non-adherence was done by dichotomizing whether or not nurses complied with clinical guidelines in providing healthcare services regarding hypertension follow-up care. Binary counts showing whether or not nurses made records in compliance with clinical guidelines were done using frequency statistics tables in SPSS. Based on clinical guidelines, adherence was affirmed present if at least 60% of sample records showed that nurses made records in line with guidelines. Conversely, non-adherence was affirmed if less than 60% of sample records showed that nurses made records as per the guidelines. The at least 60% threshold affirming adherence was derived from clinical guidelines. This study's results on nurses' adherence and non-adherence to guidelines are as follows:

Adherence: Percentages showing adherence by nurses regarding making records are as follows: Blood pressure (100%), Pulse rate (96%), Estimated glomerular filtration rate (eGFR) (70%), Cholesterol (66%) and Evaluation of oedema (64%).

Non-adherence: Percentages showing non-adherence by nurses regarding making records are as follows: Dyspnea (99%), Raised Jugular venous pressure (99%), Apex beat (100%) and Crepitations (83%). Number of pillows used to sleep at night (100%), Cyanosis (72%), Clubbing (72%), Chest pains (100%), (BMI) (82%), Waist circumference (100%), Blood glucose (77%), and Urine and eye tests in the

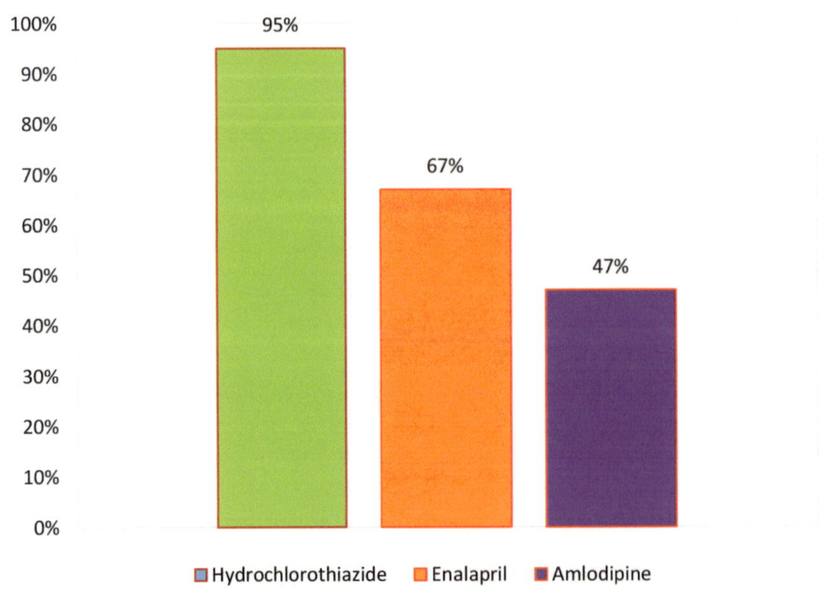

Figure 1.
Commonly used antihypertensive medications.

past 12 months (68% and 100% not recorded respectively). Adherence and side effects of prescribed medication were (100%) unrecorded. Smoking (90%), Alcohol use (91%), Exercise (99%), Salt and fat reduction (100%) were unrecorded.

Moving onwards, the test for presence of significant association between compliance by nurses to clinical guidelines (adherence and non-adherence) and categories of attributes (physical examination, physical measurements, life-style modification, routine blood tests, and history) was done using the chi-square test at 5 percent level of significance. The Pearson chi-square value = 11.654 (p-value = 0.020) and Cramer's V score = 0.634 (p-value = 0.020) indicate presence of statistically significant and strong association between compliance outcome (adherence and non-adherence) and category of attributes. The results confirm existence of significant difference between adherence and non-adherence proportions at 5 percent level.

The authors of the study conducted in Mkhondo Municipality [17] assert that the high prevalence of uncontrolled hypertension can possibly be attributed to obesity, lack of physical activity and dyslipidaemia. Moreover, the prevalence of uncontrolled hypertension and its association with low HDL-C, inadequate physical activity and obesity were reported [17].

Figure 2 below shows percentages of adherent and non-adherent attributes for this study.

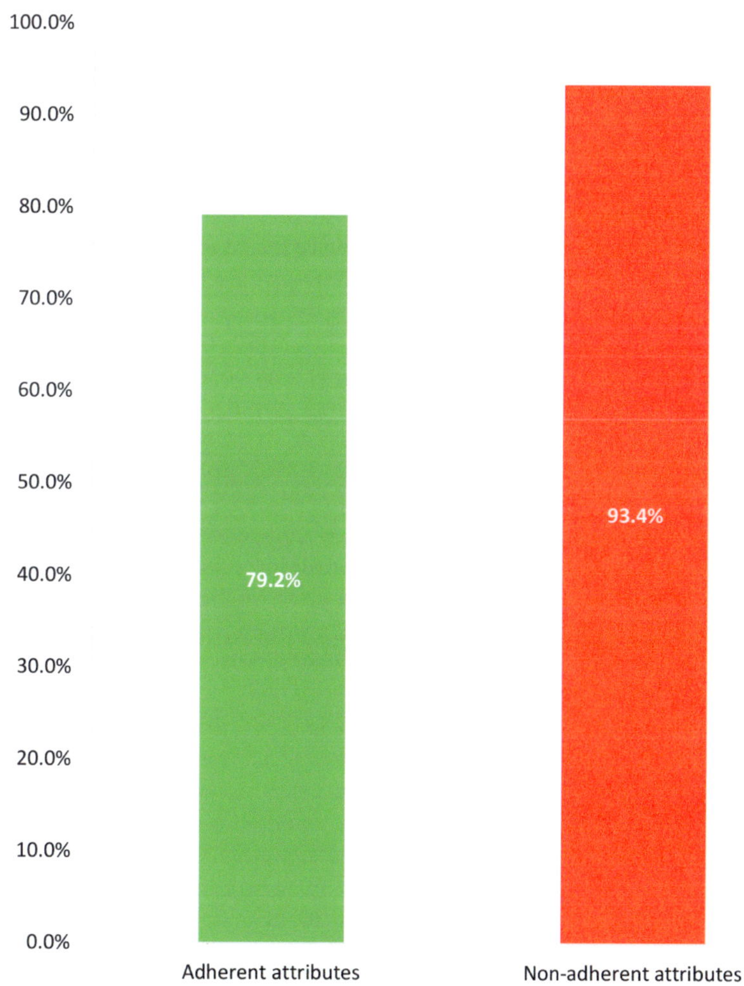

Figure 2.
Adherent and non-adherent attributes.

2.12 Discussion

The aim of the study was to evaluate the follow-up care received by patients with hypertension at PHC facilities in the Tshwane district. The study found a significant percentage (93.4%) of non-adherence to hypertension guidelines among consulting nurses at selected PHC facilities. Based on the results of this study, some professional nurses could not interpret the danger related to an elevated eGFR or cholesterol. Where the BMI was measured, it was not interpreted so that interventions could be implemented. In the follow-up visit, there was total misunderstanding of lifestyle modification and how it must be implemented in the management of hypertension. It was clear that PHC facilities require greater assistance and support from the employer, the NDoH of South Africa, to enable PHC nurses in the Tshwane district to adopt more follow-up care of hypertensive patients. Furthermore, in order to assist, guide and motivate the nurses to become active partners in their care, in-service trainings, resources and equipment are needed. There should be a remediation programme for professional nurses who have been trained but are found to be non-adherent to the guidelines. In a study conducted in Kinshasa, Congo, in which knowledge of consulting nurse's was assessed, 84% of the nurses reported to have received training [19]. The results suggest that training alone may not be enough, but continuous support and remedial actions may be necessary [19].

In addition, nurses of PHC facilities need to be supported by policy and organisational change. The results of the study [19] also supported the earlier observation made by the researcher in the research problem that chronic services are regarded as fast track and sometimes very incompetent nurses are allocated to these services since they are regarded as predominantly treatment collection with no specialised skills required. In accordance with other similar studies, most of the files of hypertensive patients that were audited for this study were found to be demonstrating positive and negative strengths regarding the follow-up care received by patients with hypertension.

A study conducted in Brazil by [16] on the association between follow-up care in health services and adherence to antihypertensive medication indicated that the level of therapeutic adherence in different populations of hypertensive patients is frequently investigated, given the severity of the problem. The adherence identified in the population was high (63%), possibly influenced by the characteristics of the participants, who had cardiovascular disease associated with arterial hypertension and, consequently, needed and sought health care more frequently. The findings indicate that higher consultation attendance has a statistically significant relationship with better medication adherence. This reinforces the notion that accessibility and frequent use of health services significantly affects the health conditions of hypertensive patients with associated cardiovascular disease [16].

Furthermore, the significance of follow-up care in clinics was analysed in relation to the level of therapeutic adherence and the prevalence of acute events [20, 21]. Patients who did not seek emergency services in the last two years had better adherence rates ($p = 0.04$). Since acute episodes usually lead to the introduction of new drugs in the treatment protocol of hypertensive patients, the lower adherence of the group that sought emergency services may be related to the problem in adapting to combination therapy, which demands post-discharge follow-up [20, 21].

In the study conducted in Brazil [16], the authors sought to advance knowledge concerning the correlation between health services and medication adherence when investigating attendance of hypertensive patients' at nursing consultations, since these are mainly focused on health education [16]. Regardless of the fact that the respondents had a greater number of medical appointments than nursing consultations, drug adherence was better among those who attended nursing consultations more frequently ($p = 0.022$). In addition, the study indicated the number of consultations necessary to improve the therapeutic adherence of hypertension patients [16].

Repeated nursing follow-up does not necessarily result in increased therapeutic adherence, and can increase health care costs [22]. The practice revealed by the present chapter of 4 to 6 nursing consultations per annum is the preferred level of nursing follow-ups, to attain better levels of antihypertensive treatment adherence. It was also observed that hypertensive patients who attended medical and nursing consultations or who had received health orientations in the last 6 months presented greater therapeutic adherence, with a statistically significant correlation ($p = 0.013$). PHC professionals have a high capability and meaningful opportunity to impact the improvement of patients' treatment adherence, through the support of guidelines and care during visits, home visits, health talk actions and tracking of non-adherent behaviours [23].

Regarding the view of impact of follow-ups in PHC services on therapeutic adherence of hypertensive patients, directed public policies are necessary to enhance this level of attention, and bring it closer to the population. Also meriting consideration is the social capital of the Brazilian population, which assists people overcome obstacles regarding the accessibility and utilisation of clinics by giving information and treatment support. For hypertensive patients, involvement into social health networks encourages them to look for specialised health care, although the decision to take part in treatment follow-up must be from the patients themselves [24]. However, treatment adherence will definitely be influenced by participation in social health networks and presence of follow-up visits in the clinics.

2.13 Limitations

The results of this chapter are valid in the specific context of the Tshwane district and cannot be generalised to the entire Gauteng province or to the whole country.

3. Conclusions

The objectives of the study were to describe the follow-up care received by patients with hypertension at PHC facilities in the Tshwane district and to determine nurses' adherence or non-adherence to the guidelines regarding hypertension follow-up care. The conclusion drawn is that follow-up care obtained by hypertensive patients in PHC facilities in the Tshwane district was found to be insufficient, and demonstrated by a trend of non-adherence to the guidelines. This showed a considerable lack of knowledge and practice in the treatment of hypertension in PHC clinics.

4. Recommendation

4.1 Nursing practice

- It is recommended that unskilled professional nurses should not be allocated to hypertension follow-up care or to a chronic section. Even if guidelines are available, they will yield better results if they are used by professional nurses who understand consultation skills such as history taking, physical examination and interpretation of investigations.

Acknowledgements

Thanks, are extended to the Tshwane district of Gauteng province, South Africa for granting permission to conducting the study and for providing support. The authors further thank the managers of the selected PHC facilities and their clerical staff for their support.

Authors' contribution

M.J.M., the author of the chapter, conducted the research.
D.S.K.H., the study supervisor, assisted in writing the chapter.

Funding information

The study was self-funded.

Conflict of interest

The authors declare that there are no competing interests regarding the writing of this chapter.

Disclaimer

The expressed ideas pertaining to the chapter are of authors and do not indicate the policy or position of any associations with them.

Data availability statement

Data sharing is inapplicable to this book chapter since no new data were formulated or interpreted.

Author details

Julia Manyelo and Debbie Habedi*
University of South Africa, Pretoria, South Africa

*Address all correspondence to: habeddsk@unisa.ac.za

References

[1] Ramsay, M, Sankoh, O. SA has the highest blood pressure in Southern Africa. Johannesburg: Wits University; 2017. Available https://www.wits.ac.zaresearch.news. [Accessed 28 June 2017].

[2] Nkosi-Mafutha NG, De Swart HC, Mogotlane S. Conveying hypertension message: an investigation into language and content used in primary health clinics in South Africa. African Journal of Primary Health Care and Family Medicine. 2020;12(1):1-7. https://doi.org/10.4102/phcfm.v12i1.2115.

[3] Nutbeam D. Health Literacy as a public health goal: a challenge for contemporary health education and communication strategies into the 21st century. Health Promotion International. 2000 Sep1;15(3):15(3):259-267. https://doi.org/10.1093/heapro/15.3.259.

[4] Seedat YK, Croasdale MA, Milne FJ. South African hypertension guidelines. South African Medical Journal. 2006 Apr;96 (4Pt2):337-62.

[5] Adedeji AR, Tumbo J, Govender I. Adherence of doctors to a clinical guideline for hypertension in Bojanala district, North-West province, South Africa. African Journal of Primary Health Care and Family Medicine. 2015. Apr 13; 7(1). http://dx.doi.org/10.4102/phcfm.v7i1.776

[6] Ernst S. Hypertension guideline adherence by private practitioners and primary health care physicians in Pretoria. SA Fam Pract. 2005 Apr 1; 47(3) :51-54. http://dx.doi.org/10.1080/20786204.2005.10873202-DOI.

[7] South Africa (Republic) Department of Health. Strategic plan 2014/15 to 2018/19. Pretoria: Government Printer; 2014.

[8] South Africa (Republic) Department of Health. 2018. Gauteng Health achieves highest percentage of ideal clinics across the country. Available: https://www.gov.za/speeches. [Accessed 28 May 2019].

[9] National Institute for Health and Care Excellence. NICE guideline. London: NICE; 2019.Available: www.nice.org.uk/guidance/ng/36.

[10] Dhungana, RR, Pandey, AR, Bista B, Joshi S, Devkota S. Prevalence and associated factors of hypertension : a community-based cross-sectional study in municipalities of Kathmandu, Nepal. Int J Hypertens, 2016. https://doi.org/10.1155/2016/1656938.

[11] South Africa (Republic) Department of Health. Primary health care standard treatment guidelines and essential medicines list. Department of Health, South Africa; 2008.

[12] Polit, DF, Beck, CT. Nursing Research. generating and assessing evidence for nursing practice. 10th ed. New York: Wolters Kluwer; 2017.

[13] Burns, N, Gray, JR, Grove, SK. The Practice of Nursing Research, Appraisal, Synthesis and Generation of Evidence. 7th ed. St Louis, Missouri: Elsevier; 2013.

[14] Brink, H, van der Walt, C, van Rensburg, G. Fundamentals of Research methodology for healthcare professionals. 4th ed. Cape Town: Juta; 2018.

[15] Bless C, Higson-Smith, C, Sithole SL. Fundamentals of Social Research Methods: An African Perspective. 5th ed. Cape Town: Juta Education (Pty) Ltd; 2016.

[16] Albuquerque NLS, Oliveira ASS, Silva JM, Araujo TL. Association between follow-up in health services and antihypertensive medication adherence. Rev Bras Enferm 2018; 71(6):3006-3012. http://dx.doi.org/10.1590/0034-7167-2018-0087.

[17] Masilela C, Pearce B, Ongole JJ, Adeniyi OV, Benjeddou M. Cross-sectional study prevalence and determinants of uncontrolled hypertension among South African adult residents of Mkhondo Municipality. BMC Public Health. 2020 Dcc; 20(1069):1. https://doi.org/10.1186/s12889-020-09174-7.

[18] Agudelo EL, Salva AR, Pinera AD, Roche RG, De Vos P, Battaglioli T, Van der Stuyft P. Assessment of hypertension management and control: a registry-based observational study in two municipalities in Cuba. BMC Cardiovasc Disord. 2019Dec; 19(1): 1-0. hptts://doi.org/10.1186/s12872-019-1006-6.

[19] Lulebo, AM, Mapatano, MA, Kayembe, PK, Mafuta, EM, Mutombo, PB Coppieters Y. Assessment of hypertension management in primary health care settings in Kinshasa, Democratic Republic of Congo. BMC Health Serv Res. 2015 June; 15(573):1-8.

[20] Kirchmayer U, Agabati N, Belleudi V. Socio-demographic differences in adherence to evidence-based drug therapy after hospital discharge from acute myocardial infarction: a population-based cohort study in Rome, Italy. J Clin Pharm Ther.2012Feb;37-44. https://doi.org/10.1111/j.1365-2710.2010.01242.x.

[21] Mathews R, Wang TY, Honeycutt E, Henry TD, Zettler M, Chang M et al. 2015. Persistence with secondary prevention medications after acute myocardial infarction: insights from the TRANSLATE-ACS study. Am Heart J. 2015 July; 170 (1): 62-69.doi: 10.1016/j.ahj.2015.03.019.

[22] Schroeder K, Fahey T, Hollinghurst S, Peters TJ. Nurse-led adherence support in hypertension: a randomized controlled trial. Fam Prac. 2005 Apr 1;22(2):144-51https://academic.oup.com/fampra/article/22/2/144/522313.

[23] Chang TE, Ritchey MD, Ayala C, Durthaler JM, Loustalot F. Use of strategies to improve antihypertensive medication adherence within United States outpatient health care practices. DocStyles 2015-2016. J Clin; Hypertens.2018Feb;20 (2):225-32. https:doi.org/10.1111/jch.13188.

[24] Palafox B, Goryakin Y, Stuckler D, Suhrcke M, Balabanova D, Alhabib KF et al. Does greater individual social capital improve the management of hyper-tension? Cross-national analysis of 61 229 individuals in 21 countries. BMJ Glob Health. 2017Dec1;2(4):e000443.

Chapter 16

The Use of the Conceptual Framework to Develop a Training Programme for Home-Based Carers Who Care for People with Cardiovascular Diseases

Mamare Adelaide Bopape

Abstract

Cardiovascular disease (CVD) is the complex disease associated with morbidity, mortality and loss of quality of life. Furthermore, it is the most significant cause of death in the diabetic population. South Africa is faced with an increasing number of people diagnosed with diabetes mellitus which intensify the burden on the health system. Home Based Carers (HBCs), also known as Community Health Workers need to undergo training before taking – up health-related jobs at the community level. HBCs who care for patients with cardiovascular diseases at the community level need to be trained on how to care for their patients at care and management. The systematic literature review method was used to review literature related to diabetes mellitus, type 2 diabetes mellitus, Community Health Workers, CHWs diabetic knowledge and diabetes mellitus, diabetic training of CHWs. The following themes and their subthemes have emerged: (1) The use of Practice orientated theory for training development which include the agent, the recipient, the context, the dynamics, procedure and terminus; (2) The use of the ADDIE model in the development of a training programme for HBCs which include Analysis, Design, Development, Implementation and Evaluation. Two conceptual frameworks to be used to guide the development of the training programme for HBCs for people with diabetes. The ideas of Dickoff and others can be used to formulate the conceptual framework that guides the development of training for HBCs for cardiovascular patients. The six concepts of the survey list include agent, recipient, context, dynamics, procedure and terminus. Instructional design system following the ADDIE model provided practical steps for organising training development project. According to Branch, ADDIE's model describes and prescribes what needs to happen during the process.

Keywords: cardiovascular disease, diabetes mellitus, type 2 diabetes mellitus, home based carers, conceptual framework, training programme

1. Introduction

Cardiovascular disease (CVD) is the complex disease associated with morbidity, mortality and loss of quality of life [1]. Furthermore, it is the most significant cause of death in the diabetic population. South Africa is faced with an increasing number of people diagnosed with diabetes mellitus which intensify the burden on the health system. The number of adults with diabetes in South Africa has increased to 4.5 million [2]. This caused the country to expand its healthcare focus to include Diabetes Mellitus. Home-Based Carers (HBCs), also known as Community Health Workers (CHWs) are involved in caring for diabetes mellitus patients in collaboration with the Primary Health Care. The previous study done in the Southern African context revealed that patients lack respect to HBCs and the HBCs lack training on chronic conditions including diabetes mellitus [3]. HBCs need to undergo training before taking – up health-related jobs at the community level. HBCs who care for patients with cardiovascular diseases including diabetes mellitus at the community level need to be trained on how to care for their patients.

In this chapter, we present conceptual frameworks that can be followed to develop training programmes for HBCs systemically. A conceptual framework is a network of interlinked concepts that can provide a comprehensive understanding of a phenomenon [4]. Furthermore, it provides an interpretative approach to reality, to express and explain ideas and also to make inferences or draw conclusions [4, 5]. A framework is a layered structure indicating the kind of programs which should be built and how they would interrelate. The conceptual framework aims to guide the development of the training programme for HBCs necessary for empowering them with knowledge and skills useful during care of People with Cardiovascular diseases including Diabetes Mellitus.

2. Systematic literature review method

The systematic literature review method was used to review literature related to diabetes mellitus, type 2 diabetes mellitus, Community Health Workers, CHWs diabetic knowledge and diabetes mellitus, diabetic training of CHWs. The theories where two themes with their subthemes that has emerged. Other related sources were used to support the themes that has emerged from the theories. The following themes and their subthemes have emerged: (1) The use of Practice orientated theory for training development which include the agent, the recipient, the context, the dynamics, procedure and terminus; (2) The use of the ADDIE model in the development of a training programme for HBCs which include Analysis, Design, Development, Implementation and Evaluation.

3. The use of practice orientated theory for training development

The issues that need to be addressed in the development of the conceptual framework are goal content, the prescriptions of the activity to attain the desired outcome, and the survey list to identify the gap between the intended activity and the prescriptions of the activity [5]. The main aim of the framework is to identify concepts that could be reflected in the training program. The concepts identified are utilised to describe the conceptual framework that guided the development of the training program for HBCs.

The ideas of Dickoff and others can be used to formulate the conceptual framework that guides the development of training for HBCs for cardiovascular patients. The six concepts of the survey list include agent, recipient, context, dynamics, procedure and terminus. The following questions are used as the basis for the formulation of the conceptual framework that informed the development training programme in this study were:

- Who is the agent? -The agent refers to the person who performs the activity which is the development of the training programme to improve knowledge, skills and attitude of the HBCs who cares for diabetes people.
- Who is the recipient? - The recipients of the activity who will benefit from the training program in this study are the HBCs who care for diabetes people.
- What is the context? - The context of the training programme is where the HBCs provide care for PWD.
- What are the dynamics? - Dynamics in this study, are the challenges and the training needs that motivated the development of the training programme.
- What is the procedure? -The procedure included the processes followed during the development of the training programme.
- What is the terminus? - Terminus refers to the end product of the activity which in this study are competent HBCs, autonomy to provide care to diabetic people and controlled blood glucose in diabetes people.

3.1 The agent

The agent is the first aspect of the survey list and refers to a person who performs the activity with the aim of Dickoff and others, which is the development and implementation of the training programme for HBCs who care for diabetes mellitus people. The agent should be the researcher who conducts needs analysis and facilitate the development of the training program for empowering HBCs who care for PWD. The agent as the facilitator in this study should possess certain characteristics. The agent is expected to develop a training programme and empower HBCs with knowledge and skills necessary for the provision of care to PWD. Therefore, the agent is expected to be competent and also required to possess personal qualities and abilities necessary to perform these activities [6]. Furthermore, the agent needs to possess the following characteristics knowledge, skills and attitude to be able to capacitate HBCs with the necessary information to be able to execute their expected tasks with ease. The following characteristics of the agent are described below: knowledge, skills and attitude.

3.1.1 Knowledge

Knowledge" refers to a body of facts or ideas acquired through study, investigation, observation or experience [7]. The role of the agent as a facilitator was to develop the training programme for the HBCs who care for PWD. The agent was required to be aware of the training needs of the HBCs to develop an effective training programme, therefore training needs analysis was necessary for the development of the training programme. The agent should possess scientific knowledge and research skills that will make it possible to explore and describe the knowledge and learning needs of the HBCs for people with diabetes. The agent should detect the challenges that inhibit quality care and management of PWD. The recipients will contribute towards the development of the training programme by pointing out their challenges and learning needs during the care of diabetes mellitus people.

3.1.2 Skills

The agent should be able to build good interpersonal relationships with the recipients and other stakeholders (dietician and the pharmacist) to relate and create an environment conducive for implementation of the training programme. An agent should be able to motivate and empower the participants to bring out the best in them through management skills. An agent listens actively to hear the participants' thoughts and messages and respond appropriately through listening skills. Good communication skills enable the agent to create a healthy interaction among the participants, communicate effectively so that he/she can understand problems, elaborates the points of the team and his own, and effectively conveys ideas and messages, clarity and confidence to the participants.

3.1.3 Attitude

The agent treats the participants equally during training and know-how to consider the differences in each one's personalities. The agent is friendly and honest to the participants to create an admirable and pleasant environment good for interaction. People love to be with a person who has a desirable attitude and a pleasant manner of dealing with other people. The agent should be patient and persevering to be able to appreciate and understand the difficulties of the participants and determined to see objectives achieved. The agent also has a sense of empathy for the participants who need to be understood. The agent should competent and demonstrate a professional attitude in carrying out their function. The agent should be respectable, reliable and committed to helping the participants learn for themselves and also confident to project a positive and purposeful atmosphere in the workshop.

3.2 Recipient

The recipients refer to a person who receives the activity [5]. The recipients were all the HBCs who care for the diabetes mellitus people and benefited from the training programme design. The HBCs have the responsibility to provide effective and efficient quality health care to people with diabetes. The agent should be informed by the recipients' experiences in the context they are providing service that the training programme is needed to address the training needs identified during situational analysis. The recipients interact with the agent by reacting during the implementation of the training programme to achieve their desired goals.

3.2.1 Characteristics of recipients

The recipients are expected to have certain characteristics that enable them to benefit from the programme and to participate fruitfully during the training. They are expected to be caring for people with diabetes to be able to participate in the training programme to achieve the desired outcomes of providing quality care. The HBCs as the recipients of the training programme in this context should be emotionally intelligent to be able to change and cope during training [8]. Attending the training programme would enhance knowledge, skills and attitudes to enable the recipients to perform their expected activities.

The HBCs as the recipients are expected to have the following characteristics of adult learners by Malcolm Knowles as outlined in Klopper (2009): self-concept, adult learner experience, readiness to learn, orientation to learning and motivation to learn. These characteristics offer HBCs a wide range of benefits, including improved comprehension of key concepts and a boost in knowledge retention.

3.2.1.1 Self-concept

HBCs as the recipients in this study and as adult learners are entitled to make their own decisions and take control of their own lives. The HBCs as adults identify the value of attending training because they want to learn what will be useful to them. The researcher role as a facilitator during the implementation of the training programme is to guide and direct them.

3.2.1.2 Adult learner experience

HBCs gain a lot of experience when working with diabetes mellitus patients on treatment at, therefore the training programme should focus on their unique training needs. HBCs as adult learners employed their learned experiences during care of diabetic people before they participated in the study to direct their learning because and to be actively involved in their learning.

3.2.1.3 Readiness to learn

HBCs as the recipients of the training were ready to challenge themselves with new learning experiences that offer some sort of social development benefit. They are ready to challenge themselves with new learning opportunities that will help them to fine-tune skills that pertain to their working environment.

3.2.1.4 Orientation to learning

As the recipients of the training, HBCs as adult learners are expected to change their perspective from one of postponed application of knowledge to immediacy of application. Their orientation towards learning was expected to shift from one of subject-centeredness to one of problem centeredness so that they will be able to solve problems related to their work problems.

3.2.1.5 Motivation to learn

HBCs need learning activities that will demonstrate how learning is going to benefit their work area.

3.2.2 Roles of the recipients in programme development

The roles of the recipients during programme development included participation during needs analysis to assess their knowledge and point out their practices, sources of information, challenges and training needs. The HBCs knowledge gaps and learning needs lead to the plan used to develop a collective training programme including the nurse, dietician and a pharmacist.

3.2.2.1 Skills of the recipients

HBCs as recipients possess different skillsets which assist in the execution of their daily tasks and to relate well with others to achieve the desired programme development goals as planned including communication skills, interpersonal skills, listening skills and patience.

3.3 Context

Context according to Dickoff and others refers to the setting in which activity took take place [5]. The context is also described as an environment where data were collected about knowledge, experiences and the learning needs of HBCs who care for PWD and also where the training programme was implemented. The functions of the HBCs in this context are mandated by the Department of Health (DoH) which operates under the legal framework of the South African government. For the development of an effective training programme, the researcher needs to take into consideration the Guidelines on the Implementation of the Three Streams of Primary Healthcare Re-engineering [9], in line with the Policy Framework and Strategy Ward Based Primary Healthcare Outreach Teams [9] which regulate the functioning of the HBCs in this context.

The agent and the recipient need to understand the context concerning legal and policy frameworks that govern the activities of the HBCs. It was necessary for the agent and the recipient to understand the policies that regulate the day-to-day activities of HBCs in this context. To support the HBCs to improve quality health care provision, it is important to establish the relationship between legal frameworks, health context policies/guidelines and procedures [10]. Context of the training programme provides learning opportunities for recipients who are the HBCs. The context of the training can be influenced by the internal sources of the agent that guides her activities including competence and communication competence and the external resources available for maintaining and supporting the agent's capacities and power.

3.4 Dynamics

Dynamics refers to the energy source or motivation for the activity inside an individual or the internal motivating factors for success [5]. Dickoff and others further explain that dynamics explore the physical, biological, psychological and chemical power sources of recipients and agents [5]. The training programme needs the dynamics that serve as the motivating factors that can be utilised to accomplish the activities of training programme development. The training programme needs to address the motivating factors as outlined by the HBCs during needs analysis to improve their knowledge, skills and attitude:

3.5 Procedure

This aspect of the survey list is the guiding procedure, technique or the protocol of the activity [5]. This refers to the general rule that guides the activity and provides steps to be followed to achieve the set goals of the programme. Dickoff and others indicate that the procedure highlights the path, steps or pattern followed when performing an activity [5]. Furthermore, Dickoff and others indicate that procedures are the guiding rules, protocols or techniques while an activity takes place and do not prescribe particular features [5]. The procedure that provided steps followed during the development of the training programme to achieve the training goals was described. The procedure that can be followed for the development of a comprehensive training programme is the ADDIE Model of instruction [11]. The procedure for the development of the training programme described steps for creation of the following: learning outcomes, subject content, assessment strategies, instructional strategies, resources and trainers. Problem-based learning encourages the recipients of the programme to solve work-related problems by completing the given activities.

DOI: http://dx.doi.org/10.5772/intechopen.95939

3.6 Terminus

Terminus refers to the last stop, end-point of the activity [5]. Terminus is the desired outcome an agent wishes to attain by implementing a particular procedure. The terminus confirms whether the desired goals have been attained or not. The participants have to express the need for diabetes mellitus training to enhance their knowledge and skills relevant to the provision of quality care to diabetes people. The training programme aims to empower HBCs with knowledge related to the management of people with diabetes mellitus. The training-related needs of the recipients should be accommodated in the training programme with the result of having competent HBCs. The HBCs are expected to be competent when providing care to diabetes people which can be achieved by attending diabetes mellitus training before commencing their duties.

Empowering HBCs may introduce the following benefits: enhancing the development of HBCs knowledge and skills, ensuring the provision of quality care to diabetes mellitus people, increase self-confidence in HBCs during provision of care, prevent diabetes mellitus complication and control of blood glucose in PWD. Training assists HBCs with relevant knowledge and proper information that will assist in coping during the provision of service to PWD and the community may develop trust in the services provided by HBCs.

4. The use of the ADDIE model in the development of a training programme for HBCs

4.1 Definition of the ADDIE model

ADDIE model is a systematic instructional design and abbreviation of the following logical steps: Analysis, Design, Development, Implementation and Evaluation [11]. These steps are sequential meaning the output of one step becomes the input for the next step [12]. It is also called an iterative feedback model because the results of the last stage are returned to the point of origin for feedback, to close the loopholes and or to refine the learning product [12]. ADDIE model is pursued to ensure that correct steps are followed to develop appropriate learning material optimally, to meet the needs of the HBCs [13]. The model was helpful because it is process-based and follows a systemic problem-solving approach that provides well defined basic and easy to follow steps [14–17]. The benefit of using this model is that it permits to refer and revisit previous steps during the process.

4.2 ADDIE steps

Instructional design system following the ADDIE model provided practical steps for organising training development project. According to Branch, ADDIE's model describes and prescribes what needs to happen during the process [11].

4.2.1 Analysis

The analysis is the first step of ADDIE's model which is used to identify training needs to develop the training programme for the HBCs and formed the basis of all other steps [18]. On this step, needs analysis should be conducted to identify gaps in diabetes knowledge and practices of HBCs. Major knowledge gaps and training topics suggested serve as the foundation for specifying the learning outcomes, content and activities, instructional strategies and assessment strategies. Knowledge gaps are identified through the needs analysis to develop training [17, 19]. The analysis provides an opportunity to complete a thorough analysis of HBCs' training needs that will guide the designing and the development of the training programme.

4.2.2 Design

The design step is the blueprint of how the training programme is created [20]. The purpose of the designing step is to define the anticipated performance and suitable evaluation methods [11]. In the design step, learning outcomes are identified and formulated because the success of the training implementation depends on clearly formulated learning outcomes, to meet the needs of HBCs. There are two types of the learning outcomes namely; critical cross-field outcomes and specific learning outcomes which should be formulated. The information gathered during the analysis step (situational analysis) should be used to create a plan to bridge the learning gaps (training needs) identified and developed the specific learning outcomes. Based on the learning outcomes, the training content, teaching/learning methods, instructional strategies and assessment criteria should be designed.

The format of the design should encompass the following elements: the name of the training programme, NQF level, Credits, Purpose of the training programme, duration of the programme, learning assumed to be in place, critical cross-field outcomes, specific outcomes and assessment criteria, Unit standard and programme assessment [21]. The HBCs have a job description that describes their activities for caring for people with chronic conditions that are context-specific and is developed by NGOs managers. The designing of the training is based on SAQA because it was established to create a single, integrated, national education and training framework for the whole nation, and to improve the quality of education and training in South Africa. The adaptation of the SAQA standards format for guiding the design of the training programme should be helpful in the planning.

The clear and precise learning outcomes are formulated using Bloom's Taxonomy to classify the following levels of learning: remember, understand, apply, analyse, evaluate and create [22]. Critical cross-field outcomes to address the participants' needs and requirements and Specific Learning Outcomes for HBCs to achieve should be included.

Content is the focal point for engaging the HBCs during the process of knowledge construction. The content which is consistent with the learning outcomes should also be established and designed at this step.

4.2.3 Development

The development step is where the researcher create and assemble the content of the programme assets created in the design phase [23]. This step is aimed to create the learning content that incorporates all the learning needs of the HBCs, and also to develop learning materials with learning outcomes that are relevant, legible and reader-friendly for the level of the HBCs. The structure and content of the training programme including learning activities, instructional and assessment strategies are aligned with developed learning outcomes.

Learning materials that covered all the SLO should be developed at this stage. During the development of the learning materials, the researcher should consider the competency level of the HBCs. The training materials should be drafted first and then submitted for evaluation for representativeness, appropriateness, completeness and importance to the research supervisors, psychologist, dietician and pharmacist before a final version can be concluded. The professional nurse, psychologist, dietician and Pharmacist should be included because they formed part of the implementation of this training programme.

4.2.3.1 Content development

The researcher should consider the following aspects during content development: the relevancy of the content included in the specific learning outcomes and objectives to achieve the SLO. The process of preparing the content should be based on the gaps identified during needs analysis and it matches the learning outcomes identified in the design step [24]. The content is divided in line with the SLO.

4.2.3.2 Instructional strategies

Learner-centred and problem-orientated strategies guide frameworks for accomplishing the learning outcomes. The instructional strategies should accommodate individual learner's rates of learning and learning style based on reviewed literature. The following instructional strategies lecturer method, discussion, active learning, and cooperative learning/group discussions, role-plays and case-based exercises can be used [25].

4.2.3.3 Assessment criteria

The strategies for assessment should be developed at this stage to measure success gained from the developed programme Assessment should be undertaken regularly throughout the implementation of the training and there is an activity interlinked with all activities. The formative assessment strategies such as open-ended questions, group discussions, and peer assessment to assess the understanding and achievement of the learning outcomes during the workshop should be used. The assessment questions should be formulated at the end of every activity to assess comprehension of the content done concerning the learning outcomes of the specific unit.

4.2.3.4 Training materials

The training materials including hard copies of training manuals should be printed for all the trainees and also the PowerPoint slides which covered all the SLO should be created.

4.2.4 Implementation

A training program for HBCs who care for people with cardiovascular diseases including diabetes mellitus is delivered at this step. The subject matter included should be based on the previously developed material and the research articles. Efforts should be made to use the most recent information about DM. All the trainees should be provided with a hard copy of the training material to use before the training commences.

4.2.4.1 Training delivery

Dates for training should be identified and arrangements made with the managers of the HBC centres to release the HBCs for teaching. The training programme is at Level 4 of the National Qualification Framework (NQF) with 11/2 credits. The contact sessions for interactive facilitation with HBCs and different facilitators should be scheduled. Training should take place at a central venue away from the HBCs workplace to avoid disturbances during training and to enhance learning.

4.2.5 Evaluation

The evaluation of the training programme was guided by Kirkpatrick four-level evaluation model [26].

4.2.5.1 Reaction (level I)

Reaction refers to the way in HBCs measure their satisfaction with the training [27]. Evaluation indicators should include training objectives, topic, content, venue, time, environment, facilitator's knowledge and preparedness, training manuals, the benefits of training on the job and what HBCs think should have been included in the training. HBCs have to be asked to rate these indicators on a 3-point Likert scale. Additionally, HBCs should also be asked to write suggestions on the training in the comment box. HBCs can be given 45 minutes to complete the evaluation tools at the end of the session.

4.2.5.2 Learning (level II)

Learning in this study refers to the extent to which the attitudes of the HBCs change, their knowledge increases and their skills broadened post-implementation of training [27, 28]. The evaluation of learning measures what the participants have learned and gained from the training programme [29]. The questionnaire can be used to evaluate learning and it can be the major focus to evaluate knowledge of HBCs post-training compared with pre-training analysis.

4.2.5.3 Behaviour (level III)

The focus of the behaviour level was on the exploration of the extent to which the knowledge and skills acquired in the training were applied back at work [29]. The trainees should report on their changes in behaviour when they returned to work after attending the training.

4.2.5.4 Results (level IV)

Results level focused on the realisation of aimed objectives and change in productivity after training [29]. HBCs should be encouraged to report on the challenges they experienced in the application of knowledge and skills learned during training.

5. Conclusion

The conceptual framework has a vital purpose in creating situations to achieve the desired goals or outcomes [5]. Development of the training programme was necessary because its availability and training of HBCs will increase disease-specific knowledge. The suggested ideas of the survey list of Dickoff and others used successfully as a reasoning map to describe the conceptual framework for the development of the training programme for HBCs. The utilisation of ADDIE's model of instructional design in the development of the training programme will benefit both the quality of the training content, teaching strategies, and assessments methods. The utilisation of ADDIE's model of instructional design in the development of the training programme can benefit both the quality of the training content, teaching strategies, and assessments methods. The six elements of the survey list of Practice orientated theory form the base of the training programme development. The training programme that would be developed based on the elements of Practice Orientated Theory to provide benefits for both the HBCs and the people with cardiovascular diseases.

Author details

Mamare Adelaide Bopape
University of Limpopo, South Africa

*Address all correspondence to: mamare.bopape@ul.ac.za

References

[1] Trikkalinou, A., Papazafiropoulou, A. K., & Melidonis, A. (2017). Type 2 diabetes and quality of life. *World journal of diabetes*, *8*(4), 120-129. https://doi.org/10.4239/wjd.v8.i4.120

[2] International Diabetes Federation. (20159. IDF Diabetes Atlas.7th ed. Brussels, IDF. 2019.

[3] Maimela, E, Van Geertruyden, J, Alberts, M, Madjadji, SEP, Meulemans, H, Fraeyman, J & Bastiaens, H. (2015). The perceptions and perspectives of patients and health care providers on chronic diseases management in rural South Africa: a qualitative study. *Biomed Central Health Services Research* Volume15:143

[4] Jobaraan, Y. (2009). Building a Conceptual Framework: Philosophy, Definitions, and Procedure. *International Journal of Qualitative Methods 2009, 8(4)*

[5] Dickoff, J., James, P. & Wiedenbach, E. (1968). Theory in a practice discipline. American Journal of Nursing Company, 17(5): 415-444.

[6] Anema, M.G. & McCoy, J. 2010. Competency-Based Nursing Education. *Guide to Achieving Outstanding Learner Outcomes:* Springer Publishing Company. New York.

[7] Ahenkorah-Marfo, M. (2012). Clarifying Concepts of Knowledge and Information - Literature Review Journal of Knowledge Management Practice, 3(2)

[8] Jooste, K. & Mothiba, T.M. (2013). A conceptual framework for cost management training in the Limpopo Province of South Africa. Journal of Nursing Management

[9] Department of Health: Republic of South Africa. Policy framework and strategy for Ward Based Primary Healthcare Outreach Teams 2018/19-2023/24

[10] Nangombe, J.P. & Justus AH. (2016). Development of the conceptual for a quality improvement training programme for health professionals in the ministry of health and social services in Namibia. International Journal of Health, 4(1) (2016) 46-53

[11] Branch, R.M. (2009). Instructional Design: The ADDIE approach. DOI 10.1007/978-0-387-09506-6_2. Springer Science and Business Media, LLC.

[12] Wetty, G. 2007. The Design Phase of the ADDIE model. Journal of GXP Compliance. 11(4), 40-48.

[13] Piskurich, G. M. 2015. Rapid Instructional Design: Learning ID Fast and Right. 3rd edition. John Wiley and Sons, Hoboken, NJ, USA.

[14] Chen, Y. Chen, T. and Tsai, L. 2011. Development and evaluation of multimedia reciprocal representation instruction materials. International Journal of Physical Sciences Vol. 6(6), pp. 1439, 18 March 2011. DOI: 10.5897/IJPS11.066

[15] He, Z. Marquard, J and Henneman, E. 2017. Model Guided Design and Development Process for an Electronic Health Record Training Program. AMIA Annu Symp Proc. 2017 Feb 10; 2016:1814-1821

[16] Hess, A. K. N. and Greer, K. 2016. Designing for Engagement: Using the ADDIE model to integrate High-Impact Practices into online Information Literacy Course. Communications in information literacy | vol. 10, no. 2, 2016

[17] Malan, Z. Mash, B. and Everett-Murphy, K. 2015. Development of a training programme for primary care

providers to counsel patients with risky lifestyle behaviours in South Africa. Afr J Prim Health Care Fam Med. 2015 Jun 5;7(1). doi: 10.4102/phcfm.v7i1.819

[18] Akkoyunlu, B. and Arkün, S. 2008. A Study on the devclopment process of a multimedia learning environment according to the ADDIE model and students' opinions of the multimedia learning environment. Interactive Educational Multimedia, ISSN 1576-4990, N°. 17, 2008,1-19.

[19] Gyawali, B. Mishra S. R. Neupane, D. Vaidya, A. Sandbaek, A. and Kallestrup, P. 2018. Diabetes management training for female community health volunteers in Western Nepal: An implementation experience. BMC Public Health. 2018;18:641. doi:10.1186/s12889-018-5562-y.

[20] Cheung, L. 2016. Using the ADDIE Model of instruction to Teach Chest Radiograph Interpretation. Journal of Biomedical Education. Volume 2016, Article ID 9502572, 6 pages http://dx.doi.org/10.1155/2016/9502572

[21] South African Qualifications Authority (SAQA). 2005. www.saqa.org.za/docs/pol/2015/National%20Policy%20for%20Assessment

[22] Krathwohl, D. R. 2002. A Revision of Bloom's Taxonomy: An Overview, Theory into Practice, 41:4, 212-218, DOI: 10.1207/s15430421tip4104-2

[23] Niari, M. and Hartofylaka, A. M. 2007. Instructional Design of the WaW e-courses. The Journal for Open and Distance Education and Educational Technology Volume 13(2)

[24] Hsu, T. Lee-Hsieh, J. Michael, A. Turton, M. A. and Cheng, S. 2014. Using the ADDIE Model to Develop Online Continuing Education Courses on Caring for Nurses in Taiwan. The Journal of Continuing Education in Nursing. DOI: 10.3928/00220124-20140219-04

[25] Gleason, B. L. Peeters, M. J. Resman-Targoff, B. H., Karr, S. McBane, S. Kelley, K. and Denetclaw, T. H. 2011. An Active-Learning Strategies Primer for Achieving Ability-Based Educational Outcomes. *American Journal of Pharmaceutical Education*, *75*(9), 186. http://doi.org/10.5688/ajpe759186

[26] Kurt, S. (2016). Kirkpatrick Model: Four Levels of Learning Evaluation, in *Educational Technology*, October 24, 2016. Retrieved from https://educationaltechnology.net/kirkpatrick-model-four-levels-learning-evaluation

[27] Farjad, S. (2012). The Evaluation of Effectiveness of training courses in University by Kirkpatrick Model (case study: Islamshahr university). Social and Behavioral Sciences 46 2837-2841

[28] Patel, S.R., Margolies, P.J., Covell, N.H., Lipscomb, C. & Dixon, L.B. (2018). Using Instructional Design, Analyze, Design, Develop, Implement, and Evaluate, to Develop e-Learning Modules to Disseminate Supported Employment for Community Behavioural Health Treatment Programs in New York State. Front. Public Health 6:113. doi: 10.3389/fpubh.2018

[29] Shek, D.T.L. & Chak, Y.L.Y. (2012). Evaluation of the Training Program of the Project P.A.T.H.S.: Findings Based on the Perspective of the Participants from Different Cohorts," The Scientific World Journal, 2012, Article ID 687198, 10 pages, 2012. https://doi.org/10.1100/2012/687198

Chapter 17

Family-Centered Diabetes Care for Better Glycemic Outcomes of Outpatients in Rural Areas

Mabitsela Hezekiel Mphasha and Tebogo Maria Mothiba

Abstract

Most of diabetes care of outpatients takes place at their families. Family members who may have inadequate or lack diabetes knowledge are expected to offer home care, predisposing patients to poor outcomes and associated health problems. To review and discuss literature related to family-centered diabetes care. Comprehensive Literature Review was used to collect data by reviewing literature related to family centered diabetes care. Literature review involved evaluating discoveries of other researchers. The results of literature review showed that family-centered care is essential for better diabetes outcomes and preventing new cases. So far, family-centered care was successful in children's diabetes care and may be beneficial for older outpatients. Family-centered diabetes care improves knowledge of both patients and families, minimize prevalence and improve diabetes outcomes of outpatients.

Keywords: family centered diabetes care, diabetes, family, outpatients, literature review

1. Introduction

The International Diabetes Federation (IDF) [1], pointed out that rising cases of Diabetes Mellitus (DM) are a threat to the public health sector and seventh leading cause of death in South Africa [2]. In Africa, South Africa (SA) is the fifth country with the highest population of diabetes patients which is estimated at 2.6 million and more than 1.5 million people with undiagnosed diabetes mellitus [3], specifically, Type-2 Diabetes Mellitus (T2DM), remains more common where 2 million persons have been diagnosed with T2DM in SA [4]. Diabetes has recently been found to be a high risk Non-Communicable Diseases (NCDs) linked to COVID deaths worldwide. Central to DM prevalence is obesity which is a leading predisposing factor to all NCDs.

Family members of diabetes patients are already at risk of developing the disease due to family history. Physical and mental health of family members may be negatively affected while taking care of diabetes patient, leading to compromised patient care [5]. Hence the introduction of Family Centered Care (FCC) to lessen the negative consequences of caregiving for individuals diagnosed with DM. Rural areas such as Limpopo Province in SA, have been progressively urbanized, which has led to adoption of unhealthy lifestyles such as physical inactivity and bad eating habits, resulting in rising prevalence of obesity which contribute to poor diabetes outcomes and complications [6].

IntechOpen

So far, family-centered diabetes care has been successful and produced better diabetes outcomes in children, who are helped by family members to carry certain relevant tasks related to self-care practices [7]. Less focus has been given to older people who are mostly affected by diabetes [3]. Therefore, this book chapter is intended on closing the gap by advocating for the family-centered diabetes care among older outpatients at rural areas.

2. Diabetes burden

Approximately 9% of people worldwide have diabetes and that 90% of the diabetic cases are Type 2 Diabetes Mellitus (T2DM) cases [8]. Over 80% of diabetes cases are those living in developing countries [9]. Type-2 diabetes is rising in Africa and threatening public health sector particularly because it is predisposing factor to various NCDs including diabetes, and its prevalence is anticipated to increase by 110% over the next two decades, from 19.8 million individuals in 2013 to 41.5 million by 2035 [1]. Inactive lifestyle characterized by lack of exercise and poor eating habits are a problem in South Africa leading obesity and subsequently increased diabetes prevalence and complications. Around 7% of South Africans aged 21 to 79 years have diabetes mellitus [1]. The prevalence of DM among South Africans aged 30 years or more has expanded since 2009, and 11 million increase are anticipated in the year 2020 [10]. Statistics SA [2] further points out that diabetes mellitus and different types of heart diseases are part of the ten leading causes of death in all parts of SA. The StatsSA [2], reported that Limpopo Province has DM prevalence rate of 5.2% and is the fourth province with highest DM prevalence, while Western Cape Province leads with of 6.9% DM prevalence.

3. Provision of diabetes healthcare services to outpatients

Diabetes outpatients receive treatment at Primary Health Care (PHC) facilities, which is nurse driven. The South African Department of Health, in an attempt to manage chronic diseases including DM introduced Chronic Disease Outreach Program (CDOP) to follow-up on patients, particularly those with NCDs [11]. In line with CDOP, health professionals such as general practitioners, dietitians, physiotherapists and psychologists regularly visit PHC facilities to see patients requiring their services. Diabetes patients are required to consult these healthcare professionals 2–3 a years. The introduction of the outpatient's services in SA helped in reducing management costs which are imposed by mere presence of diabetes, and more costly in the presence of complications. The outpatient services also helped in improving family involvement in the care of loved ones.

4. Assembling diabetes team for the care of outpatients

The diabetes team for the treatment and care of outpatients at PHC facilities with recognition of the outreach programs by other healthcare professionals who may not be full time at the PHC facilities, and are as follows:

5. Family-centered diabetes care

The FCC is defined as "provision of healthcare in partnership or in recognition that the family has a role to play in the treatment of persons living with chronic diseases and specifically diabetes" [12]. The FCC is an approach of responding to the needs, values and cultural needs of the patient and FMs [13]. The FCC begins from consultation at the healthcare facility involving healthcare professional, patients and family members, being involved in decision making and shared leadership [14]. Family Members are often asked to share responsibility in support of person living with diabetes, and such activities includes driving patients to appointments, and social and emotional support among others. The FCC in diabetes care has so far produced better outcomes in younger children who are usually cared for by their parents or families, since younger children are unable to perform certain tasks related to self-care [7]. However, the FCC have so far failed to utilize same family support for better care of older people who are mostly affected by diabetes [1].

The aim of the FCC is to maintain and strengthen family bond and roles so as to provide healthy family functioning, and at the same time improving the Quality of Life (QoL) of patients, as well as minimizing new cases involving family members who are already at risk due to family history. Despite the benefits of adequate diabetes knowledge, it is worrisome that international knowledge and awareness of diabetes stays low [15]. In SA, diabetes knowledge among T2DM patients in most affected areas is reportedly inadequate [16]. It is essential for healthcare providers to assess knowledge of patients and family members so as to design appropriate diabetes intervention and educate properly. Therefore, the FCC seeks to close the knowledge gap through family-patient consulting healthcare provider together.

6. Principles of family-centred care

The FCC principles are frequently aligned with a vision of effective health care delivery as described by Johnson and Abraham [17], and are as follows:

- **Information Sharing**: This principle acknowledges that healthcare practitioners, patients and family members all must share information for better care of patients. See **Table 1** on responsibilities of diabetes team. The process of sharing information should be open, objective and without bias [17]. Patients and family members timely are empowered with complete and accurate information for the care and decision-making [18].

- **Respect and Dignity:** Healthcare professionals need to understand that patients are vulnerable and do their best to maintain patients' dignity [19]. After healthcare professionals have discussed medical options with patients and family, they should respect that patients have final decision [17].

- **Participation:** This principle acknowledges that patients and family members have role to play in the care, after being empowered with diabetes care information [18].

- **Collaboration:** This principle acknowledges that healthcare professionals must primarily involve and engaging patients as the main consumer on the involvement or adoption of family-centered care for its successful implementation. Furthermore, once patients have been engaged and approved adoption of FCC, in the provision of ongoing diabetes self-care education and support, patients, families and healthcare professionals jointly make diabetes interventions programs together that considers the needs, strengths, values, and abilities of recipients [17].

Diabetes team	Responsibility
General Practitioners	Clinically assess the patients
	Provide required medical interventions
Nurses	Assess and refer patients and their families to multi-disciplinary team
	Establish diabetes support groups at the PHC facilities
Dietitians	Provide dietary care services
Physiotherapists	Provide exercise care services.
Psychologists	Provide psychological and behavioral care services.
Social workers	Provide services on how best to cope with the disease and also on social relief or grants for the care of diabetes patients.
Patients	Recipient of family-centred diabetes care and share experiences of living with diabetes.
Family members	Recipient of family-centred diabetes care and advocate for patients by expressing additional health challenges which the patients has omitted.
	Provides emotional support to the patient, and care at home.

Table 1.
Diabetes team and their responsibilities.

7. Diabetes self-care, self-care activities and its adherence

Diabetes self-care is explained as "evolutionary process of development of knowledge or awareness by learning to survive with the complex nature of the disease within social context" [20]. Diabetes education is critical and must be practically translated into activities for the achievement of better diabetes outcomes. The self-care activities includes adherence to dietary plan, avoidance of fatty food, regular physical activity and self-glucose monitoring, and foot care, taking of medication (insulin or an oral hypoglycaemic agent), and cessation of smoking [21]. In addition, self-care activities includes good problem-solving skills, healthy coping skills and risk-reduction practices [20]. Integrating self-care activities into patients' daily routine improves diabetes outcomes, minimizes chances of developing complications and diabetes related health problems. Compliance or adherence to diabetes treatment remains a problem, in spite of the advantages of integrating the self-care activities into patients' daily routine.

Diabetes Self-Management Education and Support, and Family as provider of home care to patients.

Diabetes Self-Management Education (DSME) is regarded as "the process of facilitating knowledge, skill, and ability necessary for diabetes self-care" [18], and is provided by healthcare providers. Multi-disciplinary team provides various diabetes care services, therefore, a clear referral system should be developed and implemented. The DSME is provided with the sole purpose of capacitating both patients and family members with skills and knowledge required in self-care practices. Adequate diabetes care knowledge may pursue both patients and their family members to follow healthy lifestyle healthy lifestyle [15], so as to prevent diabetes complications and also reduce new cases, respectively. Sufficient diabetes knowledge also minimizes risk of comorbidity which impact significantly the QoL of patients [22]. However, Ajzen et al. [23] argued that adequate knowledge alone is not sufficient for the adoption of healthy lifestyle, it should be accompanied by positive attitudes. There should be collaboration between the health sector and the family, since collaboration is one of the principles of FCC. Among the families of patients, there should be dedicated person to represent the family in the interaction and consultation with patients at the healthcare facilities [24]. Spouses and parents can be in charge of both their partners and children; respectively, however, the families may as well nominate a member to represent them. In ensuring the success of the FCC, the healthcare professionals may assure the families that they will be listened, supported and that their doors will forever be opened for any challenges encountered to ease the home caregiving. The family receives home care through consulting together with patients or DSME program. The outpatients receive their diabetes treatment at PHC facility, which is inadequately resourced with other healthcare workers such as dietitians and physiotherapists, who support the PHC facilities. Therefore, there is a need for a well-organized and structured education programme for people living with diabetes for the DSME to be fully functional at PHC level.

Whereas, Diabetes Self-Management Support (DSMS) refers to the "support that is required for implementing and sustaining coping skills and behaviours needed to self-manage on an ongoing basis, and it is provided by family members with recognition that most care happen at the families patients reside" [18]. Family plays especially significant role in diabetes care for better glycaemic outcomes. A study involving 5000 diabetes patients recognizes importance of family, relatives and colleagues in improving well-being and self-management of diabetes [25]. Home care refers to "health or social service provided by formal and informal caregivers to the recipient" [26]. Informal home caregivers are explained as "individuals actively and directly involved in the patient care and support at home without earning any salary for caring and supporting the patients" [27]. The FMs maybe distressed by diabetes status of their loved ones, particularly when they have poor knowledge of the condition or not knowing how best to provide support [25]. Families sometimes have misconceptions, like believing that their loved ones living diabetes know more about the management of the disease, than they actually report. The family as informal caregivers are usually not trained in the care of patients; and as such families are underutilized resource. The success stories related to home care for diabetes patients includes adherence to diabetes treatment and improved quality of life and reduction of prevalence. However, failures of home care which often occurs in the event of inadequate diabetes knowledge includes poor diabetes outcomes and quality of life. Hence the need for family centered diabetes care to improve knowledge of both family and patients.

8. Why adopt family-centred care in diabetes management

Lack of adequate knowledge about illness and inadequate social support contribute to poor control of diabetes [25]. The adoption of FCC is aimed at capacitating both family members through the DSME together with patients at the healthcare facility, which capacitate and empower them with knowledge on how to best become healthcare providers at home, where most of the diabetes care takes place. Adequate social support from knowledgeable family members helps in preventing, delaying and minimizing the severity of diabetes complications, as well as reducing the chances of family members from developing diabetes. Family members are informal healthcare providers at home as they primarily provide Diabetes Self-Management Support. The QoL is regarded as "an estimation of well-being as well as the measurement of health and the effects of health care" [28]. In order to achieve better QoL, it is important to adhere to diabetes treatment and adopt a healthy lifestyle [3]. Adequate family support also helps in achieving good QoL [29], particularly when the family are knowledgeable with regard to diabetes care.

9. The type of support a family can give to diabetes patients

Living alone is linked with increasing depression, poor diabetes outcomes and increased mortality [30]. The family support and care for patients, with daily living activities which includes meal preparation and consumption, physical activity, collection of medication, bathing, distribution of household chores, bathing and clothing, and honoring of medical appointments. Families also help patients cope `with the diabetes and also may be required to financially support the patients so as to daily meet the activities of daily living. Quality of life and better glycaemic outcomes have been associated with better income [31].

9.1 Supporting family

Family communication needs to be improved during DSME, and also empower them with knowledge and skills essential in positively influence patient health behaviors and subsequently diabetes outcomes. Lack of diabetes care knowledge among family members, result in stress of not knowing how best to care for loved one in need of support, hence adoption of family centred diabetes care empowers family and minimizes the negative psychological impact. Exclusion of families during consultations may lead to families having misconceptions that patients know more about diabetes management than actually patients know, relying on the patients to report to them on how to best care for them [24], leading to inappropriate care. Educating families on diabetes care needs and why the changes are necessary can aid in easing the stress brought along by inadequate knowledge. The family may as well need to be educated on the coping skills. The effective family involvement in diabetes care may help the family accept the lifestyle modifications for the patients and family members' health considering that they are already at risk due to family history [29]. Additional information which should be provided to the family during consultation includes information about the disease, possible treatment alternatives and stress management skills, as well as helping them plan for the future [32].

10. The negative ways family can affect diabetes

Actions of family members in providing support to diabetes patients may be harmful and lead to poor diabetes outcomes [33], particularly when family members who are not trained about care, are not capacitated through DSME on self-care activities. Family culture, way of living and problem-solving skills may additionally contribute in harming the patients and resulting poor diabetes outcomes. The required diabetes self-management activities may be in conflict with the traditional family way of cooking and eating, which may prompt family to not accept the lifestyle modification and new way of doing things [33].

Family members usually support the patients at home through food preparation and may compromise and sabotage patients through cooking and serving unhealthy meals, tempting patients to consume unhealthy food for the sake of peace at home [30]. Additionally, the family members may also discourage patients from regularly taking medications and its adherence, particularly when the patient relies on them for getting and taking medications and meals. Hence the need for family centred diabetes care to minimize the ways family can negatively impact on patients' outcomes for better glycaemic outcomes.

11. Barriers to family-centered Care

- **Understanding Family-Centered Care:** Lack of understanding of the concept of family-centered diabetes care by both healthcare providers and patients may negatively impact on its successful implementation. Hence, there is a need for in-service training of healthcare providers on the family-centered diabetes care for better outcomes [25]. Policy makers and legislatures develops and introduces policies, whilst healthcare providers at any setting are the drivers or implementers of the policies. The drivers of policies need to be trained on the pros and cons of FCC in diabetes care and also given guidelines on family centered diabetes care to minimize confusion and for effective implementation.

- **Support for Practices**: Loss of income and employment may affect provision of support to patients as required by the FCC. Repeated visits and honoring of medical appointments should be observed, and that the spirit of humanity must at all times prevail so as to enable consistent support and care during the loss of income [24]. The South African Government introduced Old-Aged Grant, of which diabetes patients are among the beneficiaries considering that diabetes affects mostly the elderly. The introduction of old-aged grants in SA helped the elderly persons getting and needed support from the family members. Also, the families must be empowered with diabetes care knowledge and how it could also benefit their health, so as to minimize the presence or absence of income being motivating factor for provision of support.

- **Research:** Research helps in informing policy developers, healthcare providers, patients and family members on what should be done in the provision of health formal and informally to the patients. Therefore, lack of adequate research on family centered diabetes care for outpatients may negatively impact on the adoption and implementation of the family centered diabetes care.

12. Advantages of family-centered diabetes care

- **Reduces the diabetes treatment costs:** Diabetes is costly disease to manage, and more costly in the presence of complication. It has been reported that the global diabetes management cost amount to $1.31 trillion, which accounts to 1.8% of 2015 global gross domestic product [34]. The FCC reduces diabetes associated hospital admissions and readmissions costs [35], as well as estimated lifetime health care costs.

- **Improvement of Hemoglobin:** Hemoglobin A_{1c} (HbA_{1c}) improves by 1% in T2DM patients [36].

- **Reduces/prevent complications:** The FCC prevent, delays and minimizes the severity of diabetes complications, improve quality of life and better glycaemic control through lifestyle behaviors such as healthy eating habits, regular physical activity and adherence to intake of diabetes medication.

- **Improves the clinical and psychosocial aspects of diabetes:** The presence of diabetes affect the quality of life of patients and also brings along emotional and psychological burdens resulting in stress and depression, which worsens in the presence of complications such as erectile dysfunction.

13. Conclusion

Adoption and implementation of the family-centred diabetes care can assist in improving better glycaemic outcomes in older diabetes outpatients It will also help in improving knowledge of both patients and family members for improved quality of life and reduction of new cases.

Author details

Mabitsela Hezekiel Mphasha* and Tebogo Maria Mothiba

1 Department of Public Health, University of Limpopo, South Africa

2 Faculty of Health Sciences Executive Dean's Office, University of Limpopo, South Africa

*Address all correspondence to: pitso85@gmail.com

References

[1] International Diabetes Federation. *IDF Diabetes Atlas*. Seventh Edition. Brussels, IDF. 2015.

[2] Statistics South Africa. Patterns of morbidity and mortality in older persons in South Africa, 2013. 2014. Available at: http://www.statssa.gov.za (Accessed: 19 September 2015).

[3] International Diabetes Federation. *IDF Diabetes Atlas*. Fifth Edition. Brussels, IDF. 2013.

[4] Hardy, D.S, Stallings, D.T, Garvin, J.T, Xu, H, and Racette, S.B. Best anthropometric discriminators of incident type 2 diabetes among white and black adults: A longitudinal ARIC study. *PLoS ONE*. 2017, (1):1-12

[5] Kokorelias KM, Gignac MAM, Naglie G and Cameron JI. Towards a universal model of family centered care: a scoping review. BMC Health Services Research. 2019, 19(564):1-11

[6] Ganu D, Fletcher N, and Caleb N.K. Physical disability and functional impairment resulting from type 2 diabetes in sub-Saharan Africa: a systematic review. *African Journal of Diabetes Medicine*. 2016. 24(1): 10-14

[7] Ingerski LM, Anderson BJ, Dolan LM, Hood KK. Blood Glucose Monitoring and Glycemic Control in Adolescents: Contribution of Diabetes-Specific Responsibility and Family Conflict. J Adolesc Health. 2010;47:191-7.

[8] World Health Organization. Global Strategy on Diet, Physical Activity and Health. Physical Activity [Internet]. 2017 [cited March 30, 2017]. Available from: http:// www.who.int/ dietphysicalactivity/pa/en/

[9] Morrison, Zoe, Douglas, Anne, Bhopal, Raj, Sheikh, Aziz, and Lean, Mike. *Understanding experiences of participating in a weight loss lifestyle intervention trial: a qualitative evaluation of South Asians at high risk of diabetes.* BMJ Open, 2014. 4 (6): 1-9

[10] Shilubane, H, Netshikweta, L and Ralineba, T. Beliefs and practices of diabetic patients in Vhembe district of Limpopo Province. *African Journal of Primary Health Care Family Medicine.* 2016. 8(2):1-6

[11] Mayega RW, Guwatudde D, Makumbi FE, *et al*... Comparison of fasting plasma glucose and haemoglobin A1c point-of-care tests in screening for diabetes and abnormal glucose regulation in a rural low-income setting. *Diabetes Research and Clinical Practice* 2014, 104:112-120.

[12] Baig, A.A, Benitez, A, Quinn, M.T, and Burnet, D.L. Family interventions to improve diabetes outcomes for adults. *Annals of the New York Academy of Sciences*. 2015. 1353(1): 89-112. Available in PMC 2016 September 01.

[13] Kuo, D.Z, Houtrow, A.J, Arango, P, Kuhlthau, K.A, Simmons, J.M and Neff, J.M. Family-centered care: current applications and future directions in pediatric health care. *Maternal and Child Health Journal*. 2012. 16(2):297-305. Available from: http://www.ncbi.nlm.nih.gov/pubmed/21318293

[14] Carman, K.L, Dardess, P, Maurer, M, *et al.* Patient and family engagement: a framework for understanding the elements and developing interventions and policies. *Health Affirmation (Millwood) [Internet]. Project HOPE - The People-to-People Health Foundation, Inc.* 2013. 32(2):223-231.

[15] Spronk, I.; Kullen, C.; Burdon, C. and O'Connor, H. Relationship between nutrition knowledge and dietary intake. *Br. J. Nutr.* 2014, 111:1713-1726.

[16] Mohammadi S, Karim NA, Talib RA, and Amani R.. Evaluation of quality of life among type 2 diabetes patients. Int J Community Med Public Health. 2016, 3:51-56.

[17] Johnson BH and Abraham MR. Partnering with Patients, Residents and Families: A resource for leaders of hospitals, ambulatory care settings, and long-term care communities. Bethesda, MD: Institute for Patient- and Family centred care. 2012.

[18] Powers MA, Bardsley J, Cypress M, et al. Diabetes Self-Management Education and Support in type-2 diabetes: A joint position statement of the American Association of Diabetes Educators and the Academy of Nutrition and Dietetics. *Clin Diabetes*, 2016, 34: 70-80

[19] Carter, R., Lubinsky, J. & Domholdt, E. 2013. *Rehabilitation Research: Principles and Applications.* 4Th edition. Missouri: Elsevier Saunders

[20] Cooper H, Booth K, and Gill G. Patients' perspectives on diabetes health care education. Health Educ Res, 2003. 18(2):191-206.

[21] Shrivastava SR, Shrivastava PS and Ramasamy J. Role of Self-Care in Management of Diabetes Mellitus. Journal of Diabetes & Metabolic Disorders, 2013, 12 (14): 1-5

[22] Nguyen, V.H, Tran, T.T, Nguyen, C.T, *et al.* Impact of Comorbid Chronic Conditions to Quality of Life among Elderly Patients with Diabetes Mellitus in Vietnam. *Int. J. Environ. Res. Public Health* 2014, (16) 531:1-11

[23] Ajzen I, Joyce N, Sheikh S, *et al.* Knowledge and the prediction of behavior: the role of information accuracy in the theory of planned behavior. *Basic Appl Soc Psych*. 2011, 33(2):101-117.

[24] Rosland, A.M, Heisler, M, Choi, H.J, Silveira, M.J and Piette, J.D. Family influences on self-management among functionally independent adults with diabetes or heart failure: do family members hinder as much as they help? *Chronic Illn*ess.2013, 6:22-33.

[25] Kovacs, B, Burns, K, Nicolucci, A, Holt, R. I, *et al.* Diabetes Attitudes, Wishes and Needs second study (DAWN2): Cross-national benchmarking indicators for family members living with people with diabetes. Diabetic medicine: *Journal of the British Diabetic Association*. 2013, 30:778-788.

[26] Cooper J and Urquhart C. Homecare and the informal information grapevine: implications for the electronic record in social care. *Health Informatics J.* 2008, 14 (1): 59-69

[27] Hu, J, Amirehsani, K, Wallace, D.C and Letvak, S. Perceptions of barriers in managing diabetes: perspectives of Hispanic immigrant patients and family members. *Diabetes Educator*. 2013, 39:494-503.

[28] World Health Organization. Health Promotion Glossary. Geneva: World Health Organization. 1998

[29] Baig, A.A, Benitez, A, Quinn, M.T, and Burnet, D.L. Family interventions to improve diabetes outcomes for adults. *Annals of the New York Academy of Sciences*. 2015. 1353(1): 89-112. Available in PMC 2016 September 01.

[30] Mayberry, L.S, Rothman, R.L and Osborn, C.Y. Family members' obstructive behaviors appear to be more harmful among adults with type 2 diabetes and limited health literacy. *Journal of health communication*. 2014. 19 (2):132-143.

[31] Mayberry, L.S and Osborn, C.Y. Family support, medication adherence,

and glycemic control among adults with type 2 diabetes. *Diabetes. Care. 2012.* 35:1239-1245.

[32] Martire LM, Schulz R, Helgeson VS, Small BJ and Saghafi EM. Review and Meta-analysis of Couple-Oriented Interventions for Chronic Illness. Annals of behavioral medicine: a publication of the Society of Behavioural Medicine: a publication of the society of behavioural Medicine, 2010, 40: 325-342

[33] Denham SA, Manoogian MM, and Schuster L. Managing family support and dietary routines: Type 2 diabetes in rural Appalachian families. Families, Systems, & Health; 2007, 25(36):1-12

[34] Seuring T, Archangelidi O and Suhrcke M. The Economic Costs of Type 2 Diabetes: A Global Systematic Review. *Pharmaco Economics,* 2015. 33(3): 1-16

[35] Healy SJ, Black D, Harris C, Lorenz A, and Dungan KM. Inpatient diabetes education is associated with less frequent hospital readmission among patients with poor glycemic control. Diabetes Care. 2013, 36:2960-2967

[36] Siminerio L, Ruppert K, Huber K, Toledo FG. Telemedicine for Reach, Education, Access, and Treatment (TREAT): linking telemedicine with diabetes self-management education to improve care in rural communities. Diabetes Educ. 2014, 40:797-805

Chapter 18

The Importance of Health Literacy Related to Medications Instructions to Promote Adherence in People Living with Cardiovascular Diseases at Rural Settings

Charity Ngoatle and Tebogo Maria Mothiba

Abstract

Health literacy related to prescribed medications instructions is the ability to read, understand and carry out medication instructions as directed. Being generally literate does not automatically make one to be health literate. In most cases, a person's health literacy is overlooked based on their good general literacy. A convergent parallel mixed method design was used to explore and describe the practices of diabetes mellitus patients regarding prescribed medications instructions. The results showed failure to interpret medications instructions which leads to non-adherence unaware. On the other hand, non-adherence led to complications. Enhancing health literacy includes explanation of the medication instructions in details including the exact times for medication consumption. This could be achieved through peer teaching, health talks with patients and workshops.

Keywords: health literacy, prescribed medications, instructions, non-adherence, diabetes patients

1. Introduction

Health literacy regarding medications instructions is important to people with cardiovascular diseases. Understanding medication instructions is of vital importance to people living with cardiovascular diseases for proper disease management. Taking medication properly is one of the critical aspects in the control of diabetes mellitus. Many people can read medication instructions simply because they are literate; however, patients fail to interpret the medication instructions because they are health illiterate. Even though basic general literacy plays a role in understanding phenomena in general, health literacy regarding medications instructions could be achieved even when an individual do not have general literacy. So, patients with low health literacy have shown to suffer from low medication knowledge and understanding [1]. Health literacy regarding medication instructions basically means 'an understanding of the actual meaning of the instructions on how medication should be consumed'. This chapter will be based mainly on the study conducted among diabetes mellitus patients on treatment at selected rural area in Capricorn District, Limpopo province, South Africa.

The study employed a convergent parallel mixed method research design. The total population was 144 patients; 18 participated in the semi-structured interviews for qualitative study and 137 respondents for the quantitative study. The major findings of the study were: misconceptions and misunderstanding, unclear instructions, poor explanation by medication dispensers, non-compliance, negligence, experiencing complications, lack of knowledge and need assistance. The study also outlined the demographic data of the participants as factors influencing adherence and more insight will be shared in the chapter.

2. What is general literacy, health literacy, and literacy related to medication instructions?

General literacy refers to the basic ability to read, write, and figuring things out without considering the background in which reading, and writing occurs [2]. **Health literacy** on the other hand refers to the "degree to which individuals have the capacity to obtain, process, and understand basic health information and services necessary to make proper health decisions" [3]. Although general literacy has an impact on health literacy, being generally literate does not necessarily mean one will understand the health language. However, [4] asserts that the degree of health illiteracy related to medication instructions was linked to low education level. **Medication instructions** refers to the detailed information on how medication should be taken [5]. These instructions are normally found on the medication packages, bottles, inserts etc.

2.1 Types of health literacy

Health literacy is the junction between general literacy, health, and health care, but also incorporate attributes of the other types of literacies to varying degrees [6]. The concept of health literacy stemmed from the concern that individuals need more than just having general literacy skills to be able to manage the complexities of health and health system issues. There is a considerable intersection between general literacy and health literacy. Nonetheless, there are strong health-specific demands involved in health literacy that differs from those in general literacy [6]. Therefore, having general literacy alone is not adequate if one has to live a healthy life and to be able to prevent, manage, and control diseases and illnesses.

Therefore, health literacy is divided into three levels namely; basic health literacy, communicative health literacy, and critical health literacy [3].

2.1.1 Basic/functional health literacy

Functional health literacy is characterised by adequate fundamental skills in reading and writing to enable an individual to function efficiently in everyday situations. Therefore, functional health literacy is important to access services and information required to support individual's health, such as reading information about medication on medication labels [3]. Inadequate health literacy can result in difficulty following instructions from a doctor, and taking prescribed medication incorrectly, nonetheless, medical information is well understood when provided slowly, with the use of simple words and avoiding more information at a time [7].

2.1.2 Communicative/interactive health literacy

Interactive health literacy refers to more advanced, cognitive, and literacy skills which, together with social skills, that could be employed to actively participate in everyday activities. These skills are used to excerpt information and derive meaning from different forms of communication, and to apply new information to changing circumstances [3]. The interactive health literacy approach improves individuals' capability to act autonomously on knowledge. So, patients with inadequate health literacy are less likely to understand and take part in disease prevention and health promotion programs [7]. These patients are likely to be hospitalised more often than those with adequate health literacy.

Patients who reported having confidence in the ability to take medications confirmed a lack of comprehension in understanding medication instructions [8]. Patients further indicated numerous obstacles to effective medication management embedded in poor communication. Hence, patients expressed favouritism for more clearer medication instructions which could address some of the challenges they face.

2.1.3 Critical health literacy

Critical health literacy includes advanced cognitive skills, which together with social skills can be applied to critically analyse information and to use that information to exercise greater control over life events and situations. Therefore, health literacy moves beyond communication to the development of skills necessary to effect social change to support health [3].

From these types of health literacy descriptions, [9] came up with a framework for health literacy (**Table 1**) as follows:

Types of health literacy	Nutbeam's (2000) definitions	Categories of analysis
1. Functional health literacy	An individual capability to seek and comprehend health information.	The ability to recognise the formation of physical activity patterns in daily life.
2. Interactive health literacy	An individual capability to put health information into practice to achieve good health outcomes in various daily practices.	The ability to put to practice the comprehension of how physical activity patterns are made, and to employ, and exercise a lively everyday lifestyle within the prevailing. Conditions.
3. Critical health literacy	Possessing skills to critically evaluate health information and utilise information to achieve maximum control, including addressing structural determinants of health including empowerment skills; capabilities to act to bring change in conditions for ones' health and others.	The capability to relate judgementally to physical activity recommendations, to comprehend the effect of social determinants on physical activity ranks, and to draw on these capabilities to bring change to the prevailing conditions in enhancing the acceptable everyday lifestyle for self and others.

Table 1.
Health literacy framework.

2.2 Characteristics of individuals with low health literacy

- Poor overall health status.
- Higher rates of hospitalisations, death, and longer hospital stay.
- Higher rates of hospital readmissions within three days of discharge.
- Decreased capacity to manage chronic diseases.
- More likely to make errors with medications.
- Seek medical care when they are more ill.
- Have less knowledge on own illness management [6].

2.3 Factors influencing health literacy and medication adherence

Research has shown that there are several factors which influence health literacy among individual groups.

1. **Poor labelling instructions** on medication, packaging, lack of patient teaching on medication use, and disease processes contribute to non-adherence [10]. Patients therefore do not see the importance of following correct medication therapy because they do not understand.

2. **Gender** - Sixty-eight percent (68%) of the study participants were females. This could be because most women tend to report a lot of health issues and have greater utilisation of medical services than men [11]. Furthermore, this can be due to the traditional role of caring for sick family members and children. This traditional gender anticipation offers women with more interactions with the healthcare system, providing them additional chances to build their knowledge base, and consequently resulting in increased levels of health literacy than those of men. Gender differences in health literacy among Korean adults revealed that Korean women had a significantly higher level of health literacy compared to men, in understanding instructions on medication bottles [11]. The study explored gender differences in the level of health literacy and appropriate factors linked with health literacy.

   However, women reported more depressive symptoms of chronic diseases than men [11]. A question could be raised as to why these women would suffer depressive symptoms while we expect them to be healthy and in control of their diseases since they report frequently to the health facilities. This could be that, when women are sick, they lack proper care from their spouses or anyone to care for them, or they could be inappropriately taking their medications.

3. **Educational level** – Most of the diabetes mellitus patients (47%) attended school up to high school whereas only 11% did not attend school at all.

   Observations from previous studies illustrate that individuals with higher socioeconomic status or higher education levels had a better comprehension of prescribed medications and medication labels hence leading to the minor occurrence of adverse medication occasions [12]. Despite this, failure to comprehend and interpret medication prescriptions is still prevalent through all educational levels [12]. However, it is evident that a bit of general literacy plays part in augmenting health literacy. This was observed in patients who used many sources of medication information and found to be more informed than those who relied on one information source, for instance, using medication labels only while others used also some internet, books, and leaflets [12].

Having attained higher educational qualifications together with a family history of diabetes mellitus was significantly concomitant with a better understanding of health teaching and instructions [13]. It is evident that having enough health literacy is not the only factor related to good glycaemic control, rather the effect of adequate health literacy in attaining good glycaemic control can be disguised by patients with a better understanding of health education and instructions [13]. Therefore, patients can be health literate, but still, fail to comprehend medication instructions.

4. **Age** – Eighty-two percent (82%) of the participants were 50 years and above. It is well known that the risk of diabetes mellitus especially Type 2 is associated with age. However, as people age, their memory also deteriorates which could affect medication instructions comprehension. So, age has not been identified as a feature in the misapprehension and misinterpretation of prescription medication and medication labels. Misunderstanding was common across all age groups. Hence a more specific and clearer explanation is needed for the diabetes mellitus patients to understand medication instructions. Conversely, research affirms that health literacy is a durable predictor of health outcomes than socio-economic status, age, or ethnic background [6].

5. **Complexity of medication therapy** – fifty percent (50%) of the respondents were using four and more drugs for diabetes and other comorbidities. Diabetes patients on complex regimen were three times non-adherent than those with a simple regimen [14]. Therefore, simplifying diabetic medication therapy to at least single or two medications could make it easier for patients to follow [14].

6. **Poor health literacy** - other contributory factors to non-adherence in diabetes mellitus patients were identified as follow: firstly, poor health literacy coupled with low health numeracy [15]. This is irrespective of whether an individual is generally literate or not. Secondly, deficient or unclear teaching on medication, particularly if the teaching is not personalised for the patient or on each medication. Some patients do not interpret medication labels and medication information correctly and this is common even when labelling requires minimal reading skills. For example, instructions to take medicine twice daily (which is vague since 'daily' means once per day), or every 12 hours means individuals should make further decisions to understand the instructions. "Take medication as directed" is further, more difficult to interpret since the instructions need to be further broken down. Patients are more likely to understand more specific medication administration times such as 08 A.M., 06 P.M. but instituting periods can be useful or suit some individuals better. Using multifaceted medication regimens independently predicts the probability that patients interpret medication instructions, advice, or education incorrectly.

   Health professionals are the major role players in disseminating health information and are the first and most precise sources of information in health-related matters. Although they have restricted time with patients during consultations, they fail to issue out information as expected and patients opt for sources with questionable credibility, such as the internet, television, and newspapers, for health information [16]. These defective sources mostly lead individuals into making erroneous verdicts about their health. The patients should be taught how to seek credible information sources on the media. There should be ever-ready more specific and detailed health information materials to give out to the patients to reference at home *(see appendix 1)*.

7. **Inadequate patient education related to medication use** - Research has also shown that medication non-adherence and treatment ineffectiveness can be negatively influenced by the inability to comprehend medication instructions. The problem is not with patients using medications only but also dispensing health practitioners and medication manufacturers. Most of the generally used medication label instructions are unclear, and misunderstanding takes place also in highly educated patients [17]. Poor understanding of medication instructions or misinterpretations could be a cause for patients not using their medications as prescribed. Misinterpretation of medication instructions leads to subprime medication therapy resulting from consuming less than instructed, getting insufficient medication concentrations, or increased risks of adverse effects by overdosing and medication concentration increasing interactions.

It is evident that inadequate health literacy hinders patients' understanding of medication instructions [18]. The instructions also could be written in the clearest and specific manner, however, there is limited evidence supporting the best practices for writing prescription medication instructions to enhance patients' comprehension for proper use of the medication. Therefore, a more specific wording should be used on prescription medication instructions to enhance patients' comprehension [18].

3. Impacts of poor health literacy of medication adherence

Most of the time medication dispensers think that patients understand the instructions given to them regarding their medications but that is not always the case. Health literacy regarding medication instructions is a subject on its own, which needs to be unpacked. Health literacy do not always need basic literacy skills, if the individual understands the clock she or he is covered.

3.1 Misconception and misunderstanding

Misconception or misunderstanding could lead patients to non-adherence to their medication. Diabetes mellitus patients had misconception and misunderstanding regarding the prescribed medication instructions [19]. The instructions did not have specific times at which medications should be consumed. The instructions on the medication packages are not adequate; for instance, the instructions were written as morning, noon, night, or two times a day etc. [20]. This kind of instructions may be dangerous because patients with poor health literacy would interpret them wrongly [20]. Patients end up with drug toxicity or underdose. Patients also had incorrect perception of the medication instructions where the patients do not fully understand the instructions [21].

3.2 Non-compliance

One of the major problems responsible for non-adherence is the fact that patients esteem themselves as understanding the instructions. Diabetes mellitus patients perceived themselves as understanding the medication instructions which is however contrary to how they "actually" carried them out [19]. Understanding medication instructions means taking medication correctly and that includes taking the correct dose, at the right frequency, being persistent and consistent [21]. Non-adherence is linked to increased health services utilisation and frequent hospitalisation [22]. Many of the diabetes mellitus patients demonstrated a knowledge discrepancy concerning medication use during disease treatment [23]. This lack of knowledge can aggravate the health state of people with diabetes mellitus. Subsequently, bring about a momentous increase in direct and indirect health costs.

Non-compliance is often coupled with patient's negligence. Diabetes mellitus patients often drink too much alcohol and when drunk, do not take their prescribed medications. Similar situation is recorded in [24] where non-compliance was linked to patients not giving attention to their health with double increase in non-compliance due to alcohol use.

On the contrary, most patients were non-compliant because they had poor health literacy either because of shallow explanations given by health professionals or the unclear medication instructions on medication packages, leaflets or doctor's prescriptions.

3.2.1 Shallow explanations by professional nurses

Professional nurses as medication dispensers at primary health care level need to give a full explanation of the medication instructions to the patients. *(Refer to* ***Table 3****).* Diabetes mellitus patients do however indicate that they do not get such explanations as expected. **Participant 'G'** *when asked to share how she was told to take their medications said, "No. They have never explained well to me, but they said I should take the medication in the morning, during the day, and when I go to sleep".* **Participant 'E'** also said, *"They said I should take the medication the way they are; but for the times and hours no. They just said in the morning, during the day, and at night".*

In other words, patients do adhere to what the professional nurses tell them however, that information given to them is incomplete. This incomplete explanation therefore contributes to patients not adhering to treatment.

3.2.2 Unclear medication instructions on medication packages, leaflets or doctor's prescriptions

The medication instructions on the leaflets, packaging, and doctors' prescriptions are not clear. There is a poor explanation of the time-frequency on the documents' medication instructions. **One drug is written as**, *"1mg once daily".* **Another one is written:** *"One 500mg tablet 2 to 3 times a day".* There is no time interval reflected on the doctor's prescription, medication leaflets, and packaging. The drugs are written as follows: *"One 850mg tablet twice a day".* **Another drug is written, "***40 to 80mg daily".* **Whereas another one is written**, *"Daily doses over 10mg in 2 divided doses". there are no specific times for taking medication on diabetic medication instruction documents. One drug is written as, "Doses of 160mg daily in 2 divided doses". Another one is written: "Should be taken the same time every day".*

The medication instruction does not specify the exact times for taking the medications. **One drug is written as,** *"Doses of 160mg daily in 2 divided doses".* **Another one is written:** *"Should be taken the same time every day".*

Doctors should clarify medication instructions to patients and if they fail to do so, the pharmacists and professional nurses should, when dispensing 11]. If the health professionals fail, the last resort would be the medication packages and accompanying print materials like container labels, package inserts, medication

Symptoms experienced	Agree	Neutral	Disagree
Changes in vision	59	8	70
Numbness	60	7	70
Tingling sensation	47	4	86
Burning/pain on the toes or fingers	54	3	80
Erectile dysfunction in men	17	6	34
Poor hearing	18	2	117
A wound that does not heal	7	2	128

Table 2.
The symptoms experienced by diabetes mellitus patients on treatment.

guides etc. however, the print materials have been found to be complex and written in medical language which patients do not understand irrespective of their literacy level [25]. Most the patients on diabetes medications are elderly. It will serve us right as health professionals to write or tell the patients the exact times for taking the medications. This should also include the rationale for doing so. That is, to avoid over- or under-medicating themselves.

3.3 Complications

Non-compliance due to poor literacy result in some patients experiencing complications. Most of the patients experiencing complications do not know that they are linked to the disease process and non-adherence. Patients who were not compliant experienced complications compared to those who are compliant [26]. Some of the complications experienced by diabetes mellitus patients on prescribed medications are listed on **(Table 2)**. For erectile dysfunction, women were excluded.

4. Need versus no need for assistance with adherence to medications

Most of the diabetes mellitus patients are not aware that they are not taking medications correctly. This is because patients believe they are complying with how professional nurses have told them. On the other hand, other patients think they still need further assistance on how to adhere to medications. Misunderstanding of medication instructions could be reduced through improving clarification and understanding of labeling on prescribed medications by medication dispensers [20]. That is the reason patients believe the information given to them by health professionals as they trust that they are experts in their fields. It is, therefore, health professionals' duty to fully equip themselves with the knowledge needed for patients to understand the medications instructions. This knowledge should be made clearer to the level of patients understanding.

Participant 'T' *indicated that they need assistance and said, "I feel I need assistance on how I should eat and take medication correctly. I do not have such knowledge, I need it".*

On the contrary, **participant 'V'** said, *"According to me I do not need it because every time when I collect medications here at the clinic, they teach us how we should consume them".* **Yet participant 'U'** also said, *"No, I do not need it. I see myself taking the medications correctly, I am satisfied".*

5. The importance of health literacy on disease management

Health literacy is essential for effective access to care, self-care of chronic conditions, and maintenance of health and wellness. It is also essential to healthcare, necessitating individuals to have a more active role in decision making and disease management [27]. Health literacy enables patients to accurately interpret the medication instructions to ensure proper and safe use. It is therefore linked to medication adherence and consequently contribute towards persevering life.

6. Interpretation of the medication instructions

Understanding medication instructions coupled with other treatment measures like lifestyle modification, play a major part in controlling diabetes mellitus. The instructions need to be clear such that patients will not take their medications incorrectly as a result of misunderstanding. It is important for medication dispensers to make sure that patients understand the correct meaning of these instructions before they leave the facilities. Health literacy should therefore be imparted to enhance medication instructions comprehension and medication compliance in diabetes mellitus patients [1]. **Table 3** give an outline of the prescribed medication instructions' explanation as a recommendation to assist people with cardiovascular diseases on treatment.

Area	If on your medication it is written	It means
Before or after	Before food or meal	Take your medication, then you can have your food immediately or 30 minutes before food
	After food or meals	Eat your food first then after that you can take your medication.
Daily	Take 1 tablet daily	Since a day has 24 hours; therefore, divide 24 hours by 1 = 24. So, you are going to take your medication at the same time every day. E.g., if you choose 07 h00 am, that should be your everyday time.
At night	Take 1 tablet at night	It is the same as above, but you choose a night -time. E.g., 19 h00.
In the morning	Take 1 tablet mane or in the morning.	Same as the above but you choose a morning time. Any time before 12 h00 noon. E.g., 07 h00 am.
2x a day	Take 1 tablet two times a day (BD).	You divide 24 hours by 2 = 12 hours. For every 12 hours you should take your medication. E.g., if you choose 07 h00 in the morning, the next 12 hours will be at 19 h00 in the evening
3x a day	Take 1 tablet three times a day (TDS).	You divide 24 hours by 3 = 08 hours. For every 08 hours you need to take your medication. E.g., if you take the first dose/pill at 06 h00 am, 14 h00, & 22 h00.
4x a day	Take 1 tablet 4 times a day.	You divide 24 hours by four = 06 hours. For every 06 hours you need to take your medication. i.e., 06 h00, 12 h00 pm, 18 h00 & 00 h00 am.

Table 3.
An outline of the prescribed medication instructions' explanation.

7. Conclusions

Health literacy regarding prescribed medication instructions if important to diabetes mellitus and people with cardiovascular diseases at large. Understanding prescribed medications instructions by diabetes mellitus patients could assist in alleviating some of the complications experienced by some of the patients living with this disease.

Conflict of interest

The authors declare no conflict of interest.

A. Appendices

Appendix 1 provide take home information for diabetes mellitus patients as reference guides.

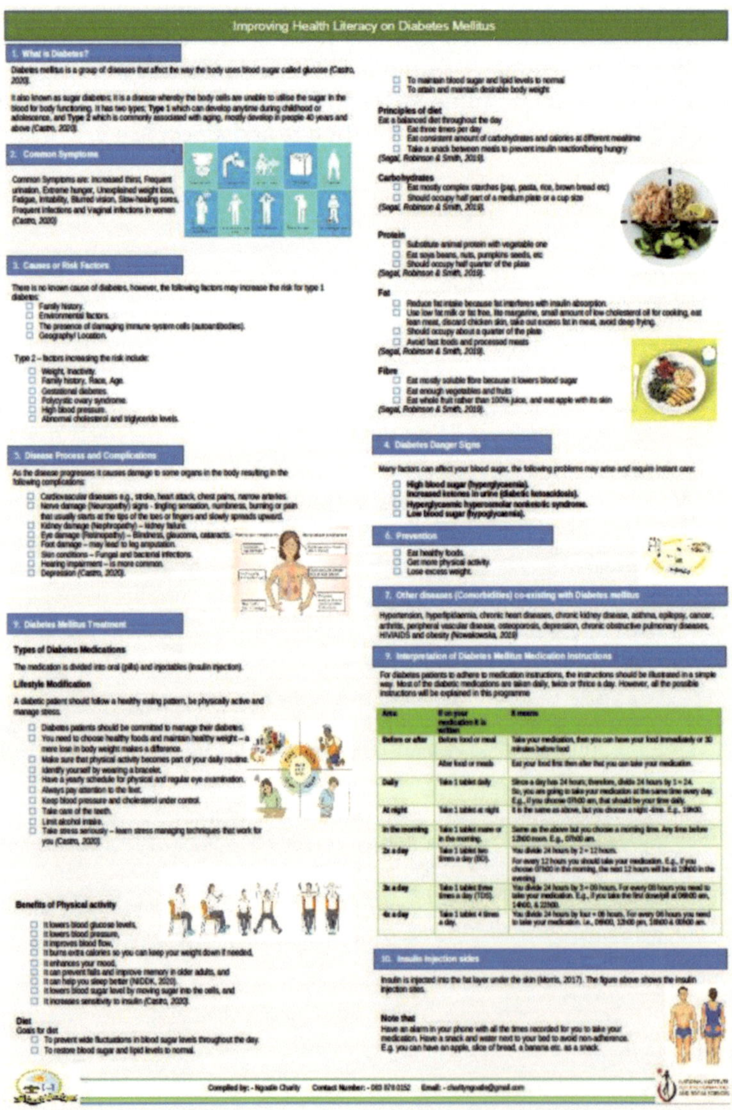

DOI: http://dx.doi.org/10.5772/intechopen.95902

B. Appendix 1

Improving health literacy on diabetes mellitus.

Author details

Charity Ngoatle and Tebogo Maria Mothiba*
University of Limpopo, Polokwane, South Africa

*Address all correspondence to: tebogo.mothiba@ul.ac.za

References

[1] Lee YM, Yu HY, You MA, Son YJ. Impact of Health Literacy on Medication Adherence in Older People with Chronic Diseases. Collegian. 2017 (24): 11-18. [Online]. Available from: http://dx.doi.org/10.1016/j.colegn.2015.08.003.

[2] Mayer GG, Villaire, M. Health Literacy in Primary Care. New York: Springer Publishing Company, LLC; 2007.

[3] Vidgen H. Food Literacy: Key Concepts for Health and Education. New York: Routledge; 2016.

[4] Alburikanh KA, AbuALrees A, Alenazi M, Albabtain H, Alqouzi M, Alawaji M & Aljadley HS. Patients' Understanding of Prescription Drug Label Instructions in Developing Nations: The Case of Saudi Arabia. Research in Social and Administrative Pharmacy. 2018; 14(5): 413-417

[5] Stevenson, A. Oxford Dictionary of English. 3rd edition. US: Oxford University Press; 2011.

[6] Johnson A. Health Literacy, does it make a Difference? Australian Journal of Advanced Nursing. 2014;31(3):39-45.

[7] Shirindi ML, Makhubele JC, Fraeyman J. Barriers to Medication Adherence Among Women Living in Rural Areas Suffering from Hypertension. The Case of Dikgale-Community. Etho Med. 2016;10(1): 76-84.

[8] Mohan AV, Riley MB, Boyington DR, Kripalani S. Illustrated Medication Instructions as a Strategy to Improve Medication Management Among Latinos: A Qualitative Analysis. Journal of Health Psychology. 2012;18(2): 187-197.

[9] Bruselius-Jansen M, Bonde AH, Christensen JH. Prompting Health Literacy in the Classroom. Health Education Journal. 2017;76(2): 156-168.

[10] Frances A, Thirumoorthy T, Kwan YH. Medication Adherence in the Elderly. Journal of Clinical Gerontology and Geriatrics. 2016;7(2): 64-67.

[11] Lee HY, Lee J, & Kim NK. Gender Differences in Health Literacy among Korean Adults: Do Women Have a Higher Level of Health Literacy than Men? American Journal of Men's Health. 2015;9(5): 370-379.

[12] Patel MJ, Khan MS, Ali F, Kazmi Z, Riaz T, Awan S, Sorathia SL. Patients' Insight of Interpreting Prescriptions and Drug Labels - A Cross-Sectional Study. PLoS ONE. 2013;8(6): e65019. DOI: 10.1371/journal.pone.0065019.

[13] Chen G.D, Huang CN, Yang YS, Lew-Ting CY. Patients Perception of Understanding Health Education & Instructions Has Moderating Effect of Glycemic Control. BMC Public Health. 2014;(14): 683. [Online]. Available from: http://www.biomedcentral.com/1471-2450/14/683.

[14] Gebrehiwat T, Jemal L, Dawit T. Non-adherence and Associated Factors among Type 2 Diabetic Patients at Jimma University Specialized Hospital, Southwest Ethiopia. Journal of Medical Sciences. 2013;13(7): 578-584.

[15] Dunning T. Care of People with Diabetes: A Manual of Nursing Practice. 4th edition. UK: John Wiley & Sons, Ltd:2014.

[16] Caylan A, Yayla K, Oztora S, Dagdeviren HN. Assessing Health Literacy, The Factors Affecting it, and Their Relationship to Some Health Behaviors among Adults. Biomedical Research. 2017;28(15): 6803-6807.

[17] Koster ES, Blom L, Winters NA, Hulten RP, Bouvy ML. Interpretation of Drug Label Instructions: A Study among Four Immigrants Groups in the

Netherlands. International Journal of Clinical Pharmacy. 2014; 36(2):274-281.

[18] Davis TC, Federman AD, Bass III PF, Jackson RH, Middlebrook SM, Parker RM, Wolf MS. Improving Patient Understanding of Prescription Drug Label Instructions. Journal of General Internal Medicine. 2009;24(1):57-62.

[19] Ngoatle C. Development and Implementation of an Educational Programme to Enhance Health Literacy on Prescribed Medication Instructions among Diabetes Mellitus Patients on Treatment at Ga-Dikgale Village Clinics in Capricorn District, Limpopo Province. [thesis]. Polokwane: University of Limpopo; 2020.

[20] Terefe A, Chanie T. Assessment of Patients Misunderstanding of Dosage Regimen Instructions Among Adolescent and Adult Outpatients in Ethiopia: The Case of a Primary Hospital. International Journal of Pharma Sciences and Research. 2014;5(8):446-453.

[21] Cecilia Health. Diabetes Medication Adherence: Understanding the Challenges to Improve Health Outcomes. New York: Cecilia Health. [internet] 2020. Available from: ceciliahealth.com/diabetes-medication-adherence.

[22] Zullig LL, Gellad WF, Moaddeb J, Crowley MJ, Shrank W, Granger BB, Granger CB, Trygstad T, Liu LZ, Bosworth HB. Improving Diabetes Medication Adherence: Successful, Scalable Interventions. Patient Preference and Adherence. 2015;(9): 139-149.

[23] Faria HTG, Zanetti ML, dos Santos MA, Teixeira CRD. Patient's Knowledge Regarding Medication Therapy to Treat Diabetes: A Challenge for Health Care Services. Acta Paul Enferm. 2009;22(5): 612-617.

[24] Aminde LN, Tindong M, Ngwasiri CA, Aminde JA, Njim T, Fondong AA, Takah NF. Adherence to Antidiabetic Medication and Factors Associated with Non-Adherence Among Patients with Type-2 Diabetes Mellitus in Two Regional Hospitals in Cameroon. BMC Endocrine Disorder. 2019; 19(35):1-9.

[25] Jeetu G, Girislı T. Prescription Drug Labelling Medication Errors: A Big Deal for Pharmacists. J Youngd Pharm. 2010; 2(1):107-111.

[26] Manobharathi M, Kalyani P, John William Felix A, Arulmani A. Factors Associated with Therapeutic Non-Compliance Among Type 2 Diabetes mellitus Mellitus Patients in Chidambaram, Tamilnadu, India. International Journal of Community Medicine and Public Health. 2017; 4 (3): 787-791.

[27] Parker RM, Jacobson KL. Health Literacy. Emory School of Medicine and Public Health. [internet]. 2012. Available from: https://www.nationalacademies.org/hmd/~/media/Files/Activity%20Files/PublicHealth/HealthLiteracy/HealthLiteracyFactSheets- Feb6- 2012-Parker-JacobsonFinal1.pdf.

Chapter 19

Self-Management Strategies to Curb the Development of NCDs in Rural Communities

Tebogo Maria Mothiba

Abstract

Prevalence of Non-Communicable Diseases (NCDs) in both Low- and Middle-Income countries is viewed as problematic and could lead to side effects when poorly managed. Therefore, serious intervention whereby People Living With the NCDs (PLWNCDs) could take a lead in controlling the side effects and managing the diseases themselves so that they maintain the QoL. To review and discuss literature related to self-management strategies to curb the development of NCDs in rural communities. Comprehensive Literature Review was used to collect data by reviewing literature related to self-management strategies to curb the development of NCDs in rural communities. The results of literature review showed that Self-management of NCDs is viewed as the only way to improve health outcomes and maintain QoL, by employing relevant strategies which will assist in achieving healthier life despite the situations at rural communities. Western World health systems have NCDs management centres at the community level to empower patients with knowledge for improving their QoL, whilst such centres do not exist in the Low-and Middle- Income countries poor communities. The PLWNCDs and residing at rural communities in Low- and Middle- Income countries can benefit from NCDs self-management strategies, despite the poor conditions.

Keywords: non-communicable diseases, people living with NCDs (PLWNCDs), low- and middle-income countries, rural communities, quality of life

1. Introduction

The prevalence of Non-Communicable Diseases (NCDs) in both Low Income and Middle Income countries is viewed as problematic. Therefore, serious intervention whereby people with the NCDs could take a lead in controlling the side effects and managing the diseases themselves so that they maintain the quality of life [1]. Self-management of NCDs is viewed as the only way to improve health outcomes and maintain quality of life. In maintaining the quality of life it is believed that the People Living with NCDs (PLWNCDs) have to employ various relevant strategies which will assist in achieving healthier life despite the situation they find themselves in especially in rural communities. In the Western World health systems there are Non-Communicable Diseases (NCDs) management centres at the community level to empower patients with knowledge on how to care for themselves to improve their quality of life [2], whilst such centres do not exist in the Low Income and Middle Income countries poor communities. Therefore, this chapter is aimed at explaining various self-management strategies that PLWNCDs could use in rural communities to raise awareness and as a means of providing information about management of the diseases.

2. Knowledge of PLWNCDs in managing the condition

It has been observed that mostly PLWNCDs in rural communities have limited knowledge when it comes to self-management of the disease including NCDs. The basic things which they understand and believe in is mostly the traditional herbs which might be used to curb the diseases' signs and symptoms. There is lack of knowledge on the lifestyle that communities and PLWNCDs could adhere to in order to minimize predisposing factors and also complications of NCDs. They lack knowledge on the type of diet, exercises they must engage in and the fact that they must avoid excessive alcohol intake and cigarette smoking. The identified lack of knowledge in managing the diseases calls for provision of basic health education at all levels of care especially at primary health care level in order to target rural communities where the problems has been identified. The following has to be included in the health education programme:

2.1 Motivational interview

The HCPs professionals have to use motivational counseling whenever they are consulting or interviewing the PLWNCDs. They should not use directive questions but make sure that the questions asked encourages the PLWNCDs to take part in planning for the health care intervention so that they have that feeling which indicates that they are fully participating in their care and are listened to by HCPs who will be encouraging them to participate and make calculated decisions. This interviewing style of asking the PLWNCDs provocative questions and discussing their responses, often helps uncover important self-management issues and has been proven that is effective in preventing relapse in patients as they will be part of the decision-making process. Motivational interview interventions have been found to be effective in enhancing adherence to intake of chronic diseases medication [3].

2.2 Identifying

The PLWNCDs will be assisted to be able to identify barriers that could be common to impede successful self-management of the disease. Mostly the barriers that exist are co-morbidities which aggravates the existing condition which needs to be self-managed. Therefore, it means that self-management strategies developed with the assistance of the HCPs must include on how to also manage the co-morbidities. A Mixed Method United States study investigating barriers to chronic disease reporting in public schools reported that improving parental education will help in improving chronic disease reporting [4].

2.3 Practice

HCPs are encouraged to support PLWNCDs in self-management of the condition by making changes in practice systems to accommodate these individuals. Group visits or support groups sessions could be arranged on scheduled times known to everyone who belongs to the group so that they can discuss on how they could self-manage their condition by getting advice from others who are in the similar situations. The HCPs could explain to PLWNCDs the disease management guidelines that could be used including patient reminders and to structure planned visits for review to suits the patients' time. A study about practice change in chronic condition care, encourages the use of theories, which must be adapted and supplemented [5].

Theory enables greater understanding of the relationships amongst factors that influence behavior change [6]. Theories which could be used. Health educational which contains behavior change are extra effective in the management of NCDs. Some of the theories which could be used in practice change includes Health Belief Model (HBF), Trans Theoretical Model (TTM) and Social Cognitive Theory (SCT). The HBF emphasizes that perceived threat as a motivating force and perceived benefits as offering desired course of action, while TTM views behavior change as a process wherein individual's progresses through a chain of awesome stages of change and lastly the SCT describes gaining knowledge as a reciprocal interaction between an individual's cognitive processes, environment and behavior (reciprocal determinism).

2.4 Community

The PLWNCDs could be assisted with improving and controlling pain and mood through participation in programmes emphasizing four efficacy-enhancing strategies: mastery of skills through learning and practice, modeling by inspirational role leaders, encouraging participants to attempt more than they are currently doing and re-interpretation of symptoms to distinguish pain caused by the disease from those that caused by therapeutic interventions. NCDs require life-long self-management with regular HCPs' support and supervision [7–9].

2.5 Telephonic helpline

The Department of Health could assist the PLWNCDs by creating a telephonic helpline where the calls could be answered and assist the PLWNCDs to manage the challenges such as symptoms they are experiencing at that moment prior going to the Primary Health Care Clinic. These telephonic helplines can also assist in clarifying issues like how to take treatment when they have forgotten the medication instructions. It has been found that the use of telephone-based patient self-management of chronic diseases is more cost-effective way to minimize healthcare expenditures [10].

3. Billboards, pamphlets, educational booklets, posters and radio talks

The Department of Health (DoH) and also HCPs have equal responsibilities in making sure that health messages which include health advise reach to individuals in need including PLWNCDs. The DoH has a responsibility of making sure that health messages are placed on billboards which are believed to be influential platform to educate people on health issues. The HCPs professionals have to write Pamphlets, Educational Booklets and Posters which can convey health messages to PLWNCDs. The pamphlets and educational booklets could be distributed at the Primary Health Care clinics and also at local shops and saloons whilst the posters could be displayed on notice boards at the clinics and also on poles along the streets. These will encourage everyone to read through as long as they are visible. Old PLWNCDs who cannot read and write can also request the children whom they are living with to read through for them. All these Billboards, Pamphlets,

Educational Booklets and Posters must also be written in local language. The DoH has to approach local radio stations to provide slots where HCPs could be able to reach out communities to provide Health Education on NCDs. These sessions must also have questions and answers sessions where listeners could be provided with an opportunity to ask questions where they could be provided with an opportunity to be clarified on issues they do not understand as far as NCDs are concerned. It has been found that the use of mass media campaigns can change health behaviors of the people in line with the communicated message [11].

3.1 Other related roles executed by HCPs to assist PLWNCDs to manage NCDs

HCPs should advise PLWNCDs to visit clinics with their families or guardians, at least quarterly, to receive health education together so as facilitate self-management. Support groups for PLWNCDs should be initiated by the facilities to promote acceptance of the condition and give health education when patients come to collect their medication. Community structures must be developed, the Home-Based Carers should be trained to facilitate the programmes to execute activities to assist the PLWNCDs to manage their condition. A South African study reported limitations and challenges to the roles of Community Health Workers (CHWs), which includes not maximally using home visit for health education and further that CHWs are most focused on the sick people and not preventing vulnerable family members [12].

4. Strategies by health care professionals (HCPS) in assisting PLWNCDS to maintain quality of life

It is evident that for the PLWNCDs to adhere to self-management strategies themselves, Health Care Professionals (HCPs) must work together with them to design, develop and implement health plan which has to focus on short and long term goals that could be sustainable, effective, efficient and could be manageable.

The following are the strategies that could be used by HCPs to assist the PLWNCDs which has been found to be successful in countries in the European Region such as Italy, Montenegro, Azerbaijan, and Tajikistan [13], and helped in adherence of self-management strategies and to control the condition:

4.1 Self-management support

Families, friends, community members and different categories of Health Care Providers (HCPs) must be educated on Self-Management Support so that they provide relevant support to PLWNCDs and their family. The support should be developed with the PLWNCDs so that he/she can own the decisions taken and focus on reducing health risk thus maintaining quality of life [14]. The following are the support that is relevant to the PLWNCDs so that they can be encouraged to take care of themselves:

Patient centred: Self-management programs should be initiated so that they empower PLWNCDs to take a lead role in planning care and should support them to work in partnership with their HCP to set goal and action plans [14]. The patients will be able to adhere to what they have planned for with HCP because they were involved from the beginning in planning their care. This will also encourage them to implement all strategies advised with in controlling the disease. It has been found that the management of chronic disease encourages patient-centered care such legitimizing lived experiences with disease and acknowledging patient expertise [15].

Psychological support: It may be necessary to provide psychological support so that people can be able to cope with the disease and also accept their self-manage which might have been changed by the disease [11]. The health care facilities in the Primary Health Care environment must have psychologists to cater for psychological problems. The advices that they give to PLWNCDs will make them to realize that they can be able to avoid the stressors in the environment that they leave in so that they cope with the disease and play a significant role in maintaining their quality of life.

Cultural-relevance: Programmes that are offered for the PLWNCDs should be context-specific because it will also be culturally sensitive and appropriate for different cultural groupings that might exists in the same community [14], provision of care to communities must be relevant and appropriate so that it could accepted by everyone. Thompson [16] recommended that medical interventions should recognize and respect diversity of religious, spiritual and cultural beliefs in the practice.

Systematic follow-up: HCP at primary health care level have to conduct clinical assessments on the people in need at community level and follow-up care system must be established [14]. Self-Management Support has been found to be the most frequently used intervention in Chronic Care Model, which is associated with improvements, particularly amongst people living with diabetes and/or hypertension [17].

4.2 Self-management responsibility

The PLWNCDs have to take responsibility to maintain their own health by making sure that they manage themselves remotely away from the HCPs.

- It is advisable that those with smartphones could be able to set up reminders on their cellphones to remind them on the time to take their medications, clinic follow-up dates and also save short messages of when to eat and the type of diet to take. These reminders have been proven to assist in adherence to medication instructions and also health advise. It is evident that all these methods of reminding a person will assist them in adhering to medication and health advise instructions.

- The PLWNCDs has to be provide with a small room at the Primary Health Care clinic where they can be able to monitor their own vital signs with simple operated machine such as Blood Pressure, Temperature, Glucometer machine and weighing scale as these will assist them with self-monitoring without calling any HCP to assist.

- Initiating support groups at Primary Health Care level when visiting the clinics will assist PLWNCDs in advising one another on how to adhere to all health and medication advise and instructions so as to achieve health outcomes when living with NCDs, share experiences and also share strategies they use to adhere to health instructions.

- The PLWNCDs must commit themselves to behavioral change as this is key in making sure that they eliminate what is harmful to their bodies and maintain behaviors that will promote quality of life which include amongst other things adherence to correct diet, engaging in physical activity, cessation of smoking and drinking an acceptable amounts of alcohol.

Disclosing the disease to family members who will in turn play a role in treatment supporter and also encouraging to adhere to health advice such making sure that the whole family control salt intake and engage in physical activity just to support PLWNCDs that they are living with. The family members will also do more in making sure that they support their loved ones [1].

5. Strategies that could be adhered to at community level to manage NCDS

The following are the NCDs management strategies that could be used at community level to manage the disease:

5.1 Establishment of trust within community members

Interpersonal positive relationships amongst community is key for management of NDCs because they can support and adhere to reasonable self-management strategies in controlling and maintaining quality of life whilst living with the disease. Establishment of mentors within the communities to promote maintenance of healthy lifestyle and encourage PLWNCDs to adhere to health care and medication instructions. An American Study pointed out that the structural collaboration between health system and community organizations helps in improving healthcare access at community level and also promoting preventive culture [18].

5.2 Establishment of community forum

These types of forum will assist in bringing PLWNCDs together and support one another by sharing their experiences and how people are managing challenges they come across. Additionally, the forum sessions will assist in discussing which specific strategy could be used to solve and adapt to what PLWNCDs are experiencing. More knowledge will be acquired from these forums related to the disease. The health professionals are expected to form part of this forum to provide medical advice always through workshops and health education sessions. This forum could also assist in reaching out for community members who are unable to travel to hospitals due to lack of financial resources to cater for transport. The community members could also be able to identify amongst themselves people who will be able to assist with daily support to PLWNCDs so that they are able to adhere to appropriate self-management strategies. Furthermore, the community forums could engage with the local businesses so that they paste posters and distribute pamphlets that have self-management strategies for PLWNCDs. The health interventions programmes to control risk factors at community levels requires trained NCDs nurses, functional equipments and community forums [19].

5.3 Involve of partners in managing NCDs

Partners of PLWNCDs can play a significant role in management of NCDs by making sure that resources needed are always to adhere to healthy life style, supporting them to adhere to medication, assisting in household responsibilities amongst other things raising children and others so as to alleviate them from stressors that could aggravate the disease. Supporting their partners to adhere to health education instructions and supporting them during medical consultations is significant. Spousal support has been found to positively influence health outcomes and improve quality of life of patients [20].

5.4 Common transportation to hospital for follow up visits

The communities could be able to arrange common transport during the days allocated by nearest clinics and or hospitals to manage chronic diseases. This will assist in such a way that PLWNCDs will be able to budget for the transport money which might be cheaper than arranging own transport or even using public transport. This might also promote the sense of belonging to a group which might even serve as a support of group of PLWNCDs. It has been found that the strong and well-organized community involvement can positively influence provision of healthcare at primary healthcare level [18].

5.5 Fighting stigma associated with NCDs

Stigmatization is regarded as public health issue faced by PLWNCDs leading to their discrimination, isolation and social rejection from the society [21]. Stigmatization may negatively impact on the health of PLWNCDs and further increase the overall burden of the disease. The HCPs needs to take actions to help PLWNCDs on ways to fight the stigma through hearing experiences of the patients and further raising community awareness.

6. Strategies that could be used to support self-management for PLWNCDS

The self-management strategies that could be used are inclusive of that the PLWNCDs have to realize that they have responsibility to take care of self in managing the chronic condition which has to go beyond identifying the challenges they are experiencing but to solve problems they have. The perception is that if PLWNCDs practice healthy lifestyle to mitigate predisposing factors therefore they will be able to also manage the condition later in life [22]. Self-management of chronic condition calls for the PLWNCDs to work together with family, community and also the HCP to manage the condition in facilitating care this will be focusing on promoting wellness and lessening deterioration of health.

Self-management strategies must include the following:

6.1 The importance of knowledge acquisition related to the disease

The PLWNCDs must seek knowledge related to the condition, treatment they are taking and lifestyle to maintain. This will enhance how they management the condition because they will be able to know all aspects related to the disease condition including the complications, the type of treatment and its side effects. These will assist them to adhere to health advise and medication instructions. The existence of knowledge about the condition and all related aspects will enable them to take a lead in making lifestyle changes to promote quality of life.

6.2 Development of self-management plan

The PLWNCDs are expected to develop a self-management plan which is inclusive of strategies which will assist in coping with psychological effects caused by the condition. They need to request for the psychological assistance with problem solving and decision-making skills related to daily life experiences and or challenges. Given the problem solving and decision-making skills they would have acquired they will be assisted in adherence to health advise and medication instructions.

The PLWNCDs must draw a self-management plan that include action plan of enhancing health advise and medication adherence because if they draw the plan themselves with short- and long-term goals, they will own that decision and make sure that they achieve what was planned.

6.3 Cessation of smoking and alcohol intake

The PLWNCDs who are smoking have to stop and those who are drinking excessively alcohol are encouraged to minimize. The reasons for the importance of the changed behavior must be clear to PLWNCDs so that they do not return back to old habits ever again. The importance of cessation of smoking that must be known to PLWNCDs is that the risk of developing acute myocardial infarction drops immediately when one stops smoking and continues to decline each year until ones' health is the same as those who are not smoking within the period of 5 years. Smoking cause the development of atherosclerotic disease, acute coronary disease and has an effect on platelets and for PLWNCDs to smoking will save them from ill health adding to already what they are experiencing [22].

The importance of not drinking alcohol for the PLWNCDs is that they will be saving themselves from liver diseases such as alcoholic hepatitis and pancreatitis [23]. Therefore, it will be valuable for PLWNCDs to quit than to continue smoking and or drinking alcohol as there are more complications that may arise.

6.4 Monitoring of ones' vital signs and symptoms

The PLWNCDs must be taught and know how to monitor vital signs and symptoms of the condition so that they could seek for medical help and or control them timeously to prevent severe complications. This will also assist them to adhere to a lifestyle that bring about improvements in their daily living. Self-monitoring of vital signs and symptoms is useful because it leads to reduction of hospitalization and re-admissions to hospitals because PLWNCDs can be able to identify problems and deal with them timeously [24]. Cardiovascular diseases, cancer, chronic respiratory diseases and diabetes are amongst the leading cause of NCDs with specific signs and symptoms [25], however, common signs and symptoms of NCDs includes pain, fever, headaches, swelling, inflammations, and stiffness of joints.

6.5 Minimize salt, sugar sweetened and unhealthy food

Salt and sugar sweetened intake need to be controlled as it influences the functioning of the cardiovascular systems resulting in worsening the condition for PLWNCDs. The regular consumption of salt intake and sugar-sweetened food is discouraged for PLWNCDs because they contribute to an increase in blood glucose and blood pressure. Many guidelines recommend that patients with NCDs should reduce both sugar-sweetened and sodium intake. PLWNCDs need to know the type of drinks that should not be taken as they could raise blood sugar levels and also high blood. The PLWNCDs need to know that they can improve their blood sugar levels when their carbohydrates intake is between 5–35% of their calories. The key to eating well when living with NCDs is to eat a variety of healthy food from each of the food groups that is Proteins, Carbohydrates, Fruits and Vegetables. PLWNCDs have to avoid food such as cakes, cookies, refined grains, muffins or anything made of white flour [26]. Therefore, changes in diet involve PLWNCDs' greater commitment and introducing changes in lifestyle that are not necessarily happily accepted but to give up consuming foods that they truly enjoy but which they are forced to exclude in their diet [24]. A healthy eating includes intake of 400 g or five portions of fruits and vegetables, 30% of total energy intake of fats [27], less than 10% of total energy intake from free sugars, which is equivalent to 50 g or about 12 teaspoons [28], less than 5 g of salt per day which is half a teaspoon [29] and consumption of variety of food.

6.6 Engage in healthy habits

The PLWNCDs has to stop to engage in unhealthy activities and modify their lifestyle in totality in order to promote quality of life [30]. The by PLWNCDs must engage in physical activity, adhere to diet, medical and health advise which is good for their condition [31]. It must also be clear to PLWNCDs that adherence to correct diet, medical and health advise is important because what one eats and do influence how the body reacts to a condition.

The PLWNCDs must engage in physical activity so that they can keep lower blood pressure and cholesterol levels lower, improve blood flow and keep body weight under control. Furthermore, they must know that physical activity boosts energy level that will assist in getting work done without feeling exhaustion, it promotes positive attitude in an individual that resulting in relieving someone stress of not appreciating oneself and it promote sleep thus resulting in a good rest. The PLWNCDs need to know that engaging in household chores does not not replace in engaging in physical activity.

6.7 Management of own stress levels

Another self-management strategy that PLWNCDs must adhere to is to **manage own stress levels** to avoid falling into depression that could worsen their condition to an uncontrollable state. Stress is one of the main problems amongst PLWNCDs and this led to development of chronicity which must be avoided by the people. In other words, stress can be considered as a cause and as well as a consequence of NCDs. On the other hand, stress increase glucose and glycosylated hemoglobin which may increase stress levels amongst individuals with Type 2 diabetes, as well as causing other physical, behavioral and mental disorders [32], this must be avoided, and HCPs need to skill up by PLWNCDs.

NCDs management must be known to by PLWNCDs as a constant process; it is an ongoing challenge that maybe complicated by the impact of stress. Excessive stress is a major barrier to effective control of the condition and a danger to PLWNCDs' general health. Whether or not you have NCDs, stress is harmful because it causes so much wear and tear on the body. The ability to think clearly and to make good decisions is impaired when the mind is burdened therefore, it is advisable to PLWNCDs to seek professional help when they feel stressed and be able to know when they are stressed [33]. Stress management and avoidance of stressors is key when leaving with NCDs to promote quality of life.

6.8 The importance of adherence to prescribed medication and Health advise to maintain quality of life

The PLWNCDs are dependent on treatment they collect from the health facilities therefore it is important that they are encouraged to collect their medications as instructed so that they do not miss the treatment. However, in rural areas sometimes medications are not always available when they arrived to collect in Primary Health Care clinics therefore, the PLWNCDs are advised to go 3 days or prior finishing the medications that they are having so that if they do not find them they will be having enough to visit the nearest hospital to get the medications. They are also encouraged to have treatment buddies who ae relatives who will encourage and monitor them to take treatment as prescribed. It is also important that PLWNCDs have knowledge of the importance of adherence to treatment such as its efficacy, pharmacological action and complications when it is not taken correctly. The fact NCDs management is complex, requiring a life-long commitment and drastic changes to the patient's lifestyle the PLWNCDs has to make sacrifices and adhere to various lifestyle changes which have been mentioned. Social support from family members is also key therefore, PLWNCDs have to disclose their diagnosis to family members so that they can provide them with practical help and can reduce lack of adherence to health advise and medication instructions [34]. Quality of life is about how good or bad a person regards their life to be, and not what other people necessarily imagine it to be [35], and it is maintained through adherence to treatment, exercise and healthy eating.

6.9 Self-care activities

Patients exhibit poor self-care behaviors. This is significantly associated with the level of education and not having knowledge about the NCDs which emanated from low levels of education of PLWNCDs. Therefore, PLWNCDs must be educated of self-care activities which will assist them in maintaining quality of life that is taking care of their selves to be clean, in the era of pandemic such as COVID-19 consistent washing of hand with soap and water, wearing of face musk and staying in a well ventilated space must be maintained. Taking acceptable portion of well-balanced diet without must be an option always for PLWNCDs [36].

Adequate knowledge of foot care to those who have diabetes because if this is not done, they need to know that it might contribute to ulceration that could result in amputation that could increase stress levels in ones' life and further increase financial burden [37].

7. Other related important information for self-management that PLWNCDS could adhere to

The information includes the following:

7.1 Existing knowledge related to medication taken for NCDs

A chronic disease, such as NCDs is taken as a burden for the person who lives with it therefore to accomplish good self-care so that one can be able to accept decisions and self-manage the disease in daily basis. The level of knowledge about the disease empowers the patient to act as an equal partner in the management of the disease [38]. Patient education for NCDs control was found to be the cornerstones of their disease management.

7.2 Self-management programme

The establishment of the education workshops as part of NCDs medical management could assist the PLWNCDs and controlling the disease. The annual meeting and health days whose purpose is to provide a regular forum of communication on management of NCDs will be important to assist the PLWNCDs to manage their condition. In order to accomplish good self-care, patients need to be qualified and able to accept decisions and self-manage a disease on a daily basis and these workshops and meetings could achieve that. The level of knowledge about the disease empowers the patient to act as an equal partner in the management of the disease.

7.3 What need to be done to promote adherence

Low health literacy of PLWNCDs must be addressed through educating them to understand the treatment and also health instructions. These teachings must be personalized for each patient and for each medication. Teach them on how to interpret medication labels and medication information correctly. This is common even when labelling requires minimal reading skills. For example, instructions to take medicine twice daily (which is vague since 'daily' means once per day) or every 12 hours means individuals must make further decisions about what the words actually mean.

"Take medication as directed" is even more difficult to interpret and the instructions need to be broken down further. Patients are more likely to understand more specific medication administration times such as 08 a.m., 06 p.m. but indicating times may be useful to or suit some individuals better than others. These instructions, advice or education must be clear to PLWNCDs to promote adherence.

8. Conclusion

People Living With NCDs from low- and middle- income countries and residing in rural communities can adopt and employ various relevant NCDs self-management strategies for controlling side effects, improve health outcomes and general wellbeing, including maintenance of quality of life.

Author details

Tebogo Maria Mothiba
Faculty of Health Sciences, University of Limpopo, South Africa

*Address all correspondence to: tebogo.mothiba@ul.ac.za

References

[1] Hearn, J., Ssinabulya, I., Schwartz, JI., Akiteng, AR., Ross, HJ. & Cafazzo, JA. Self-management of non-communicable diseases in low- and middle-income countries: A scoping review. *PLoS ONE*, 2019, 14(7): e0219141.https://doi. org/10.1371/ journal.pone.0219141

[2] Xiao, Y. The "expert patient" approach for non-communicable disease management in low- and middle-income settings: When the reality confronts the rhetoric. *Journal of Chronic Disease and Translational Medicine,* 2015, 1(3):145-151.

[3] World Health Organization. Country experiences in integrated policy development for the prevention and control of noncommunicable diseases. Regional Office web site (http://www. euro.who.int/pubrequest). 2015, 1-38, ISBN 978 92 890 5105 7

[4] Herve T, Vignon Z, Line G, Jean-Pierre G, Lauzier S, Lawani AM, Huirat CFL, and Moisan J. Effectiveness of motivational interviewing interventions on medication adherence in adults with chronic diseases: a systematic review and meta-analysis, International Journal of Epidemiology, 2017, 46 (2): 589-602

[5] Rivkina V, Tapke DE, Cardenas LD, et al.. Identifying barriers to chronic disease reporting in Chicago Public Schools: a mixed methods approach. BMC Public Health, 2014, 14, 1250: 1-8

[6] Harris M, Lawn SJ, Morello A, et al. Practice change in chronic conditions care: an appraisal of theories: BMC Health Serv Res, 2017, 17(170): 1-14

[7] Contento IR. Nutrition education: Linking research, theory and practice. Sudbury, Massachusetts: Jones & Barlett; 2007.

[8] Thoesen, M. & Newton, K. Supporting Self-Management in patients with chronic illness. School of medicine: University of Louisville, 2005

[9] McGowan, P., Fredericks, S., Gail, B. & Des Roseirs. Guidelines of strategies to support self-management in chronic conditions: Collaboration with clients. *Clinical Guideline,* Ontario Ministry of Health: Canada, 2009

[10] Boxer, H. & Snyder, S. Family Practice Management. American academy of family physicians, 2009

[11] Avery G, Cook D and Talens S. The impact of a Telephone-Based Chronic Disease Management Program on Medical Expenditure. Popul Health, 2015 (3): 156-162

[12] Wakefield MA, Loken B and Hornik RC. Use of mass media campaigns to change health behaviour. Lancet. 2010, 376 (9748): 1261-1271

[13] Tsolekile LP, Puoane T, Schneider H, Levitt NS and Steyn K. The roles of community health workers in management of non-communicable diseases in an urban township. Afr J Prim Health Care Fam Med.2014, 6(1): E1-E8

[14] Brake, L.C., Muere, R.H. & Kehl, K.A. *Self-management support for people with long term conditions*. 2ndedition. Wellington: Ministry of Health. 2015.

[15] Deter HC. Psychosocial interventions for patients with chronic disease. Biopsychosocial Med, 2012 (6)2: 1-10

[16] Thompson G. Chronic illness, spirituality, and healing: diverse disciplinary, religious, and cultural perspectives, Disability & Society, 2014, 29:8, 1335-1336, DOI: 10.1080/09687599.2014.934063

[17] Reynolds R, Dennis S, Hasan L, et al. A systematic review of chronic disease management interventions in primary care. BMC Farm Pract, 2018, 19(11):1-8

[18] Vidal, N., León-García, M., Jiménez, M. *et al.* Community and health staff perceptions on non-communicable disease management in El Salvador's health system: a qualitative study. *BMC Health Serv Res* **20,** 474 (2020). https://doi.org/10.1186/s12913-020-05249-8

[19] Maimela, E., Alberts, M., Bastiaens, H. *et al.* Interventions for improving management of chronic non-communicable diseases in Dikgale, a rural area in Limpopo Province, South Africa. *BMC Health Serv Res* **18,** 331 (2018). https://doi.org/10.1186/s12913-018-3085-y

[20] Baig, A.A, Benitez, A, Quinn, M.T, and Burnet, D.L. 2015. Family interventions to improve diabetes outcomes for adults. *Annals of the New York Academy of Sciences*. 1353(1): 89-112. Available in PMC 2016 September 01.

[21] Elliot VL, Morgan D, Kosteniuk J, Froehlich Chow A, Bayly M. Health-related stigma of non-communicable neurological disease in rural adult populations: A scoping review. Health Soc Care Community. 2019;27:e158–e188. https://doi.org/10.1111/hsc.12694

[22] Grady, PA. & Gough LL. Self-management: A Comprehensive approach to management of chronic condition. *American Journal of Public Health, 2014,* 104(8): e25-e31

[23] Parry, C., Patra, J. & Rehm, J. Alcohol Consumption and non-communicable disease: Epidemiology and policy implication. *Addiction, 2011,* 106(10): 1718-1724

[24] McBain, H., Shipley, M. & Newman, S. The impact of self-monitoring in chronic illness on healthcare utilization: A systematic review of reviews. *BMC Health Services Research*, 2015, 15:656

[25] Joseph N, Srinath R, Ramanathan A, Gupta AK, Nandan P, Afnan R. Awareness of risk factors, warning signs, and immediate management measures of noncommunicable diseases: A multihospital-based study. J Nat Sc Biol Med 2018;9:227-235

[26] Nicholas, H. Foods to avoid for people with diabetes, reviewed by N Butler. Medical news. 2017

[27] World Health Organization. Guidelines: Sodium intake for adults and children. 2012

[28] World Health Organization. Guidelines: Sugars intake for adults and children. 2015

[29] World Health Organization. Diet, nutrition and the prevention of chronic diseases: report of a joint WHO/FAO Expert Consultation. WHO Technical Report Series, No. 916. Geneva. 2003

[30] Jawarski, M., Panczyk, M., Cedro, M. & Kucharska, A. Adherence to dietary recommendations in diabetic mellitus: Disease acceptance as a potential mediator. 2017, From: http://doi.org/10.2147/ppa.s147233

[31] Dineen-Griffin, S., Garcia-Gardenas, V., William, K.& Benrimoj, SI. Helping patients help themselves: A systematic review of self-management support strategies in primary health care practice. *Plos One, 2019,* 14(8): e0220116

[32] Brammon, L., Feist, J. & Updegraff, J.A. *Health psychology: An introduction to behaviour and health.* Boston Cengage Learning, 2013

[33] Joseph, P.N. Managing stress and diabetes. Diabetes forecast magazine, 2013

[34] Miller, T.A. & Dimatteo, M.R. Importance of family/social support and impact on adherence to diabetic therapy: Diabetes, metabolic syndrome, 2013

[35] Raghavendra N, Viveki RG, Gadgade A. 2017. An observational study to assess the health-related quality of life of type 2 diabetes mellitus patients attending a tertiary care hospital, Belagavi. Int J Community Med Public Health; 4:3347-53.

[36] Glantz, S. & Gonzalez, M. Effective tobacco control is key to rapid progress in reduction of non-communicable diseases. *Lancet,* 2021, 379(9822): 1269-1271.

[37] Cgang, L., Chen, C. & Chen, M. 2013.The devil in the detail. *Prevention of diabetic foot ulceration in rural areas is possible. Open j knurs,* 3:257-264

[38] McElfish, P.A., Bridges, M.D. & Hudson, J.S. 2015. Family model of diabetes education with a pacific Islander community. Diabetes education. 41(6): 706-715

Chapter 20

Exploring Cardiovascular Diseases Treatment in Africa

Masebata Ramathebane, Lineo Maja and Molungoa Sello

Abstract

This topic explores current treatments of cardiovascular diseases; what treatment outcomes emanate from current drug treatment. It also covers the reasons why many studies show poor treatment outcomes. It deals with adverse drug reaction and their drug management where necessary. Current cost effective interventions including prevention strategies including drug treatments are discussed. Issues relating to patients' knowledge about medication and benefits of adhering to treatment, method of delivery of patient information, are dealt with in detail. It highlights the issues of barriers to adherence to drug treatment and non-drug life style modifications. It also deals with dispensing models that encourage adherence to medication. It explores reasons for late diagnosis and treatment. This chapter will be informed by current studies published in Africa and elsewhere.

Keywords: treatment, adherence, knowledge, cost – effective analysis, dispensing models, late diagnosis, treatment outcomes

1. Introduction

According to the World Health Organization (WHO), Non-Communicable Diseases (NCDs) refers to the non-infectious and the non-transmissible medical conditions or diseases. These diseases generally progress slowly and are of long duration. The prevalence of NCDs and risk factors varies considerably between countries, urban/rural location and other sub-populations [1]. The four main types of NCDs are cardiovascular diseases, cancers, chronic respiratory diseases and diabetes. Globally, NCDs are the leading causes of deaths; accounting for over 70% of world deaths (56 million in 2015). Some of these deaths are regarded premature as 27% of these deaths occur in people aged between 30 and 70 years. It has been found that 80% of these premature deaths occur in the low-and middle-income countries.

The World Health Organization estimates that mortality due to NCDs will rise by 17% globally in the next decade; while the African region only will experience 27% increase by 2030. Some African countries such as Algeria (76%), Egypt (84%), Libya (72%), Mauritius (89%), Morocco (80%), Sao Tome and Principe (55%), Seychelles (81%), South Africa (51%), Sudan (52%) and Tunisia (86%) have already witnessed over 50% deaths attributed to NCDs since 2018 [2]. Deaths solely attributed to cardiovascular disease (CVD) are the leading almost globally of all other NCDs. The implications to the increasing prevalence of NCDs are that NCDs will soon be the leading causes of illness, disability and death (including premature deaths) in Africa.

There are eight behavioral and physiological risk factors associated with high and continually increasing burden of NCDs, namely, tobacco use, harmful use of alcohol, consumption of unhealthy diet, physical inactivity, overweight and obesity, high blood pressure, raised blood glucose and raised total cholesterol in blood [3]. Since 2011, NCDs have been elevated onto global, regional and national development agendas through a series of political commitments. These include the 2011 United Nations (UN) Political Declaration on NCD Prevention and Control, 2011 Brazzaville Declaration on NCD Prevention and Control in the WHO African Region, WHO Global NCD Action Plan 2013–2020, 2025 Global NCD targets and 2015 Sustainable Development Goals [4, 5].

With the above global and regional background of NCDs and initiatives, the aim of this chapter is to.

2. Cardiovascular diseases

Cardiovascular diseases (CVDs) refers to a group of disorders affecting the heart and the blood vessels supplying the heart itself (coronary heart disease, rheumatic heart disease, and congenital heart disease), the brain (cerebrovascular disease), the arms and legs (peripheral artery disease, deep vein thrombosis and pulmonary embolism) [6]. Cardiovascular diseases are usually associated with a build-up of fatty deposits inside the arteries (atherosclerosis) and increasing the risk of blood clotting and vessel damage; leading to heart attacks and strokes [7]. Depending on the organ by which blood vessels are damaged, CVDs are also associated with eye, brain, kidney and heart diseases.

More often, CVDs may not have symptoms relating to underlying disease to blood vessels; but heart attack and stroke as usually the first warning of underlying CVD. Heart attack, also known as myocardial infarction, occurs because of failure to supply oxygen-rich blood to a certain part of the heart muscle due to blockade of the blood vessels supplying that part; leading to muscle cell death in that oxygen deprived area (infarct) [8]. Heart attack manifests as sharp chest pain and discomfort at the center of the chest; radiating to the arms, left shoulder, elbows, jaw and back. During the attack episode, the person may also have trouble in breathing. According to Centers for Disease Control, similar to heart attack, stroke occurs because of failure to supply oxygen-rich blood to a certain part of the brain due to blockade of the blood vessels supplying that part; and bursting of the blood vessel in the brain; leading to death of that part of the brain that is deprived of oxygen-rich blood [9]. Strokes are characterized by sudden symmetrical weakness of the limbs, face. The person experiences confusion, difficulty in speaking, vision, walking and there is loss of balance, coordination and unconsciousness may happen.

According to Plotnikoff and Dusek, hypertension (HTN) is the most important risk factor to getting ill and dying from a CVD [10]. The World Health Organization defined hypertension, also known as high blood pressure (BP), as the condition in which the blood vessels have persistently high pressure. The blood pressure is increased by the sympathetic nervous system and the renin-aldosterone-angiotensin system (RAAS). A drop in blood pressure is detected by pressure-sensitive receptors (baroceptors) which send signals to the cardiovascular centers in the spinal cord. This prompts a reflex response of increased sympathetic nervous system activity on the heart and blood vessels; resulting in increased cardiac output and vasoconstriction. The baroceptors in the kidneys respond to a decrease in blood pressure by releasing the enzyme hormone called renin. Renin converts angiotensinogen component of blood to angiotensin I; that ultimately gets converted to angiotensin II by angiotensin converting enzyme (ACE). Angiotensin II is a potent vasoconstrictor, constricting both arteries and veins. The activity of both sympathetic nervous system and RAAS result in increase in blood pressure [11].

The seventh report of the Joint National Committee on Prevention, Detection, Evaluation and Treatment of High Blood Pressure (JNC 7) define a normal BP as less than 120 mm Hg systolic and less than 80 mm Hg diastolic. If left uncontrolled and untreated, high blood pressure can result in an enlargement of the heart, heart attack, heart failure and eventually to death. Hypertension is also associated with loss of vision, cognitive and erectile dysfunction. The higher the pressure above normal, the greater is the risk of complications [12]. Hypertension is the culprit with end-organ damage in terms of all CVDs (stroke, kidney failure and peripheral vascular disease).

3. Current treatments of CVDs

Despite advances made to the treatment and prevention, CVDs are still the leading causes of death of all NCDs. Nevertheless, majority of CVDs are preventable with just lifestyle changes alone. An integrative approach has been adopted to the prevention and treatment of CVDs; as the approach address the root causes influenced by lifestyle. The approach acknowledges that the great value and potential life-saving benefits of modern pharmacology and procedures cannot use only one approach since each has own limitation [13]. The combinatory approach allows for counteracting limitations of one approach with the other approach. The goal of treating CVDs is to improve cardiovascular health and reduce deaths from heart disease and stroke.

4. Therapeutic lifestyle changes (TLCs)

Therapeutic lifestyle changes are the foundation for non-drug management of HTN and/or CVD. These include smoking cessation, reduced intake of sodium diet, the Dietary Approach to Stop Hypertension (DASH), body weight management, moderation of alcohol consumption and physical activity. The American Diabetes Association (ADA) 2020 standards of medical care recommend that for patients with blood pressure > 120/80 mmHg, lifestyle intervention consists of weight loss if overweight or obese, DASH-style eating pattern including reducing sodium and increasing potassium intake, moderation of alcohol intake, and increased physical activity [14].

4.1 Smoking cessation

Smoking increases the risk of developing serious health problems and death. It is estimated that there are 1.1 billion people who smoke and 80% of them come from the low-to-middle income countries (LMICs). Further estimates reveal that smokers are likely to develop heart disease and stroke 2–4 times higher compared to non-smokers. The **Table 1** below is a summary of the health benefits of quitting smoking from 20 minutes to 15 years adapted from the forefront UChicago Medicine [15].

4.2 Reduced intake of sodium diet

High sodium intake, estimated at >2 grams per day which is equivalent to 5 grams of table salt per day, contributes to high blood pressure and increases risk of heart disease and stroke. If global salt intake could be reduced to recommended levels, an estimated 2.5 million deaths could be prevented [16]. In a systematic review and meta regression done on salt intake in sub-Saharan Africa, the results of the study revealed high sodium intake in many adult population (and some populations of children) above the 2 g intake recommended as the upper limit established by WHO [17].

Time of quitting smoking	Extent of body recovery
20 minutes	Heart rate and blood pressure drops
24 hours	Chance of heart attack decreases
2–12 weeks	Blood circulation improves and lung function improves
1–9 months	Cough, difficulty in breathing and sinus congestion are lowered
1 year	Risk of heart disease drops to half compared to that of a smoker
5 years	Risk of cancers of the mouth, throat, gullet and bladder are cut by half. Stroke risk is reduced to that of a nonsmoker 5 to 15 years after quitting.
10 years	Risk of lung cancer drops to half compared to that of a smoker and risk of cancer of the mouth, throat, esophagus, bladder, cervix, and pancreas decreases.
15 years	Risk of heart disease is equal to that of a non-smoker

Table 1.
Time of quitting smoking and extent of body recovery.

There is a strong content-dependent relationship between raised blood pressure and consumption of high amounts of sodium. Dietary guidelines recommend a daily intake of sodium at less than 2.3 grams in the general population and less than 1.5 grams in people with high blood pressure, diabetes, kidney disease and those aged 50 years old or more. Salt reduction initiates a decline in average blood pressure in a week time. It also improves the body response blood pressure medicines. Lowering blood pressure reduces risk of heart disease, stroke and death due to salt related CVDs.

4.3 The DASH eating plan

The pioneer trial that examined the role of diet in the management of hypertension was the DASH trial in 1997. The results of the trial revealed that after approximately 3 g sodium intake per day on both control and interventional group; within 2 weeks of the intervention, blood pressures reduced and the results sustained for another 6 weeks. Systolic blood pressure (SBP) reduced by 5.5 mm Hg and diastolic blood pressure (DBP) by 3.0 mm Hg more than the control diet [18].

The DASH eating plan entails a diet rich in fruits and vegetables (8–10 servings/day); and low-fat dairy foods (2–3 servings/day), coupled with reduced saturated and total fat [19]. DASH is a flexible and balanced eating plan that helps create a heart-healthy eating style for life. The DASH eating plan requires no special foods and instead provides daily and weekly nutritional goals. DASH eating plan recommends that the choice of foods should also be based on food that are:

- Rich in potassium, calcium, magnesium, fiber (roughage) and protein
- Low in saturated fat (animal fat) and trans-fats (from snacks)
- Lower in sodium (table salt, flavourants, spices, processed foods including water)

Globally, calories obtained from Proteins, Sugars and Fats have been increasing and those from roughage-rich foods have been declining. Consumption of processed foods continues to rise rapidly in low- and middle-income settings. This nutrition transition affects dietary patterns and nutrient intake, which influence the risk of developing NCDs.

DASH diet is one among such healthy dietary patterns, which emphasizes on;

- Consumption of fruits, vegetables and low-fat dairy foods.
- Whole grains, poultry, fish, and small quantities of red meat, sweets and drinks containing sugar.
- The increased risk of cardiovascular diseases associated with higher sodium intake (>5 g/day) is most prominent in those with high blood pressure.

4.4 Body weight management

Overweight and obesity are major risk factors for a number of chronic diseases, including CVDs such as heart disease and stroke, which are the leading causes of death worldwide. Globally, obesity is one side of the double burden of malnutrition, and today more people are obese than underweight in most regions of the world. A body mass index (BMI) over 25 kg/m^{-2} is considered overweight, and over 30 kg/m^{-2} is obese. The issue has grown to epidemic proportions, with over 4 million people dying each year as a result of being overweight or obese in 2017 according to the global burden of disease [20]. Nevertheless, modest weight losses of 5 to <10% were associated with significant improvements in CVD risk factors at one year, but larger weight losses had greater benefits [21].

4.5 Moderation of alcohol consumption

The Centers for Disease Control and Prevention (CDC) define alcohol moderation as having up to one drink per day for women and up to two drinks per day for men. The definition refers to the amount consumed on any single day and is not intended as an average over several days [22]. However, it is not recommended that that people who do not drink alcohol start drinking for any reason. Excessive alcohol intake includes binge drinking, heavy drinking and any alcohol use during pregnancy. Binge drinking corresponds to five or more drinks in men and four or more drinks in women on a single occasion, generally within two hours; while heavy drinking is defined as consuming 15 drinks or more per week for men and eight drinks or more per week in women. In 2019, top nine African countries with high alcohol consumption in liters per capita were in the order of Nigeria, Eswatini, South Africa, Lesotho, Zimbabwe, Zambia, Malawi, Ghana and Morocco [23]. Excessive alcohol consumption increases the risk of developing heart disease by increasing BP and weakening heart muscles [24].

4.6 Physical activity

Globally, lack of sufficient physical activity is the fourth risk factor to development of NCDs. While physical inactivity is attributed to prevalence of diabetes at 27%, heart diseases caused by heart vessels blockage at 30% and breast and colon cancer at 21–25%; 3.2–5 million deaths globally are associated with physical inactivity [25]. The World Health Organization defines physical activity as a bodily movement produced by muscular and skeletal body systems which require energy expenditure. In other words, physical activity encompasses all activities undertaken while working, playing, carrying out household chores, traveling, recreation; in addition to exercise activities. Physical activity is further classified as moderate- and vigorous-intensity physical activity. Also, physical activities are sub-classified as aerobic (those that engage large muscles of the hands and legs; making the heartbeat and breathing rate to be faster than normal), muscle-strengthening (those that improve the strength, power, and endurance of your muscles) and bone-strengthening (those that strengthen feet, legs arm to support body weight) [26].

In order to gain health benefits of physical activity; it is recommended that children and adolescents should do at least 60 minutes of moderate to vigorous-intensity physical activity daily; while adults should do at least 150 minutes of moderate-intensity physical activity throughout the week, or at least 75 minutes of vigorous-intensity physical activity throughout the week. Those with poor mobility should perform physical activity to enhance balance and prevent falls, three or more days per week. The general rule is that two minutes of moderate-intensity activity counts the same as one minute of vigorous-intensity activity and the exercise should continue up to sweating [27].

Regular and sufficient levels of physical activity are attributed to the following cardiovascular benefits;

- Strengthened heart
- Reduced risk of heart attack
- Reduced risk of hypertension (high blood pressure), heart diseases, stroke, diabetes, various types of cancer (including breast and colon) and depression.
- Maintained healthy body weight control
- Reduced blood cholesterol level

5. Pharmacological treatment of CVDs in Africa

According to Rizos and Elisaf [28] hypertensive patients with African ancestry are a distinctive population of patients that presents with some unique characteristics. These patients commonly have increased incidence and early onset of hypertension and often-poor BP control. They often present at healthcare facilities with additional concomitant CVD risk factors.

The ADA 2020 standards on pharmacological interventions to CVDs recommend the following:

Patients with confirmed office based blood pressure ≥ 140/90 mmHg should, in addition to lifestyle therapy, have prompt initiation and timely titration of pharmacologic therapy to achieve blood pressure goals.

This is strongly emphasized in the African ancestry population that appropriate TLCs and combination of diuretic and/or calcium channel blocker (CCB) should be initiated promptly. In African black populations, patients receive aggressive treatment at lower BPs compared to non-African, non-black counterparts who are recommended initial combination therapy when they fit the requirement below.

Patients with confirmed office based blood pressure ≥ 160/100 mmHg should, in addition to lifestyle therapy, have prompt initiation and timely titration of two drugs or a single-pill combination of drugs demonstrated to reduce cardiovascular events in patients with diabetes.

Treatment for hypertension should include drug classes demonstrated to reduce cardiovascular events in patients with diabetes (ACE inhibitors, angiotensin receptor blockers, thiazide-like diuretics, or dihydropyridine calcium channel blockers).

Whites generally responded better to β-blockers and ACE inhibitors whereas blacks generally responded better to diuretics and calcium channel blockers [29].

Multiple-drug therapy is generally required to achieve blood pressure targets. However, combinations of ACE inhibitors and angiotensin receptor blockers and combinations of ACE inhibitors or angiotensin receptor blockers with direct renin inhibitors should not be used.

Pharmacologically ACE inhibitors, angiotensin receptor blockers and renin inhibitors act on the renin-aldosterone-angiotensin system to lower the cardiac pre- and after-load. So giving one class will be sufficient; although black populations generally respond poorly to ACE inhibitors [29].

An ACE inhibitor or angiotensin receptor blocker, at the maximum tolerated dose indicated for blood pressure treatment, is the recommended first-line treatment for hypertension in-patients with diabetes and urinary albumin-to-creatinine ratio $\geq$ 300 mg/g creatinine or 30–299 mg/g creatinine. If one class is not tolerated, the other should be substituted.

For patients treated with an ACE inhibitor, angiotensin receptor blocker, or diuretic, serum creatinine/estimated glomerular filtration rate and serum potassium levels should be monitored at least annually [11].

The insufficiencies associated with availability of necessary resources to monitor treatment of CVDs in Low-Middle Income Countries (LMICs) are major barriers to having integrated healthcare system with an effective data flow. These resources include technological infrastructure, financial and human resources [30].

6. Phamacovigilance of antihypertensive medications

According to the World Health Organization definition, an adverse drug reaction (ADR) is 'a response to a drug that is noxious and unintended and occurs at doses normally used in human for the prophylaxis, diagnosis, and treatment of disease, or for modification of physiological function' [26]. Also, pharmacovigilance (PV) defined by WHO as "the science and activities relating to the detection, assessment, understanding and prevention of adverse effects or any other drug-related problem [31].

In Africa, countries differ in terms of a having fully functional PV systems due to differing capacities of national medicines regulatory authorities and performance levels with respect to conducting various pharmacovigilance activities. Therefore, the system for reporting adverse drugs reactions has significant gaps to be strengthened from one country to another [32, 33]. However, in some settings within African countries, the following suspected ADRs were documented as indicated in **Table 2** [34].

Adverse drug reaction	System organ classifications (Medical Dictionary for Regulatory Activities)	Drugs class(es)
Frequent micturition	Renal and urinary disorders	Diuretics, CCBs,
Dizziness	Nervous system disorders	Diuretics, CCBs, ACEIs, Centrally acting, β-blockers, α- blockers
Headaches	Nervous system disorders	Diuretics, CCBs, Centrally acting,
Diarrhea	Gastrointestinal disorders	ACEIs
Weakness	Musculoskeletal and connective tissue disorders	Diuretics, CCBs, Centrally acting
Dry cough	Respiratory, thoracic and mediastinal disorders	ACEIs

Table 2.
ADRS, system organ classifications and suspected causal drug classes.

7. Cost effectiveness of cardiovascular disease prevention and treatment

The highest age standardized death rate from non-communicable diseases (NCDs) (779 per 100, 000) occur mostly in the African Region [35]. In sub Saharan Africa, the probability of dying from NCDs between 30 and 70 years is very high. It is also indicated that behavioral risk factors are estimated to be responsible for about 80% of coronary heart disease and cerebrovascular disease and these include tobacco use, physical inactivity, unhealthy diet and harmful use of alcohol. The cost of implementing reduction measures for tobacco control (smoke-free policies, raise tobacco taxes, package warnings, advertising bans), harmful alcohol consumption, and physical activity and diet modification is found to be low [36]. Usually these costs include media campaigns and overall program management. It is feasible to deliver cardiovascular risk reduction interventions in primary care, even in low-resource settings with non-physician health workers [37]. Currently, there are major gaps in access to these essential primary care interventions in developing countries including in those in sub-Saharan Africa [38].

There are other strategies that can be employed to prevent cardiovascular diseases. This becomes attractive to providers and can lead to policy change. According to recent surveys there is high prevalence of salt consumption [39] in South Africa. The burden of cardiovascular disease (CVD) in the same country is rising, and to address this, the government recently developed policies to reduce salt consumption in the population [39]. Population-based salt reduction strategies have been found to be a cost-effective approach to lowering the prevalence of hypertension and preventing cardiovascular disease (CVD). The cost saving for both household and providers was significantly different. The extended cost-effectiveness analysis (ECEA), which models the health gains, financial risk protection and distributional effects of public policies.

Mathers [40] states that cardiovascular diseases are responsible for about 30% of all deaths worldwide, and total deaths occurring in developing countries amount to about 80% [41]. Several authors have suggested that the combination of several preventive treatments could cut more than half the occurrence of cardiovascular disease [41–43]. The analyses have shown that two multidrug regimens of four highly effective drugs could lead to cost-effective prevention and treatment for patients with cardiovascular disease in all developing regions [44]. Wald and Law [41] specifically proposed a polypill, consisting of a statin, aspirin, a β blocker, an angiotensin-converting-enzyme inhibitor (ACEI), a thiazide, and folic acid. Suggested primary preventive therapy consists of aspirin, ACEI, calcium-channel blocker, and statin. While secondary preventive therapy consists of aspirin, ACEI, β blocker, and statin [41]. If two polypills, consisting of the same drug combinations as the primary and secondary prevention strategies, would also improve adherence, the results would be even more favorable.

In conclusion, these lifestyle modification strategies such as tobacco use control, reduction in harmful effects of alcohol, diet and physical activity and salt intake reduction are perceived to be cost-effective. Primary and secondary preventive treatments are also found to be cost-effective in preventing cardiovascular disease. This can improve on patients quality of life with cost savings.

8. Patients knowledge about cardiovascular diseases and medicines

An individual must know at least 75% of the items used in the summary variables to qualify as having acquired adequate knowledge [45]. For those patients who can achieve adequate knowledge, this should be the target for having comprehensive knowledge. However, in cardiovascular diseases, this may be affected by age, agility, and cognitive skills particularly in elderly patients.

According to Mugomeri and colleagues, nearly 36% had inadequate knowledge about hypertension while 44% had inadequate knowledge about their medicines [46]. In this study, in total, 52.4% of the patients did not turn up for appointment dates while 64.6% failed to take their medications according to the prescription at least once. It was also stated that inadequate knowledge of antihypertensive medicines was significantly associated (P = .028) with having uncontrolled hypertension [46]. Inadequate knowledge of antihypertensive medicines is an important determinant of uncontrolled hypertension [46].

The study carried out on village health workers (VHW) in Lesotho, as health workers, determining adequate knowledge and translation of knowledge to offered services indicated that among household members aged 15 years and above, only a third was advised by the VHW to go for HIV testing [47]. Communities served by VHWs with adequate knowledge did not only demonstrate better knowledge compared to their counterparts served by VHWs with inadequate knowledge, in utilization VHWs' services were high [47]. The finding confirmed what was suggested by the literature of Hirsch-Moverman [48]. Community health workers (CHWs) form part of the primary health care system [47]. The community health workers who have adequate knowledge can play a very important role in their communities in terms of education, monitoring adherence and referrals [47]. It is therefore, recommended that training of CHW on cardiovascular diseases, treatment and prevention of complication be taken as a priority in the African continent.

Information is crucial to promote patients' knowledge which increases the sense of control, decrease emotional distress, support effective self-management, and eliminate disruptions of daily activities [49, 50]. Patients want to have control over their symptoms therefore, they need as much information as possible about their symptoms and strategies to manage these symptoms. The patient knowledge about cardiovascular diseases leads to good management of the diseases. Bandura [51] reiterates that a contributing factor to the difference in symptom self-management is a person's perceived self-efficacy. Perceived self-efficacy forms the basis of any decision to act on and is defined as the perception of one's own ability to implement behavior(s) to achieve designated types of outcomes such as symptom management. Bandura [52] further explains that perceived self-efficacy beliefs are considered to be central and influential factors in determining the course of action to be chosen, the degree of effort applied, and the perseverance to continue in the face of problems and obstacles.

Intervention is required in order to improve the knowledge of patients regarding cardiovascular diseases, hypertension, and associated medications [53, 54]. This intervention comprises of the patient essential educational topics and method of delivery of patient education. Patient education topics should include pathophysiology and etiology, symptoms and signs, pharmacological treatment, risk factor modification, diet and exercise, sexual activity, immunization, sleep and breathing disorders, adherence, psychosocial aspects and prognosis associated with certain skills or self-management behaviors [54–56]. However, patient education alone is not enough, the delivery of patient education content should consider level literacy, age, and other cognitive measures. Medium of delivery of patient education must be individualized according to the needs of the patient. Some patients benefit from one-on-one sessions, while others benefit from group sessions, some still can benefit from both sessions.

The guidelines recommend patient education and counseling targeting patient skills and behavior [57]. For patient education to be effective Meng and colleagues [53] recommend outcome and measurement strategies to enlighten on primary and secondary outcomes. The primary outcome entails self-management competencies which are measured through self-monitoring and insight, skill and technique acquisition, and self-efficacy. While secondary outcomes are measured through self-management health behavior (symptom control, physical activity, medication adherence), health-related quality of life, and treatment satisfaction. Meng and colleagues [53] concluded that a patient-centered self-management might be more effective regarding certain self-management outcomes than a lecture-based usual care education.

Hinderlang [58] suggests that the material for patient education should be developed bearing in mind patients' cultural and language barriers. Patients' preferences should also be considered before embarking on patient education that may not be effective [59]. The content of patient education material should be broken down into concise, manageable sessions that do not overwhelm with vast amounts of facts and details and be free of medical jargon. The learning environment should be free of stress, environmental distractions, cultural conflicts, and value judgments all should be eliminated if possible. Timing should be based on the available time, attention span, and readiness for learning without rushing or taking too much time. The patients have to be actively involved in the process of learning and understand the value of the information and procedures being taught for improving the quality of his or her life [58]. Patients increasingly demand access to medical information, this has improved the patient-physician relationship and consequently improved patient care.

The disease management education plan should also include practical skills for patients and caregivers to participate in their own care. These may include:

a. Gargets to use and how to use them and what readings mean (BP machine etc.)

b. Assess patients understanding and their educational needs

c. Identify patients' barrier to receive information

d. Need to involve a caregiver

e. How to take one's own pulse;

f. How to take weight accurately (at the same time each day, with the same clothing on);

g. How to measure one's blood pressure correctly (if appropriate);

h. How to manage one's medications (which includes the name of drug; purpose it is used for when to take it, what to avoid and how it is stored)

i. Return with the remaining medicines in each clinic visit

j. How to lift one's feet to reduce swelling

k. How to manage food and fluids;

l. How to manage with stress and

m. How to keep a record of weight, blood pressure and any other information on the diary or calendar and share with healthcare workers

n. Self-referral and preferred method of communication

In summary self-efficacy and self-management of cardiovascular diseases will encourage patients to be in control of their diseases, and their treatment. This will improve their treatment outcome. The community health workers can provide education, support and referral roles particularly in rural settings.

9. Adherence to medications

Non-communicable diseases (NCDs) are chronic diseases where adherence to medication is essential to controlling these diseases. Patients with NCDs such as cardiovascular diseases, diabetes mellitus and hypertension are put on long-term therapy to manage their conditions. The health outcomes of these patients depend mainly on how they adhere to medication as well as on lifestyle modification. The World Health Organization (WHO) defined adherence as the extent to which the behavior of a person, such as taking medication, following a diet or lifestyle modification, corresponds with the agreed recommendations from a health care provider [60].

Although adherence is important to patients with NCDs who are on medication, non-adherence to medications is a concern in Africa. In a study conducted among patients with NCDs in Puducherry, South India, the prevalence of low adherence to medication was 32.7% [61]. In contrast, prevalence of poor adherence to diabetes mellitus medication in rural Kerala, South India was 74% [62]. A study conducted in a health facility in a peri-urban district in the Ashanti region of Ghana found that the overall prevalence of medication noncompliance among patients with chronic diseases was 55.5% [63]. Inadequate medication possession ratios and thereby treatment adherence was observed in hypertensive patients at two private outpatient health clinics in Sierra Leone, with more than 80% of patients assessed not having medication for more than 40% of the time period studied [64]. In a specialist clinic and general outpatient clinic in Nigeria, the overall self-reported high medication adherence was low among Nigerian hypertensive subjects [65]. Adherence level of hypertensive patients at Jimma University specialized hospital, Ethiopia, to antihypertensive medications was found to be sub-optimal due to daily alcohol intake, co-morbidity, number of antihypertensive medications and availability of medications without fee [66]. A study conducted in Kampala (Uganda) among hypertensive stroke patients found that 17% of the patients were adherent to antihypertensive medications, and the main cause of non-adherence was lack of knowledge [67].

Non-adherence is when patients do not take their medications at all, are taking reduced amounts, or are taking doses at the prescribed frequencies but not taking into consideration medication to food requirements [68]. Non-adherence can either be intentional or unintentional. Intentional non-adherence is when a patient makes a rational decision not to use treatment or follow treatment recommendations [69–72]. Intentional adherence includes patient-related, therapy-related, and condition-related factors [69–72]. Unintentional non-adherence is unplanned patient behavior and is less strongly associated with beliefs and the level of cognition as compared to intentional non-adherence [69–72]. Unintentional non-adherence may be caused by forgetfulness and not knowing when and how to take medicines [69–72]. Factors affecting adherence of patients to their medicines such as therapy-related and condition-related factors are associated with unintentional non-adherence [69–72].

Barriers of adherence to medication are discussed in the subsequent subsection and mainly include categories of factors affecting patients' adherence to their medicines.

10. Barriers of adherence to medication

There are barriers of adherence to medication that affect patients with cardiovascular diseases, diabetes mellitus and hypertension thus, leading to non-adherence. These barriers are classified into different categories of factors affecting adherence of patients to their medication. Categories of factors affecting patients' adherence to medication in Africa include sociodemographic, economic, environmental, condition-related factors, therapy-related, health care team and system-related factors, and patient-related factors [73–79]. Sociodemographic, economic and environmental factors are composed of low-income, poverty, minority race-ethnicity, social support, copayments, and health literacy [73, 77]. Health care team and system-related factors include patient-clinician relationship, communication style, lack of team-based care, clinician burn out, lack of knowledge, lack of policies, lack of ad hoc screening and proper referral systems, and poor universal health insurance coverage [73, 74, 76, 77, 80, 81]. Complex regimen, treatment changes, failure and duration, adverse effects, and refill frequency and consolidation are therapy-related factors [73, 78]. Condition-related factors include multiple chronic conditions, depression, psychoses, drug or alcohol abuse, dementia, major disability, severity of symptoms, and quality of life [73]. Patient-related factors include perception of illness and treatment efficacy, denial of diagnosis, fear of dependence or adverse effects, lack of knowledge, forgetfulness, and low self-efficacy [73, 80, 81].

Several interventions can be put in place to curb factors affecting patients' adherence to medication. Therapy-related and condition-related factors could be minimized by prescribing few medications which can be implemented using once daily single-pill combinations [71]. Use of once daily single-pill combinations is associated with better adherence and hypertension control [71, 82]. Also, clinicians can prescribe a larger number of medications with each prescription to reduce refill frequency [69, 71]. Patients with NCDs frequently have co-morbidities requiring additional medication to their medicines for NCDs thus, refill consolidation so that multiple medications are obtained at the same time can improve adherence [69, 71].

To curb some of the health care team and system-related factors, patients should trust and be confident that the clinician is competent and has their best interest when making management decisions [73]. Patients, especially racial-ethnic minorities, should actively participate in decisions about the management of their NCDs and what medication to take [69, 73]. Policies addressing procurement process of medication and control of NCDs should be developed and implemented in health systems [74]. Also, the use of generic medicines for NCDs and improvement of health insurance coverage will reduce the cost of care for patients with NCDs therefore, solving some of the barriers to adherence [74].

Dispensing models can be implemented to assist with monitoring adherence to medicines and the treatment outcome.

11. Dispensing models to assist with adherence and treatment outcome

Poor adherence to medication is a major contributor to uncontrolled cardiovascular diseases, diabetes mellitus and hypertension. Monitoring and detection of adherence of patients to their medication using different dispensing models assist with assessing the treatment outcome. Medication adherence can be measured directly or indirectly using several measurements either separately or together [83, 84]. Indirect measurements include pill count, patient interviews, prescription refills data, electronic monitoring system, directly observed technique, and questionnaire [83, 84]. Direct measurements include measurement of drug levels and digital medicine [83, 84]. Prescription refills data, pill count, directly observed technique, and electronic monitoring system are objective measurement whereas, questionnaires and patient interviews are subjective measurements [83, 84]. Biomedical measurements consist of measurement of drug levels and digital medicine [83, 84].

12. Different dispensing models used to measure adherence

Dispensing models include interviewing patients, questionnaires, pill count, prescription refills data, electronic monitoring system, measurement of drug levels, digital medicine, and directly observed technique [73].

Patient's interview is when a physician questions the patient about adherence to medicines. The physician asks the patient questions related to medicine-taking behavior thus, communication skills of the physician and the ability to conduct nonjudgmental discussion is important [73]. The health care professional asks the patient to estimate their own medication-taking behavior, such as which percentage of dose that they may miss within a designated period or the frequency that they are unable to follow the medication regime [83]. On the other hand, questions asked to the patient by the health care professional can be based on the patient's knowledge on the prescribed regime, including drugs' name, schedule, and indications [83]. Health care professionals then evaluate their response to determine the level of adherence [83].

Questionnaires are forms which can be completed by patients, trained nurses or healthcare professionals as a tool to monitor adherence [73]. Types of questionnaires used to measure adherence are the Brief Medication Questionnaire, Hill-Bone Compliance Scale (Hill-Bone), Eight-Item Morisky Medication Adherence Scale (MMAS-8), Medication Adherence Questionnaire (MAQ), Self-Efficacy for Appropriate Medication Use Scale (SEAMS), and the Medication Adherence Report Scale (MARS) [85, 86]. A well-known and mainly used questionnaire to measure adherence is the Morisky questionnaire [69, 83].

Pill count is a frequently used dispensing model to monitor adherence where counting returned pills by a patient gives an overview of what has been taken by the patient [73]. The health care provider counts the number of dosage units that have been taken by the patient between two scheduled appointments or clinic visits [83]. This number would then be compared with the total number of units received by the patient to calculate the adherence ratio [83]. The equation for calculating pill count is as follows: (Number of dosage units dispensed – Number of dosage units remained) / (prescribed number of dosage unit per day × number of days between 2 visits) [83].

Prescription refill data requires availability of electronic monitoring of drug prescriptions in pharmacies [73]. Prescription refill data assists with obtaining a rough estimate of medicines adherence and persistence by calculating the percentage of days covered by the prescriptions [73]. When measuring adherence using prescription refills, it is assumed that prescription-refilling patterns correspond to the patient medication-taking behavior and that the medication is taken exactly as prescribed [83].

Electronic monitoring system consists of a device in which a microcircuit is incorporated into medication packages and any removal of a dose of the medicine is detected in real time, time stamped, analyzed, stored, and communicated [73, 83]. Commonalities of different electronic monitoring devices include (i) recorded dosing events and stored records of adherence, (ii) audiovisual reminders to signal time for the next dose, (iii) digital displays, (iv) real-time monitoring, and (v) feed-back on adherence performance [83]. The commonly used electronic monitoring device is the Medication Event Monitoring System (MEMS) [73, 83].

Measurement of drug levels involves the measurement of the medicine or its metabolite concentration in body fluids, such as blood or urine, and evaluation of the presence of a biological marker given with the medicine and direct observation of patient's medication-taking behavior [73, 83]. Complete absence of medicine in a sample indicates that the medicine has not been taken by the patient for a duration equivalent to half-lives of the medicine [73].

Directly observed technique is an approach when medicine is given and taken by the patient under supervision of a member of the clinical staff every day for a certain period of time [73].

Digital medicine consists of ingestible sensors incorporates in the pill during manufacturing process, which will be ingested by the patient [73]. After ingestion, an electrochemical reaction is triggered in the stomach leading to an activation of the sensor and generating a unique message coded for the medication name and dose to a wearable patch worn by the patient on the torso and recorded the date and time of the sensor ingestion [73]. The information collected by the patch is encrypted and transmitted wireless to a designated device using Bluetooth. The sensors are then eliminated as solid waste within 72 hours [73].

There are other dispensing models used to monitor patient medication adherence thus, treatment outcome. Modern technology can be used to monitor adherence and includes the use of internet, real time medication monitoring (such as electronic pill boxes), and mobile phones [69]. The use of electronic pill boxes combined with Short Message Service (SMS) reminders are specifically designed to improve unintentional adherence [69]. These interventions have resulted in an increase in refill adherence in diabetic patients with suboptimal adherence [68]. Mobile phones can be used to send alerts to take medication to patients, track doses, and provide appropriate medication instructions [86]. Automatic home medication dispenser (AHMD) integrated with a smartphone application can be used to address adherence issues especially for elderly patients [86]. The AHMD holds up to 90 day's supply of several medications, and addresses cognitive impairment and age-related changes using components such as counter, clock dispensing mechanism, power source, input/output interface, locking system, transceiver and antenna, and physical indicators for alarms [86]. The AHMD also notifies the patient of due dosage per set dosage time or due refills through audio/visual reminders, and notifies the caregiver of missing dosages through calls or text messages [86–88].

In conclusion, it is important to monitor adherence of patients with chronic diseases to their medicines using appropriate dispensing models (either alone or in combination) as uninterrupted life-long consumption of medicines will prove patients' health outcome. In instances where non-adherence has been identified, it is essential to note factors affecting adherence of patients to their medicines and address those factors.

Author details

Masebata Ramathebane*, Lineo Maja and Molungoa Sello
National University of Lesotho, Maseru, Lesotho

*Address all correspondence to: mv.ramathebane@nul.ls; mvramathebane@gmail.com

References

[1] Dalal S, Beunza JJ, Volmink J. Mint: Non-communicable diseases in sub-Saharan Africa: what we know now. International Journal of Epidemiology. 2011;40:885-901.

[2] World Health Organization. Noncommunicable diseases country profiles 2018 [Internet].2018. **https://www.who.int/nmh/countries/en/** [Accessed: 2020-12-03]

[3] World Health Organization. Report on the status of major health risk factors for noncommunicable diseases: WHO African Region 2015. [Internet].2015. **https://www.afro.who.int/sites/default/files/2017-06/15264_who_afr-situation-ncds-15-12-2016-for-web.pdf** [Accessed: 2020-12-03]

[4] The NCD Alliance.NCDs. [Internet].2015. **https://ncdalliance.org/sites/default/files/resource_files/ncda_advocacytoolkit_en_0_0.pdf** [Accessed: 2020-12-03]

[5] World Health Organization. United against NCDs: The time to act is now; The Brazzaville declaration on noncommunicable diseases prevention and control in the WHO African region. [Internet].2011. **https://www.afro.who.int/sites/default/files/2017-06/ncds-brazzaville-declaration20110411.pdf** [Accessed: 2020-12-02]

[6] World Health Organization. Cardiovascular Diseases. [Internet].2011. **https://www.afro.who.int/health-topics/cardiovascular-diseases** [Accessed: 2020-12-21]

[7] National Health Service. Cardiovascular disease. [Internet]. 2018. **https://www.nhs.uk/conditions/cardiovascular-disease/** [Accessed: 2020-12-21]

[8] National Heart, Lung and Blood Institute. Heart attack. [Internet]. 2020. **https://www.nhlbi.nih.gov/health-topics/heart-attack** [Accessed: 2020-01-06]

[9] Centers for Disease Control and Prevention (CDC). About stroke [Internet]. 2020. **https://www.cdc.gov/stroke/about.htm** [Accessed: 2020-01-06]

[10] Plotnikoff GA, Dusek J. Hypertension. In: Rakel D. Integrative medicine 3rd ed. Philadelphia; Elsevier Saunders: 2012 p. 208-216.

[11] Harvey RA, Lippincott's Illustrated Reviews: Pharmacology 5th ed. Philadelphia; Lippincott Williams & Wilkins

[12] Chobanian AV, Bakris GL, Black HR. Mint: Seventh report of the Joint National Committee on Prevention, Evaluation and Treatment of High Blood Pressure. Hypertension. 2003;42:1206-1252.

[13] Devries S. Coronary heart disease. In: Rakel D. Integrative medicine 3rd ed. Philadelphia; Elsevier Saunders: 2012 p. 227-236.

[14] American Diabetes Association. 10. Cardiovascular disease and risk management: standards of medical care in diabetes-2020. Diabetes Care 2020;43(S1):S111–S134 DOI: **https://doi.org/10.2337/dc20-s010**

[15] Chicago Medical Center. What happens when you quit smoking. [Internet]. 2020. **https://www.uchicagomedicine.org/conditions-services/psychiatry-and-psychology/smoking-cessation** [Accessed: 2020-12-21]

[16] World Health Organization. Salt reduction. [Internet]. 2016. **https://www.who.int/news-room/fact-sheets/detail/salt-reduction** [Accessed: 2020-12-21]

[17] Oyebode O, Oti S, Chen Y, Lilford, RJ. Salt intakes in sub-Saharan Africa: a systematic review and meta-regression. Population Health Metrics 2016, 14:1:1-14 DOI: 10.1186/s12963-015-0068-7

[18] Appel LJ, Moore TJ, Obarzanek E, Mint: A clinical trial of the effects of dietary patterns on blood pressure. New England journal of medicine. 1997;336(16):1117-1124.

[19] National Heart, Lung and Blood Institute. DASH Eating Plan. [Internet]. 2020. **https://www.nhlbi.nih.gov/health-topics/dash-eating-plan** [Accessed: 2020-12-21]

[20] World Health Organization. Obesity. [Internet]. 2020. **https://www.who.int/health-topics/obesity#tab=tab_1** [Accessed: 2020-12-21]

[21] Wing RR, Lang W, Wadden TA. Benefits of modest weight loss in improving cardiovascular risk factors in overweight and obese individuals with type 2 diabetes. Diabetes care. 2011;34:1481-1482 DOI: 10.2337/dc10-2415

[22] Centers for Disease Control and Prevention (CDC). Alcohol and Public Health. [Internet]. 2020. **https://www.cdc.gov/alcohol/index.htm** [Accessed: 2020-03-10]

[23] Statista. Consumption of alcohol per capita in Africa in 2019, by country. [Internet] 2020. **https://www.statista.com/statistics/1038427/alcohol-per-capita-consumption-african-countries/** [Accessed: 2020-12-21]

[24] British Heart Foundation. Alcohol. [Internet]. 2020. **https://www.bhf.org.uk/informationsupport/support/healthy-living/healthy-eating/alcohol** [Accessed: 2020-12-21]

[25] World Health Organization. Physical activity: Background. [Internet]. 2020. **http://www.emro.who.int/health-education/physical-activity/background.html** [Accessed: 2020-12-21]

[26] Victoria state government. Physical activity - its important. [Internet]. 2020. **https://www.betterhealth.vic.gov.au/health/healthyliving/physical-activity-its-important** [Accessed: 2020-12-21]

[27] Rizos CV, Elisaf MS. Antihypertensive drug therapy in patients with African ancestry. Expert Opinion on Pharmacotherapy. 2014;15(8):1061-1064

[28] Sehgal AR. Overlap between whites and blacks in response to antihypertensive drugs. Hypertension. 2004;43(3):566-572.

[29] Jayatilleke K. Challenges in implementing surveillance tools of high-income countries (HICs) in low middle income countries (LMICs). Current treatment options in infectious diseases. 2020;1(1):191-201

[30] World Health Organization. Quality of Care: Patient Safety; 2002. [Internet]. 2020. **http://www.who.int/medicines/areas/quality_safety/safety_efficacy/ewha5518.pdf** [Accessed: 2020-12-21]

[31] Uppsala Monitoring Center. Definitions; May 2015. [Internet]. 2020 **http://www.who.int/medicines/areas/quality_safety/safety_efficacy/trainingcourses/definitions.pdf** [Accessed: 2020-12-21]

[32] Barry A, Olsson S, Minzi O. Mint: Comparative Assessment of the National Pharmacovigilance Systems in East Africa: Ethiopia, Kenya, Rwanda and Tanzania. Drug Safety. 2020;43(1):339-350

[33] Olowofela AO, Isah AO. A profile of adverse effects of antihypertensive medicines in a tertiary care clinic in

Nigeria. Annals of African medicine. 2017;16(3):114-119

[34] Aggarwal A, Patel P, Lewison G. The Profile of Non-Communicable Disease (NCD) research in the Middle East and North Africa (MENA) region: Analyzing the NCD burden, research outputs and international research collaboration. Public library of science one. 2020;15(4):1-12.

[35] World Health Statistics. Part II highlighted topics. Geneva: World Health Organization. 2012. [Internet]. 2020 **https://www.who.int/gho/publications/world_health_statistics/EN_WHS2012_Part2.pdf.** [Accessed:2020-12-21]

[36] World Health Organization. Global status report on non-communicable diseases 2010. Geneva: World Health Organization. 2010. [Internet]. 2020. **https://www.who.int/nmh/publications/ncd_report2010/en/.** [Accessed:2020-12-21]

[37] Abegunde DO, Shengelia B, Luyten A, et al. Mint: Can non-physician health-care workers assess and manage cardiovascular risk in primary care? Bull World Health Organization. 2007;85:432-440.

[38] Mendis S, Al Bashir I, Dissanayake L, et al. Mint: Gaps in capacity in primary care in low-resource settings for implementation of essential non-communicable disease interventions. International Journal of Hypertension. 2012;58:40-41.

[39] Charlton KE, Steyn K, Levitt NS et al. Mint: Diet and blood pressure in South Africa: intake of foods containing sodium, potassium, calcium, and magnesium in three ethnic groups. Nutrition. 2005;21: 39-50.

[40] Mathers CD, Lopez A, Stein C, et al. Mint: Deaths and disease burden by cause: global burden of disease estimates for 2001 by World Bank Country Groups. Working paper 18. Bethesda, MD: Disease Control Priorities Project, 2005.

[41] Wald NJ, Law MR. Mint: A strategy to reduce cardiovascular disease by more than 80%. *BMJ.* 2003;326:1419.

[42] Yusuf S. Two decades of progress in preventing vascular disease. Lancet. 2002;360:2-3.

[43] Murray CJL, Lauer JA, Hutubessy RC, et al. Effectiveness and costs of interventions to lower systolic blood pressure and cholesterol: a global and regional analysis on reduction of cardiovascular-disease risk. Lancet. 2003;361:717-25.

[44] Gaziano TA, Opie LH, Weinstein MC. Mint: Cardiovascular disease prevention with a multidrug regimen in the developing world: a cost-effectiveness analysis. Lancet. 2006;368:679-86.

[45] Nachega JB, Lehman DA, & Hlatshwayo D. et al. HIV/AIDS and antiretroviral treatment knowledge, attitudes, beliefs and practices in HIV infected adults in Soweto, South Africa. Journal of Acquired Deficiency Syndrome. 2005;38(2):196-201.

[46] Mugomeri E , Ramathebane MV, Maja L , Chatanga P, Moletsane L. Knowledge of disease condition and medications among hypertension patients in Lesotho. Journal of the American Society of Hypertension, 2014;96(2):165-70. doi: 10.1016/j.pec.2014.05.007.

[47] Thetsane R, Ramathebane M, Makatjane TJ. Village health workers' HIV/AIDS knowledge and service provision among rural communities in Lesotho. International Journal of Current Research. 2018;10(9):73420-73424.

[48] Hirsch-Moverman Yl; Daftary A, Yuengling KA, Saito S, Ntoane M,

Frederix K, Maama LB, Howard A A. Mint: Using mHealth for HIV/ TB treatment support in Lesotho: Enhancing patient–provider communication in the START Study. Journal of acquired immune deficiency syndrome. 2017;74:S37–S43.

[49] Institute of Medicine. Patients charting the course: Citizen engagement and the learning health system: Workshop Summary. Washington, DC: The National Academy Press; 2011.

[50] Balmer C. The information requirements of people with cancer. Cancer Nursing. 2005;28:36-44. [PubMed: 15681980] 28.

[51] Bandura, A. Social foundations of thought and action. Englewood Cliffs, NJ: Prentice-Hall; 1986. 34.

[52] Bandura, A. Self-efficacy: The exercise of control. New York, NY: W.H. Freeman and Company; 1997

[53] Meng K, Musekamp G, Schuler M, Seekatz B, Glatz J, Karger G, Kiwus U, Knoglinger E, Schubmann R, Westphal R, Faller H. Mint: The impact of a self-management patient education program for patients with chronic heart failure undergoing inpatient cardiac rehabilitation. Patient Education and Counseling. 2016;99:1190-1197.

[54] McMurray JJV, Adamopoulos A, Anker SD, Auricchio A, Böhm M, Dickstein K, Falk V, Filippatos G, Fonseca C, Gomez-Sanchez MA, Jaarsma T, Køber L, Lip GYH, Maggioni AP, Parkhomenko A, Pieske BM, Popescu BA, Rønnevik PK, Rutten FH, Schwitter J, Seferovic P, Stepinska J, Trindade PT, Voors AA, Zannad F, Zeiher A. Mint: ESC guidelines for the diagnosis and treatment of acute and chronic heart failure 2012. European Journal of Heart Failure. 2012;14:803-869.

[55] Meng K, Musekamp G, Seekatz B, Glatz J, Karger G, Kiwus U, Knoglinger E, Schubmann R, Westphal R, Faller H. Mint: Evaluation of a self-management patient education program for patients with chronic heart failure undergoing inpatient cardiac rehabilitation: study protocol of a cluster randomized controlled trial, BMC Cardiovascular Disorders. 2013;13:60.

[56] McMurray JJV, Adamopoulos A, Anker SD, Auricchio A, Böhm M, Dickstein K, Falk V, Filippatos G, Fonseca C, Gomez-Sanchez MA, Jaarsma T, Køber L, Lip GYH, Maggioni AP, Parkhomenko A, Pieske BM, Popescu BA, Rønnevik PK, Rutten FH, Schwitter J, Seferovic P, Stepinska J, Trindade PT, Voors AA, Zannad F, Zeiher A: Mint: ESC guidelines for the diagnosis and treatment of acute and chronic heart failure 2012. European Journal of Heart Failure. 2012;14:803-869.

[57] Dickstein K, Cohen-Solal A, Filippatos G, McMurray JJV, Ponikoski P, Poole- Wilson PA, Strömberg A, van Veldhuisen DJ, Atar D, Hoes AW, Keren A, Mebazaa A, Nieminen M, Priori SG, Swedberg K. Mint: ESC guidelines for the diagnosis and treatment of acute and chronic heart failure 2008. European Heart Journal 2008;29:2388-2442.

[58] Hindelang M. *Cardiac Care Teaching/Learning Strategies for the Home Healthcare Nurse.* Patient Education: Ever So Important. Home Healthcare Nurse; 2006, 24(1):1-16. http://www.homehealthcarenurseonline.com Date of access: 15/12/2020.

[59] Watermeyer J, Penn C. Working across language and cultural barriers: communication skills for pharmacists. Cape Town. 2009.

[60] World Health Organization. Adherence to long-term therapies evidence for action [Internet]. 2003. Available from: https://www.who.int/chp/knowledge/publications/

adherence_full_report.pdf [Accessed: 2020-12-03]

[61] Yuvaraj K, Gokul S, Ganesh Kumar S. Mint: Prevalence of medication adherence and its associated factors among patients with non-communicable diseases in rural Puducherry, South India – A facility-based cross-sectional study. Journal of Family Medicine and Primary Care. 2019;8(2):701-705.

[62] Sankar UV, Lipska K, Mini GK, Sarma PS, Thankappan KR. Mint: The adherence to medications in diabetic patients in rural Kerala, India. Asia Pacific Journal of Public Health. 2015;27(2):NP513–NP523. DOI: https://doi.org/10.1177%2F1010539513475651

[63] Addo B, Sencherey S, Babayara MNK. Mint: Medication noncompliance among patients with chronic diseases attending a primary health facility in a periurban district in Ghana. International Journal of Chronic Diseases. 2018;2018:1-10. DOI: https://doi.org/10.1155/2018/7187284

[64] Herskind J, Zelasko J, Bacher K, Holmes D. Mint: The outpatient management of hypertension at two Sierra Leonean health centres: a mixed-method investigation of follow-up compliance and patient-reported barriers to care. African Journal of Primary Health Care and Family Medicine. 2020;12(1):a2222. DOI: https://doi.org/10.4102/phcfm.v12i1.2222

[65] Akintunde AA, Akintunde TS. Mint: Antihypertensive medication adherence among Nigerian hypertensive subjects in a specialist clinic compared to a general outpatient clinic. Annals of Medical and Health Sciences Research. 2015;5(3):173-178.

[66] Asgedom SW, Atey TM, Desse TA. Mint: Antihypertensive medication adherence and associated factors among adult hypertensive patients at Jimma university specialized hospital, southwest Ethiopia. BMC Research Notes. 2018;11:27. DOI: https://doi.org/10.1186/s13104-018-3139-6

[67] Mugwano I, Kaddumukasa M, Muganyi L, Kayima J, Ddumba E, Sajatovic M, Sila C, DeGeorgia M, Katabira E. Mint: Poor drug adherence and lack of awareness of hypertension among hypertensive stroke patients in Kampala, Uganda: a cross-sectional study. BMC Research Notes. 2016;9:3. DOI: 10.1186/s13104-015-1830-4

[68] Altice FL, Friedland GH. Mint: The era of adherence to HIV therapy. Annals of Internal Medicine. 1998;129(6):503-505.

[69] Hugtenburg JG, Timmers L, Elders PJM, Vervloet M, van Dijk L. Mint: Definitions, variants, and causes of nonadherence with medication: a challenge for tailored interventions. Patient Preference and Adherence. 2013;7:675-682. http://dx.doi.org/10.2147/PPA.S29549

[70] Wroe AL. Mint: Intentional and unintentional nonadherence: a study of decision making. Journal of Behavioral Medicine. 2002;25(4):355-372. DOI: 10.1023/a:1015866415552

[71] Lehane E, McCarthy G. Mint: Intentional and unintentional medication non-adherence: a comprehensive framework for clinical research and practice? A discussion paper. International Journal of Nursing Studies. 2007;44(8):1468-1477. DOI: 10.1016/j.ijnurstu.2006.07.010

[72] Clifford S, Barber N, Horne R. Mint: Understanding different beliefs held by adherers, unintentional non-adherers, and intentional non-adherers: application of the Necessity-Concerns Framework. Journal of Psychosomatic Research. 2008;64(1):41-46. DOI: 10.1016/j.jpsychores.2007.05.004

[73] Burnier M, Egan BM. Mint: Adherence in hypertension a review of prevalence risk factors impact, and management. Circulation Research. 2019;124:1124-1140. DOI: 10.1161/CIRCRESAHA.118.313220

[74] Dzudie A, Rayner B, Ojji D, Schutte AE, Twagirumukiza M, Damasceni A, Ba SA, Kane A, Kramoh E, Kacou JBA, Onwubere B, Cornick R, Sliwa K, Anisiuba B, Mocumbi AO, Ogola E, Awad M, Nel G, Otieno H, Toure AI, Kingue S, Kengne AP, Perel P, Adler A, Poulter N, Mayosi B. Mint: Roadmap to achieve 25% hypertension control in Africa by 2025. Global Heart. 2018;13(1):45-59

[75] Gast A, Mathes T. Mint: Medication adherence influencing factors – an (updated) overview of systematic reviews. Systematic Reviews. 2018;8:112. DOI: http://doi.org/10.1186/s13643-019-1014-8

[76] Jimmy B, Jose J. Mint: Patient medication adherence: measures in daily practice. Oman Medical Journal. 2011;26(3):155-159. DOI: 10.5001/omj.2011.38

[77] Waari G, Mutai J, Gikunju J. Mint: Medication adherence and factors associated with poor adherence among type 2 diabetes mellitus patients on follow-up at Kenyatta national hospital, Kenya. Pan African Medical Journal. 2018;29:82. DOI: 10.11604/pamj.2018.29.82.12639

[78] Unni E, Farris. Mint: Determinants of different types of medication non-adherence in cholesterol lowering and asthma maintenance medications: a theoretical approach. Patient Education and Counseling. 2011;83:382-390. DOI: 10.1016/j.pec.2011.02.017

[79] Aminde LN, Tindong M, Ngwasiri CA, Aminde JA, Njim T, Fondong AA, Takah NF. Mint: Adherence to antidiabetic medication and factors associated with non-adherence among patients with type-2 diabetes mellitus in two regional hospitals in Cameroon. BMC Endocrine Disorders. 2019;19:35. DOI: https://doi.org/10.1186/s12902-019-0360-9

[80] Nyaaba GN, Masana L, de-Graft Aikins A, Beune E, Agyemang C. Mint: Factors hindering hypertension control: perspective of front-line health professionals in rural Ghana. Public Health. 2020;181:16-23. DOI: https://doi.org/10.1016/j.puhe.2019.11.007

[81] Chang H, Hawley NL, Kalyesubula R, Siddharthan T, Checkley W, Knauf F, Rabin TL. Mint: Challenges to hypertension and diabetes management in rural Uganda: a qualitative study with patients, village health team members, and health care professionals. International Journal for Equity in Health. 2019;18:38. DOI: https://doi.org/10.1186/s12939-019-0934-1

[82] Egan BM, Bandyopadhyay D, Shaftman SR, Wagner CS, Zhao Y, Yu-Isenberg KS. Mint: Initial monotherapy and combination therapy and hypertension control the first year. Hypertension. 2012;59:1124-1131. DOI: 10.1161/HYPERTENSIONAHA.112.194167

[83] Lam WY, Fresco P. Mint: Medication adherence measures: An overview. Biomed Research International. 2015;2015:217047. http://dx.doi.org/10.1155/2015/217047

[84] Arafat Y, Ibrahim MIM. The use of measurements and health behavioral models to improve medication adherence. In: Ibrahim MIM, Wertheimer AI, Babar Z, editors. Social and administrative aspects of pharmacy in low- and middle-income countries. Academic Press; 2018. p. 53-69. https://doi.org/10.1016/B978-0-12-811228-1.00004-2

[85] Luga, AO, McGuire MJ. Mint: Adherence and healthcare costs.

Risk Management and Healthcare Policy. 2014;7:35-44. DOI: https://doi.org/10.2147/rmhp.s19801

[86] Ogungbe O, Dennison Himmelfarb CR, Commodore-Mensah Y. Mint: Improving medication adherence in cardiovascular diseases prevention: what's new? Journal of Cardiovascular Nursing. 2020;35(1):6-10. DOI: 10.1097/JCN.0000000000000645

[87] Morisky DE, Ang A, Krousel-Wood M, Ward HJ. Mint: Predictive validity of a medication adherence measure in an outpatient setting. Journal of Clinical Hypertension (Greenwich). 2008;10:348-354. DOI: https://doi.org/10.1111/j.1751-7176.2008.07572.x

[88] Hoffmann C, Schweighardt A, Conn KM, Nelson D, Barbano R, Marshall F, Brown J. Mint: Enhanced adherence in patients using an automated home medication dispenser. Journal for Healthcare Quality. 2018;40(4):194-200. DOI: 10.1097/JHQ.0000000000000097